SECOND
EDITION

EVIDENCE-BASED NURSING

The Research–Practice Connection

SARAH JO BROWN, PHD, RN

Evidence–Based Practice Consultant
Norwich, Vermont

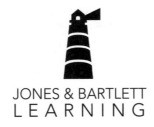

JONES & BARTLETT
LEARNING

World Headquarters

Jones & Bartlett Learning
40 Tall Pine Drive
Sudbury, MA 01776
978-443-5000
info@jblearning.com
www.jblearning.com

Jones & Bartlett Learning
Canada
6339 Ormindale Way
Mississauga, Ontario L5V 1J2
Canada

Jones & Bartlett Learning
International
Barb House, Barb Mews
London W6 7PA
United Kingdom

Jones & Bartlett Learning books and products are available through most bookstores and online booksellers. To contact Jones & Bartlett Learning directly, call 800-832-0034, fax 978-443-8000, or visit our website, www.jblearning.com.

Substantial discounts on bulk quantities of Jones & Bartlett Learning publications are available to corporations, professional associations, and other qualified organizations. For details and specific discount information, contact the special sales department at Jones & Bartlett Learning via the above contact information or send an email to specialsales@jblearning.com.

The author, editor, and publisher have made every effort to provide accurate information. However, they are not responsible for errors, omissions, or for any outcomes related to the use of the contents of this book and take no responsibility for the use of the products and procedures described. Treatments and side effects described in this book may not be applicable to all people; likewise, some people may require a dose or experience a side effect that is not described herein. Drugs and medical devices are discussed that may have limited availability controlled by the Food and Drug Administration (FDA) for use only in a research study or clinical trial. Research, clinical practice, and government regulations often change the accepted standard in this field. When consideration is being given to use of any drug in the clinical setting, the health care provider or reader is responsible for determining FDA status of the drug, reading the package insert, and reviewing prescribing information for the most up-to-date recommendations on dose, precautions, and contraindications, and determining the appropriate usage for the product. This is especially important in the case of drugs that are new or seldom used.

Production Credits
Publisher: Kevin Sullivan
Acquisitions Editor: Amy Sibley
Associate Editor: Patricia Donnelly
Editorial Assistant: Rachel Shuster
Production Manager: Carolyn F. Rogers
Marketing Manager: Meagan Norlund
V.P., Manufacturing and Inventory Control: Therese Connell
Composition: Paw Print Media
Illustrations: diacriTech
Cover Design: Scott Moden
Cover Image: © Markus Gann/ShutterStock, Inc.
Printing and Binding: Malloy, Inc.
Cover Printing: Malloy, Inc.

To order this product, use ISBN: 978-1-4496-2406-4

Library of Congress Cataloging-in-Publication Data
Brown, Sarah Jo.
  Evidence-based nursing : the research-practice connection / Sarah Jo Brown. — 2nd ed.
    p. ; cm.
  Includes bibliographical references and index.
  ISBN 978-0-7637-9465-1 (pbk.)
  1. Evidence-based nursing. 2. Nursing—Research—Methodology. I. Title.
  [DNLM: 1. Nursing Research. 2. Evidence-Based Medicine—methods. 3. Nursing Care—methods. WY 20.5]
  RT81.5.B82 2011
  610.73—dc22
                              2010026810

6048

Printed in the United States of America
15 14 13 12 11   10 9 8 7 6 5 4 3

Contents

Contributor

Chapter 12: Searching for Research Evidence
Ellen F. Hall, MALS, AHIP
Library Director and Professor
Norwich University
Northfield, VT

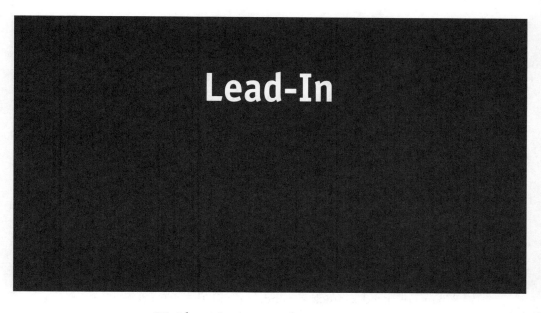

Lead-In

"Evidence is stronger than argument."
—FROM THE CELEBRITY BY WINSTON CHURCHILL, 1897

In our modern world, opinions abound. However, when much is at stake, it is essential to get beyond opinion to reliable knowledge and information. That is the case with the health care given to patients. And that is why all the healthcare professions are committed to evidence-based practice.

Evidence-based practice involves seeking out and incorporating into care the most reliable sources of evidence available—and knowledge produced by research is one of the most reliable. Scientific knowledge is reliable because it is systematically developed and open to review by all interested parties, in the form of journal articles and presentations at professional congresses.

In nursing, we have an ever-increasing body of research-derived knowledge to use in designing care for populations of patients and for individual patients. Nursing departments and agencies use research-derived knowledge when developing clinical policies and standards of care. At the point of care, individuals seek out research-derived knowledge to guide them when they are confronted with situations in which routine knowledge is insufficient.

Importantly, scientifically based care has the highest likelihood of producing desired patient outcomes. To contribute to and give scientifically based care, the 21st century nurse must be able to read research reports and decide whether and how to use research evidence in clinical decisions and care planning.

This book is offered to assist nursing students to acquire the knowledge required to engage in evidence-based practice. This knowledge includes knowledge about research methods and knowledge about how to incorporate credible research evidence into practice—both are included in this book.

Features of Note

- First, I would call your attention to the companion website for this book, which is available at 🖰 ***go.jblearning.com/brown***. Formatted by chapter, it includes study guides, supplementary papers, and links to resources.
- When you need a quick reminder about the definition of a term, a rather extensive glossary is provided at the end of the book. In addition, terms included in the glossary are printed in bold color where first introduced in the text.
- Then, there is the old she-he/her-him conundrum. There are various ways to deal with it, but I have chosen to sometimes refer to the nurse as *she* accompanied by the possessive *her* when needed. Other times I refer to the nurse as *he* accompanied by the possessive *him* when needed.

Sarah Jo Brown, PhD, RN

PART I
Nursing Research

The level of knowledge required to understand research reports published in clinical journals is somewhat akin to being a savvy computer user. To be a competent computer user, you don't have to understand binary arithmetic, circuitry, program architecture, or how central processing units work. You just need to know some basic computer language, and be familiar with the features of the hardware and software programs you use.

Similarly, as a professional nurse in clinical care, you do not need to know all the different ways of obtaining samples, how to choose an appropriate research design, or how to decide on the best statistical test. But you do need to know the basics of how various types of research are conducted and what results mean. You also need to know how good data is obtained and how incorrect conclusions are avoided.

The goal of the first part of the book is to introduce you to research methods and different kinds of research evidence. To accomplish this, seven research articles have been reprinted. I chose this learning strategy because I have found that most students prefer to learn about research methods by having the particulars of an actual study pointed out and explained—as opposed to explaining methods in more general terms.

Importantly, a grasp of the basics of research methodology lays the ground-work for evidence-based practice, which is introduced in the first chapter and described in depth in Part II.

CHAPTER ONE

The Research–Practice Connection

Effective nursing practice requires knowledge, information, judgment, skills, and art. This book is about the knowledge component—more specifically, about knowledge used to make decisions regarding the nursing care patients should receive. An important part of the knowledge used in making decisions about nursing care is produced by research. Ideally, all key decisions about how patients are cared for should be based on **research evidence** (Institute of Medicine, 2001). Although this is not a completely attainable goal, large bodies of healthcare research provide considerable guidance for the design of nursing care. The goal of this book is to help you learn how to read research articles and, along with other nurses, use the findings to plan nursing care for patients.

Research to Practice

The research **findings** of a study are "raw materials," like petroleum and iron ore that must undergo transformations to become everyday products such as gasoline and steel. Similarly, research findings undergo several transformations before they become the basis for **clinical protocols** that guide clinicians' decisions and actions. Consider the following sequence of events that leads up to development of a clinical protocol.

1. First, a study examining the clinical issue must have been conducted; however, the findings of a single study rarely provide certain and complete guidance for how to provide care for patients.

2. Thus, clinicians often wait for several (or many) studies to be conducted on the issue.
3. Eventually, a summary of all the research findings pertaining to the issue is performed. The summary identifies findings that have support from more than one study.
4. Then, using the dependable findings from the summary, a group of experts formulates clinical recommendations in the form of a **clinical practice guideline**.
5. The staff of a healthcare agency decides how the research-based guideline should be implemented in their setting; that is to say, they adapt the guideline in the process of developing a clinical protocol specific to their agency.
6. And finally, the clinical staff provides care according to the protocol, making research-based practice a reality.

These transformations must be carefully performed, and when they are, the care given is scientifically based.

Evidence Used to Develop Clinical Protocols

To produce effective and useful clinical protocols, research evidence must be used in combination with other sources of information. Thus, when developing nursing protocols, project teams actually use several different sources of evidence, including the following:

- Research findings
- Agency quality monitoring data
- Data from national databases
- Expert opinion

There is wide agreement among healthcare providers that clinical protocols should be based on research findings whenever possible; however, they must be used along with the other forms of evidence. In recognition of the fact that multiple sources of knowledge and information are used to develop clinical protocols, they are commonly called *evidence-based* protocols. Thus, from here forward I will use the descriptor evidence-based, rather than research-based, to describe protocols and practice that rest to a large degree on research evidence.

Having said this, the focus of the book is on research evidence. The fact that this book focuses on research evidence is not meant to devalue the other forms of evidence; rather, a focus on research evidence allows a close consideration of this very important source of information for clinical practice. The integration of research evidence with the other sources of evidence is described in considerable detail in Chapter 17.

Evidence-Based Clinical Protocols

Clinical protocols are standards of care in that they define care that should be given to patients who are part of a defined population. (A **population** is a group of patients who have the same health condition, problem, or treatment. A population can be defined broadly, for example, persons having surgery, or narrowly as elderly persons having hip replacement surgery.) Some clinical protocols set forth a comprehensive plan of care for the specified population, for example, perioperative and postoperative care of elderly persons having hip surgery, whereas others address just one aspect of care such as body temperature maintenance in the elderly having hip surgery. Still others are even narrower and could be called a clinical procedure, for example, blood salvage and transfusion during hip surgery.

Generally, multidisciplinary groups produce protocols that address many aspects of care, whereas nursing staffs produce protocols that address clinical issues that nurses manage. Clinical protocols can be set forth in various formats: plans of care, standard order sets, clinical pathways, care **algorithms**, decision trees, **bundles** of recommended care actions, and procedures—all are guides for clinicians regarding specific actions that should be taken on behalf of patients in the specified population. An appropriate committee or authority in the hospital, nursing department, or care-providing agency endorses each clinical protocol.

In short, clinical protocols are tools for achieving consistent, high-level care; they set forth clear standards of care for a defined patient population by specifying the care actions that should be performed. Many protocols also specify how, when, and by whom the actions should be done. Others set forth guidance for the decisions that nurses make while giving care.

Evidence-Based Care

When research findings are used to develop a protocol and the protocol is followed in daily practice, everyone involved (patients, healthcare professionals, the agency, third-party payers, and accrediting agencies) can be confident that patients in that population are receiving nursing care that is based on the best available scientific evidence.

The protocol approach to **care design** and delivery is in contrast to each nurse deciding what care she or he will give to patients—an approach to care giving that often results in considerable variability in care because of omissions and differing opinions regarding the best method of care. Evidence-based protocols are increasingly being used as standards of care and being integrated into computerized clinical information systems.

Using Clinical Protocols

In any care agency, there is not a care protocol for every patient population and every care situation. Agencies develop protocols to reduce the variability in care of their "high-volume" and "high-risk" patient groups. If a protocol exists, it should be followed unless there is a good reason for not following it. Generally, following scientifically based protocols is in the best interest of patients because doing so increases the likelihood that patients will achieve good outcomes. This is the case because the recommended actions have been scientifically studied, and people with expertise in the field have considered their application.

Protocols Are Not Recipes   Protocols should be adhered to when they exist, but they should not be blindly followed. Nurses are patient advocates, and as such look out for patients' welfare; this requires that nurses be constantly aware of patients' responses to protocols. If a nurse observes that a protocol is not producing good results with a patient, she should discuss this with a nurse leader and decide if a different approach to care should be used. A protocol may be evidence-based and it may work well for most patients, but it may not be right for every patient.

Consider this scenario: You are providing care to a postoperative patient and recognize that he does not seem as comfortable as he should be even though the pain protocol is being followed. This recognition should cause you to ask yourself questions such as, "Why isn't he getting good pain relief? Should we be doing something different?" The advisable course of action would be to talk with a nurse leader so as to get better pain relief for the patient.

If, however, you notice the same problem with two or three similar patients, you would have cause to wonder if the protocol is sound. You would then look into when the protocol was written and on what information it was based. If further investigation reveals that the recent research literature indicates that a different positioning approach is helpful or a different medication dosing schedule is more effective for this population, you should bring this information to the attention of your nurse manager or the quality improvement council for your unit.

Even when a protocol is being carried out and is effective for most patients, there are still many aspects of care that nurses do at their discretion. Some of these discretionary acts are nursing art, that is, personal style, whereas others are actions taken to fulfill a protocol's recommendations. For instance, a protocol regarding fall prevention required assessing newly admitted elderly patients for orthostatic hypotension. However, the protocol did not spell out exactly how to do this assessment. The staff nurse asked an advanced practice nurse, who told her about a recent research article comparing two procedures for evaluating positional/orthostatic hypotension in older people. It reported that one method of detecting blood pressure drop upon standing was better than the other. Thus, the gap in the protocol's recommendation could be filled by a research-informed decision made by the individual nurse. The take-away message is that care protocols are not detailed recipes for care, rather they are guides to care that should be followed in conjunction with patient preference, attentive observation, clinical judgment, and additional research information.

> ### Protocols ≠ Recipes

As a Student   At this point in your career, as a student nurse with placements in several hospitals, clinics, and agencies, you will find that some clinical settings have care protocols that clearly are based on research evidence, whereas others have care protocols but their rationale isn't clear. You might wonder: Do the required actions represent the opinions of nurses on a practice committee? Were they based on an article someone read in a professional journal? Did the chief doctor on that service stipulate how things should be done? Did the salesperson for a piece of medical equipment recommend the care actions?

To illustrate this dilemma, suppose a nursing home facility has a protocol addressing care of incontinent patients that includes the standard, "For patients who do not recognize when their bladder is full, assist the patient to a commode or toilet every four hours." However, the rationale of the standard is not stated in the protocol document. You might wonder, "Who decided that every four hours is the best interval; why not every three hours or every six hours?" As the person who will enact the protocol, you have a right to information about its basis, and for that reason clinical protocols are more frequently being written in ways that provide a description of the amount of research support for the recommended actions and/or references of supporting research articles.

Staff Nurses and Protocol Development

After you start to work as a professional nurse, you may be asked to participate in a project to develop or update a care protocol or procedure. Often, your agency will be adapting an evidence-based guideline that was issued by a professional association, leading healthcare system, or government organization. Other times, an evidence-based guideline will not be available but a research summary relative to the clinical issue has been published, and its conclusions will be used in developing the protocol. To contribute to a protocol project, you will need to know how to read and understand research articles published in professional nursing journals and on trustworthy healthcare Internet sites.

Let's assume that you are working in a well-baby clinic, and are asked to be a member of a work group revising the protocol for preventing and managing diaper dermatitis in infants. You may be asked to read, appraise, and report to the group about an evidence-based clinical guideline produced by a nursing specialty association. To do this assignment, you should be able to formulate a reasonably informed opinion as to the extent to which the guideline recommendations are evidence-based and were produced in a sound manner. If the recommendations are deemed credible, then the work group will incorporate them into the new protocol.

Another scenario could be that you read in the specialty journal for your area of practice a research report about an effective way of maintaining placement of gastric tubes in young children. Thinking about it, you realize that quite a few children on the pediatric unit where you work have pulled out their tubes. This should cause you to reflect on the effectiveness and safety of the way gastric tubes are being secured. You decide to look online

GUIDELINE: A set of recommendations for care of a patient population that is issued by a professional association, leading healthcare center, or government organization. Guidelines are not agency-specific.

PROTOCOL: A set of specific care actions for a patient population that has been endorsed by the hospital, agency, clinic, or healthcare facility. Protocols are agency-specific.

and find a research summary article about the issue that brings together the findings from four studies. It offers the conclusion that the tubes should be secured and protected in a certain way—and that way is different from the standard of care on the unit on which you are working. You and your colleagues now have an opportunity to improve the care you give to these children by designing care that is based on nursing research.

Regardless of whether you come to question the effectiveness of the care being provided through clinical observation, by reading a research article in your professional journal, or by learning of a possibly better way at a conference, the next step is to act on your insight. Talk with your nurse manager, advanced practice nurse, or a member of the unit's quality council. From this discussion you will learn how the protocol came to be as it is and stimulate dialogue regarding its effectiveness.

Short History of Evidence-Based Nursing Practice

The nursing profession, *discipline* to use the more academic term, has been conducting scientific research since the 1920s when case studies were first published in the *American Journal of Nursing*. Now nursing research is being conducted in countries around the world and reports of clinical research studies are published in research journals and clinical journals in many languages. In many countries, nursing research is funded by the government, and a handful of countries have doctoral programs educating nurse researchers. The growing cadre of doctorally educated nurses has jettisoned both the quantity and quality of clinical nursing research being conducted. In the United States, the National Institute of Nursing Research (www.ninr.nih.gov), a component of the National Institutes of Health, is a major source of funding for nursing research.

In the mid-1970s, visionary nurse leaders realized that even though clinical research was producing new knowledge indicating which nursing methods were effective and which were not, practicing nurses were not aware of the research. As a result, several projects were started to increase the utilization of research-supported actions by practicing nurses. These projects gathered together the research that had been conducted on issues such as preoperative teaching, constipation in nursing home residents, management of urinary drainage systems, and preventing decubitus ulcers. Studies were critiqued, evidence-based guidelines were developed, and considerable attention was paid to how the guidelines were introduced into nursing departments (Horsley, Crane, & Bingle, 1978; Krueger, Nelson, & Wolanin, 1978). These projects stimulated interest in the use of nursing research in practice throughout the United States; at the same time nurses in other countries were also coming to the same recognition. By the 1980s and 1990s, many research utilization projects using diverse approaches to making nurses aware of research findings were under way (Kirchhoff, 2004).

During this time, interest in using research findings in practice was also proceeding in medicine. In the United Kingdom, the Cochrane Collaboration at Oxford was formed in 1992 to conduct rigorous research summaries with the goal of making it easier for clinicians to learn what various studies found regarding the effectiveness of particular healthcare interventions. At the McMaster Medical School in Montreal, Canada, a faculty group started the **evidence-based practice** movement. This movement brought to the forefront the responsibility of the individual clinicians to seek out the best **evidence** available when making clinical decisions in everyday practice. The evidence-based practice (EBP) movement in medicine flowed over into nursing and re-energized the use of research by nurses. Three other things were happening in the late 1990s and early 2000 years:

- Considerably more clinical nursing research was being conducted.
- The EBP movement was proceeding in a somewhat multidisciplinary way.
- National governments in the United States, United Kingdom, Canada, and other countries funded efforts to promote the translation of research into practice.

Today, high-quality evidence-based clinical practice guidelines and research summaries are being produced by healthcare organizations around the world, and nursing staffs are increasingly developing agency clinical protocols based on those guidelines and summaries. Also, individual clinicians are increasingly seeking out the best available evidence to use as a guide for the care they provide to patients.

Your Path to Evidence-Based Practice

Clearly, there is a lot for you to learn. As you read this book, you will learn how to do the following:

- Locate evidence-based guidelines and research summaries
- Get comfortable reading research articles
- Develop basic skills in judging if a clinical practice guideline or research summary was soundly produced

- Decide if the research evidence available is strong enough to use as a basis for nursing care
- Participate in the development of protocols in the agency or unit in which you work

This book and your classroom experiences should help you acquire a solid base of research knowledge to launch you into becoming a 21st-century professional nurse. I would emphasize that the point of this book and of the course you are taking is not to make you into a nurse researcher, rather to help you be an informed consumer of nursing research.

Part I

Your learning path to the ultimate goal of being a nurse who contributes to scientifically based care in your work setting begins with learning about how scientific nursing studies are conducted. Thus, the main goal of the first part of the book is to help you understand the key features of five different types of research—that is, research with five different purposes and methods. For each of the five types of research, you will first read an introduction about how that type of research is done. Then, you will read an actual study report of that type of research, followed by a commentary calling attention to important features of the study. The commentary will help you to delve deeply into the study. In this part of the book, you will also examine a research summary and an evidence-based clinical practice guideline.

Most of the research articles you will be reading were published in clinical journals, not research journals. They were written for clinicians, thus they emphasize the clinical implications of the findings, not the fine points of research methodology. In Part I of the book, your goal in reading the reports is to grasp how the study was done and what was found. Then, in Part II, you will revisit these same studies, learn to critically **appraise** their soundness, and consider their **applicability** to a particular setting.

Because the book is a primer, only the most widely used and important types of research are presented. Also, the information provided is basic and selective, which means that it is not a comprehensive reference source regarding research methodology. It does not delve deeply into methodological issues; it does not explain all research designs, methods, and statistics. However, it does provide an introduction to methodological issues that must be appreciated to understand most nursing research reports.

Part II

In the second part of the book, you will learn about using research evidence in nursing practice. You will also learn about how to use research evidence in your own individual clinical practice. I call this individual use of research evidence *research-informed practice*. Most often, individual practice is *informed* by research, not *based* on it—much more about this later.

> Evidence-based practice is designed by clinical project teams.
>
> Research-informed practice is engaged in by individual clinicians.

Assumptions About the Reader

The exploration of evidence-based nursing in this book assumes that you (1) have had an introduction to statistics; (2) have some experience in clinical settings; and (3) are committed to excellence in your professional practice. Becoming a nurse who contributes to evidence-based quality improvement on your unit or in your agency requires that you be an active learner by developing the following professional habits:

- Questioning what you see in practice
- Seeking additional knowledge when care protocols seem less than effective
- Reading research articles in clinical journals
- Thinking about the application of new knowledge to your practice
- Participating in evidence-based quality improvement projects on your unit or in your agency
- Adopting evidence-based protocols when they are introduced into your work setting

Use of Other Learning Resources

Additional learning material is available online at the companion website for this book, which can be accessed at *go.jblearning.com/brown*. Some of this material guides your learning or assists you in determining if you have understood the material presented in the book. Other material is supplemental in that it provides in-depth information not considered essential but of interest to some students.

In reading this book, and indeed in your later reading of research articles, you undoubtedly will want to have a statistics book handy to look up statistical terms and tests you have forgotten or never learned. You may also want to have handy as a reference source a traditional, basic research text organized around the steps in the research process. Such a text, with its focus on research designs and methods, will be useful later when you read research reports of studies conducted using designs and methods other than those you will learn about in this book. Reference texts can also provide greater depth of information about issues that are just introduced in this book.

Your reference research text and statistics text need not be new. Slightly outdated editions of these texts are often available very inexpensively—and research design and statistics do not change much from edition to edition. Do make sure you use a basic book, not an advanced one written for researchers. If in doubt, ask your instructor for a suggestion. And don't sell them when you are finished with this course! Later in your educational program or in your first position as a staff nurse, when you read a research article and the author states that a factorial design was used, you will recognize right off that this design was not covered in this book. Then, you can go to your research reference text and read the section about this design—it will take about five minutes. This "small-bite approach" to learning about research methods can over time help you become a more sophisticated consumer of research.

REFERENCES

Horsley, J. A., Crane, J., & Bingle, J. (1978). Research utilization as an organizational process. *Journal of Nursing Administration, 8,* 4–6.

Institute of Medicine. (2001). *Crossing the quality chasm: A new health system for the 21st century.* Washington, DC: National Academy of Sciences. Retrieved from http://www.nap.edu/html/quality_chasm/reportbrief.pdf

Kirchhoff, K. T. (2004). State of the science of translational research: From demonstration projects to intervention testing. *Worldview on Evidence-Based Nursing, 1*(S1), S6–S12.

Krueger, J. C., Nelson, A. H., & Wolanin, M. O. (1978). *Nursing research: Development, collaboration, and utilization.* Germantown, MD: Aspen.

SUGGESTED READING

Good article about evidence-based practice: Melnyk, F. M., Fineout-Overhold, E., Stillwater, S. B., & Williamson, K. M. (2009). Igniting a spirit of inquiry: An essential foundation for evidence-based practice. *American Journal of Nursing, 109*(11), 49–51.

CHAPTER TWO

Research Evidence

In Chapter 1, reference was made to research evidence, but it was not explained in full. That needs to be done. As a student new to the science of nursing, when mention is made of research evidence, you will naturally think of the findings of a scientific study. However, as you proceed through this course, you will come to see that research evidence can take several forms:

- Findings from a single, original study
- Conclusions from a summary of several (or many) original studies
- Research-based recommendations of a clinical practice guideline

Types of Research Evidence

Building Knowledge

A finding of a single original study is the most basic form of research evidence. Most studies produce several findings, but each finding should be considered as a separate piece of evidence because one finding may be well supported by the study while another finding may be on shaky ground. Although a finding from an original study is the basic building block of scientific knowledge, knowledge is really more like a structure made up of many different kinds of blocks (see Figure 2–1).

Findings from many soundly conducted studies are necessary to build a reliable body of clinical knowledge regarding an issue. Insistence on confirmation of a finding from more than one study ensures that a knowledge claim is not just a fluke unique to the patients, setting, or research methods of that one

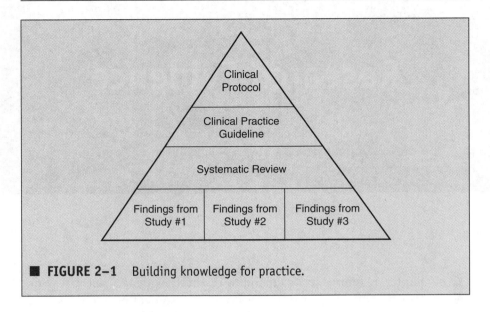

■ **FIGURE 2–1**   Building knowledge for practice.

study. If a finding is confirmed in several different studies, clinicians have confidence in that knowledge because it held up across diverse settings, research methods, patient participants, and clinician participants.

There are several recognized ways of combining findings from two or more studies; as a group these methods are called **systematic reviews.** Conclusions from systematic reviews may then be translated into evidence-based recommendations by expert panels. A group of recommendations is called a *clinical practice guideline.* Although evidence-based recommendations are not technically research evidence, if they were directly derived from research findings and summaries, they are considered so for practical purposes. In this chapter, each of these forms of research evidence is introduced briefly in turn. Later in the book, each is considered in depth.

Findings From an Original Study

Most people think of a research study as involving (1) a large number of "subjects" who are (2) randomly assigned to be in one of several study groups; (3) research environments that are tightly controlled; and (4) data that is meticulously obtained and then analyzed using statistics to produce results. In fact, research using these methods is common and valuable; however, it is only one type of scientific study—there are many other kinds of scientifically sound studies. The most common way of thinking about research methods is to categorize them as qualitative and quantitative.

Qualitative Research   Qualitative research methods collect data in the form of what people say, observations of events, and written material. The data is *not* quantified by scales or number values; rather verbal descriptions that convey the meanings in the data are constructed. The goal of qualitative research is understanding—not counting, averaging, or quantifying in any way.

Qualitative research is used to study what it is like to have a certain health problem or healthcare experience such as being a physically disabled parent or recovery after a major head injury. Qualitative research methods are also used to study social settings, social interaction, and social processes. The following are examples of situations a nurse researcher might study using qualitative methods:

1. The interpersonal support dynamics at a social center for persons with chronic mental illness (a subculture setting);
2. How intensive care unit (ICU) staff members interact with family members of unconscious patients (social interaction); and
3. How a family who has entered a family weight loss program makes changes in eating and physical activity over time (social process).

These kinds of social situations are typically tangles of issues, forces, perceptions, values, expectations, and aims. They can be understood and sorted out best by a researcher embedding herself in the situation and using methods of inquiry that will get at participants' perceptions, feelings, daily thoughts, beliefs, expectations, and behavior patterns. Data collection methods such as indepth conversations, diary keeping, extensive interviewing, extended observation, and focus groups are used to acquire insights regarding these subjective realities. The data is analyzed in ways that preserve the life-meanings of the stories and comments the participants offer.

Qualitative research is described in more depth in Chapter 4.

Quantitative Research   Quantitative research methods are also used to examine how the world works. However, numerical measurement is used to explore and confirm the level at which the phenomena are present and the nature of **relationships** among them. I realize I introduced a new word in that last sentence, so a bit of a diversion is needed here because the word is used in research articles. The word *phenomena* (the plural word) is used throughout the research world as a catchall phrase to describe the realities that exist in a field of study. The phenomena of interest in nursing can be grouped into five categories (adapted from Kim, 2000). The categories and examples of phenomena within each are:

- The client as a person
  (motivation, anxiety, hope, and adherence to treatments)
- The client's environment
  (social support, financial resources, and peer group values)
- Nursing practice
  (risk assessment for skin breakdown, patient teaching, and wound cleansing)
- The nurse–patient relationship and communication
  (person-centeredness, mutuality)
- The healthcare system
  (access to health care, quality of care)

In brief, nursing phenomena are personal, social, physical, and system realities that exist or occur within the realm with which nursing is concerned. When phenomena are examined in a quantitative research study, they are called the research *variables*.

Getting back to types of research, exploring the nature of phenomena can be done using qualitative research methods. However, the workings of many phenomena can be explored more extensively when the phenomenon is measured quantitatively. For instance, body temperature could be described using the qualitative words cool, warm, and hot, but using the quantitative standard of thermometer degrees is a more precise way of conveying and tracking body temperature.

Moreover, quantifying phenomena allows exploration of how a change in one relates to a change in another, as when the relationship between body temperature and white blood count is analyzed using a correlation statistic. Quantitative methods are also used to test how well a nursing intervention works compared to another intervention. In intervention studies, the outcomes expected to be produced by the intervention are carefully measured in each patient participant or a determination is made regarding how many patients in each group attained the outcomes of interest.

Study Purpose and Study Method   The researcher's decision to use either a qualitative method or a quantitative method is determined by the nature of the question. As just described, qualitative methods yield better understanding for some types of research questions, whereas quantitative methods provide better answers to other questions. Together, qualitative and quantitative methods serve a range of purposes:

- Understand a health, illness, or healthcare experience
- Develop a theory about responses to an illness condition
- Describe a health-related situation (e.g., mother–infant interaction)
- Measure the strength of relationships between several health-related phenomena (e.g., hours worked outside the home and mother fatigue)
- Test a **hypothesis** about the effectiveness of an intervention

Generally, each of these purposes requires a different research strategy and approach, although researchers sometimes use qualitative and quantitative methods in combination with one another. Using mixed methods may produce a more complete portrayal of an issue than can one method alone.

Qualitative research methods are generally inductive, meaning researchers produce findings by working from observations to more general statements. Qualitative researchers have strategies and plans before they enter the settings in which they will make observations and inquiries, but they are also flexible to revise their investigative approach and to follow leads that arise.

In contrast, quantitative researchers tend to have specific research questions and choose a research design that will produce answers to those questions. A **research design** is a framework or general guide regarding how to structure studies conducted to answer a certain type of research question. The four quantitative research designs used most often in nursing research are:

1. **descriptive designs,**
2. **correlation designs,**
3. **experimental designs,** and
4. **quasi-experimental designs** (Burns & Grove, 2005).

You will be learning about each of these.

Researchers choose the design that will provide the best approach to their research question or purpose and that is feasible given the resources available. Using the design features as a template, they develop a detailed **study plan** that spells out specifically how their study will be conducted. A study plan includes the following:

- The theoretical framework that will be used (if any)
- Sites and settings that will be involved
- How the sample will be obtained
- Ethical protections that will be put in place
- Information that will be provided to participants
- Design of the interventions (if any)
- Measuring instruments that will be used

- The sequence of study activities
- Data collection procedures
- How unwanted influences will be controlled
- How data analysis will be performed

In summary, the two major categories of research methods used in clinical nursing studies are qualitative and quantitative. Both methodological approaches are needed to develop the full range of knowledge needed by clinical nurses.

Conclusions of a Systematic Review

Systematic reviews are an important and useful form of research evidence. A systematic review is a research summary that produces conclusions by bringing together and integrating the findings from all available original studies. The integration of findings from several or many studies can be done using tables and logical reasoning and/or with statistics. The cumulative findings are formulated as new knowledge claims, which are unifications of the separate findings of the original studies. The methods for accomplishing the unification are widely agreed upon and serve to reduce bias resulting from the process used to summarize the findings.

Systematic reviews, when well done, bring to light trends and nuances regarding the clinical issue that are not evident in the findings of individual studies. I suggest that now you take a look at an abstract of a systematic review. I suggest this because reading and using the conclusions of systematic reviews is one of the destinations on your learning path, and looking at one will give you a sense of this learning destination.

1. Go to the CINAHL database in your library's website or online to PubMed (http://www.ncbi.nlm.nih.gov/pubmed). PubMed is a free, online database of healthcare articles.
2. Type the following text in the search box: infants sucrose Leef 2006.
3. That should bring up the citation and abstract for a systematic review of 16 studies about oral sucrose administration to decrease procedure-related pain in newborn infants (Leef, 2006).
4. Note that the abstract provides information about how many articles were included in the review, how many infants were included in the studies and what was found. Remember: You are reading a short synopsis of the review, not the entire report.

From this quick look at the abstract of a systematic review, you should get a sense of the groundwork that has been done by the person who did this review. In the process of doing the review, she did the following:

- searched for articles,
- sifted through them for relevant studies,
- extracted information from each study report, and then
- brought the findings together in a coherent way.

Clearly, this saves clinical nurses a great deal of time when they are looking for the research evidence about an issue in care. You will delve more deeply into systematic reviews in later chapters.

Recommendations of an Evidence-Based Clinical Practice Guideline

The third form of research evidence is the recommendations of an **evidence-based clinical practice guideline**. A clinical practice guideline consists of a set of recommendations, and when the recommendations are based on research evidence, the whole guideline is referred to as an *evidence-based clinical practice guideline*. These guidelines are most often developed by organizations with the resources (money, expertise, time) required to produce them. Again, I suggest taking a look at one, as follows:

1. Go to the website of the Registered Nurses' Association of Ontario (RNAO; http://www.rnao.org).
2. Click the *Nursing Best Practice Guidelines* tab, and then follow the tab and links to a list of guidelines (*Clinical Practice Guidelines Program* → *Guidelines and Fact Sheets*; scroll down and open *Oral Health: Nursing Assessments and Intervention*).
3. Scroll down until you come to *Related Downloadable Files*; open the second file, *Recommendations*.
4. The developers of this guideline looked at the research evidence regarding nursing hygiene actions and self-care actions that promote oral health in adults with special needs, such as: persons receiving cancer therapies, stroke survivors, and persons who are cognitively impaired. Based on the evidence, they derived the recommendations listed. (I suggest that you look at the Practice Recommendations [1–12] and ignore the Education and Organization and Policy Recommendations that follow.)

The strength of the evidence supporting each recommendation is indicated in the right column; don't get caught up in that right now, except I will tell you that level I is very strong research evidence whereas level IV evidence was obtained from expert opinion evidence (i.e., no research exists, so consensus of an expert panel was the best available evidence). The fact that the recommendations in this guideline were supported only by level III evidence (findings from nonexperimental studies) and level IV evidence (expert opinion) indicates that very limited research has been conducted on this issue.

Remember that you are looking at part of a much larger report. The other document, the complete guideline, presents a detailed review of the evidence that led to each recommendation. It also informs the reader that electronic database searches and Internet searches identified 1163 potential articles, however after careful review only 26 research articles and three guidelines were deemed relevant and of sufficient quality to be used as evidence sources for development of the guideline.

Research Evidence

- Findings from original studies
- Conclusions of systematic reviews
- Recommendations of evidence-based clinical practice guidelines

As you can see, evidence-based clinical practice guidelines are much more ready-to-go for clinical application than tracking down the original research articles and working forward from there to discover what the evidence-based actions would be. And they are more ready-to-go than systematic reviews. For time-pressed protocol development teams, evidence-based clinical practice guidelines and systematic reviews are the short roads to evidence-based protocols (see Figure 2–2).

If starting the development of a care protocol by retrieving individual research articles is like baking a cake from scratch, and systematic reviews are like using a cake mix, then starting with an evidence-based clinical practice guideline is like buying a cake at the bakery and adding a personalized topping or presentation.

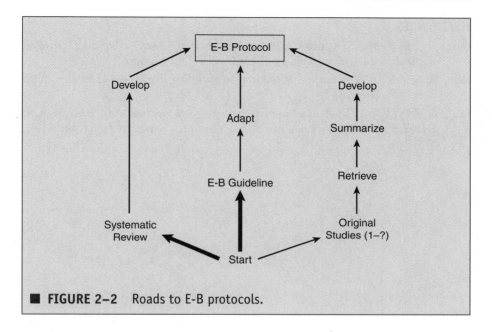

■ FIGURE 2–2   Roads to E-B protocols.

Going Forward

In the next chapter, you will learn how to read research reports of individual studies. Then, in Chapters 4 through 8, you will be guided through reading of exemplary articles reporting five different types of research (one qualitative study and four types of quantitative studies). In Chapter 9, you will read a systematic review and learn how one type of systematic review is conducted. And in Chapter 10, you will read an evidence-based clinical practice guideline and learn how they are produced.

Note that this order is the reverse of the order in which care design project teams actually **search** for research evidence—they first look for evidence-based guidelines and systematic reviews. If they exist and are well done, the team can build on them rather than reinventing the wheel. The reason for the reversal in this book is that proceeding from original studies, to systematic reviews, to evidence-based clinical practice guidelines is a more natural learning order.

REFERENCES

Burns, N., & Grove, S. K. (2005). *Practice of nursing research: Conduct, critique, and utilization* (5th ed.). St. Louis, MO: Elsevier Saunders.

Kim, H. S. (2000). *The nature of theoretical thinking in nursing* (2nd ed.). New York, NY: Springer.

Leef, K. H. (2006). Evidence-based review of oral sucrose administration to decrease the pain response in newborn infants. *Neonatal Network, 25*(4), 275–284.

CHAPTER THREE

Reading Research Articles

Although some kinds of reading are intended to be a passive experience, reading professional articles, especially research reports, should be anything but passive. One way to be an active reader is to annotate or mark your copy of the article: underline, circle phrases, highlight, or jot comments in the margin—whatever helps you keep track of important information and connect the various parts of the study. Some people prefer to make notes in a file on their laptop—fine, whatever works for you.

I annotate right on my paper copy of articles. I write something like "n = 54" in the margin so I can quickly locate the **sample** size. I underline important definitions, outcomes, or findings. I circle abbreviations that will be used in the report and the parts of a table that are most important to me or unexpected. I put question marks where a statement doesn't fit with what was said earlier or doesn't make sense. Of course, it's possible to overannotate and in so doing produce a clutter. However, if you annotate selectively, you'll be able to find important information easily when you return to the article at a later time.

In this chapter, I make suggestions about how to read reports of individual studies. At this point in your learning, the goals in reading a research article about a study are to: (1) identify why the study was done, (2) how it was conducted, and (3) what was found. After you are comfortable reading research articles, you will add the goals of determining if the study was soundly conducted and relevant to the care of patients to whom your agency or unit provides care (see text box).

> ## Goals in Reading a Research Report
>
> 1. Determine the purpose of the study
> 2. Understand how the study was done
> 3. Understand what was found
> 4. Appraise the credibility of the findings
> 5. Determine if the findings are relevant to the care of your patients

The emphasis in this chapter and in all of Part I of the book is on goals 1, 2, and 3 in the text box, although goals 4 and 5 may pop into your thinking as you read. For instance, you will undoubtedly note if the patient groups that were studied are similar to a patient you have taken care of. You may make a mental note about this; however, serious consideration of the applicability of the study to a particular patient group is on hold until Part II of the book.

In reading this chapter, you may see a few terms that are unfamiliar to you. For now, just look them up in the glossary to get a sense of what they mean. Most of them are explained in full as you proceed through the first part of the book.

Starting Point

Is this a report of an original research study? This seems like it should be an easy question to answer, but at times it is not. Some articles read like research articles, but they are in fact other kinds of reports. When you see tables with numbers and percentages, you may think you are reading a research study, but the article may just be providing numerical data to describe a clinical program. Such data is anecdotal and naturally occurring with no **control** over its quality or the conditions under which it was collected. As you will learn, it takes more than numerical data to call an evaluation report "research."

Most often, the author of a research article will refer to "the study" early in the report, but sometimes you have to read quite far into an article to determine that it has the essential elements of a study. The essential elements of a research study include the following:

- A specified research question, hypothesis, or purpose
- Specified, systematic methods of data collection and analysis

- Results of data analysis
- Findings (interpreted **results**)
- Conclusions

If all these elements are present, then the likelihood that you are reading a research study report is very high. Remember, however, that there are many types of research methods and designs, and the essential elements of each type look quite different. Most quantitative studies address specific research questions or hypotheses, whereas qualitative studies may have a broad aim or purpose. Quantitative studies report results with tables, graphs, and statistics, whereas the findings of qualitative studies consist of extended quotes, narratives, descriptions, or themes. Qualitative studies often have small sample sizes (e.g., N = 6); some quantitative studies use a very large number of participants (e.g., N = 3,200). In short, research articles are diverse but should include at a minimum a clear purpose statement, a description of methods used to collect and analyze data, results and/or findings, and conclusions.

Format of Study Reports

Research reports of original studies are organized in a very logical way, and the formats used are similar from one journal to another. This standardization can help you as a reader because you will learn where to expect, and later locate, various kinds of information about the study. The following is a brief orientation to the format of research reports.

Title and Abstract

The title tells the reader what the study examined and often the patient group of interest. These are your first clues as to whether the report is likely to be of interest to you. However, titles can be misleading because a phrase or term used in the title may be different from the one used in your practice setting.

Abstracts almost always precede the main body of the article. An abstract provides a brief summary of the study—typically 300 words or less. Note the section headings used in the abstract because they are useful in beginning to organize your thinking about the study. The abstract distills the main points of the study, and after reading it you should know if the study is of interest.

Let's assume that you've decided to read the whole study. Rather than read straight through the first time, you might want to read the Introduction and then jump to the Discussion section. The Discussion summarizes the important findings and places them in the context of findings from earlier studies. Having read the Introduction and the Discussion, you should have a sense for the context of the study—and be ready to read the article from start to finish in its entirety.

Introduction

In the Introduction of a research report, the researcher presents his view of the current state of knowledge regarding the issue or problem being investigated; this includes what is known and what the gaps in knowledge are. In addition, the researcher may discuss theories or conceptual frameworks that are used to organize thinking about the issue. This background serves as a lead-in to the statement regarding the purpose of the study that is being reported. A study purpose may be stated as: a purpose statement, aims, objectives, research questions, or as hypotheses that will be tested by the study.

Theoretical Frameworks   In the Introduction section of a research report, there may be a discussion of a theory that served as an organizing framework for the study. A theory is made up of assumptions, concepts, definitions, and/or propositions that provide a cohesive, although tentative, explanation of how a phenomenon in the physical, psychological, or social world works. Propositions are suggested linkages among the concepts of the theory that have not yet been proven.

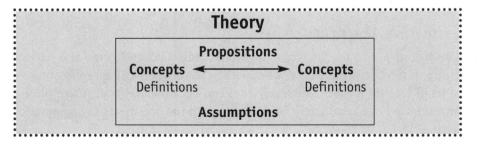

To make the proceeding paragraph a bit more rooted in the real world, consider the following illustration. The *Theory of Community Empowerment* was developed to provide direction for improving health in communities (Persily & Hildebrandt, 2008). Consider two propositions from this theory:

1. Involving lay workers in a community health promotion program extends access to health promotion opportunities.
2. Access to health promotion information leads to adoption of healthy behaviors.

Lay workers, *access*, *health promotion opportunities*, and *adoption of healthy behaviors* are concepts of the theory.

A researcher conducting a study about improving the health of elders living in their own homes might use the *Theory of Community Empowerment* as a source of ideas for the study. By translating the two theoretical propositions into more concrete terms, two study hypotheses are formed:

1. Trained volunteers who collect "healthy living" questions from elders once a month at the weekly senior lunch and deliver answers the following week will increase access to health promotion information.
2. Health promotion information of personal interest will produce changes in health-related behaviors.

The questions submitted are given to a nurse practitioner who answers them via video recording at the next week's lunch. Adoption of new health behavior outcomes will then be measured at 3-month intervals. Thus, the theory has served the research by bringing into a trial program a component that otherwise might not have been included and by providing a knowledge context for the findings. At the same time, the study acts as a test of the theory because the study has translated the abstractions of the theory into concrete realities that can be examined. If the study hypotheses are supported, the study is supported because the hypotheses represent the theory.

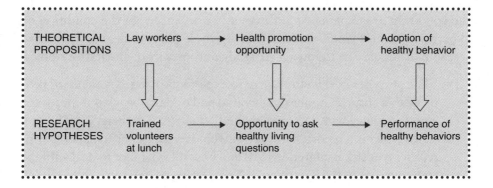

Not all study reports stipulate a theoretical framework; many researchers, particularly those testing physiological hypotheses, do not locate their studies within a theoretical framework; instead, they locate their study in a review of what is known from previously conducted research and what is still not known with certainty.

Clearly, much more could be said about the relationship between theory and research; however, doing so would be a diversion from the topic of this chapter, which is how research articles are formatted. For those who have a greater interest in the relationship among theory, research, and practice (and for those whose curriculum does not address this issue elsewhere), a paper about theory and research is available online at the companion website for this book, which can be accessed at ⊕ *go.jblearning.com/brown.*

Study Purposes   Each discipline has a set of words it uses to describe the purposes of studies, and the words do not always mean the same thing to every researcher. Purpose words and phrases you will encounter in nursing study reports include:

- Acquire insight
- Understand
- Explore
- Examine
- Describe
- Compare
- Examine the relationship/association between
- Predict
- Test the hypothesis that

In the early stages of studying an issue, research is directed at acquiring understanding of the various aspects of the issue: the problems people with the condition are experiencing, forces at work, and what the condition or experience means to individuals. Generally, these early studies use qualitative research methods. The following are study purposes from qualitative studies:

- "The purposes of this study were to explore the lived experience of people with a chronic, nonhealing wound and to describe what it means for a person to live with a chronic wound" (Beitz & Goldberg, 2005).
- "This paper is a report of a study of what fatigue means to patients with recent myocardial infarction (MI) and how they manage to deal with the consequences of this symptom" (Alsén, Brink, & Persson, 2008).

Note how both purposes set forth issues that will be examined, but they don't get highly specific about what they are looking for because they want the study participants to highlight the important aspects of their and experiences.

After the condition or situation is well understood at the experiential or social process level, other researchers may determine the frequency with which it occurs in different populations or measure the degree to which aspects of the condition or situation are present. Later, when several studies have been done and the situation is fairly well mapped, researchers will propose and quantitatively test associations between aspects of the situation or effectiveness of interventions directed at it. The following examples illustrate several way of stating quantitative research purposes:

- "The specific aims of this study were to (1) describe factors related to fatigue in older women after MI (myocardial infarction) and (2) examine the relationship of fatigue to physical activity after MI" (Crane, 2005).
- "The specific objectives of this pilot study were to (a) evaluate the effects of a culturally sensitive symptom-focused intervention on symptom distress, diabetes knowledge, perception of quality of life, glycosated hemoglobin levels, and self-care practices of older rural African-American women with type 2 diabetes" (Skelly, Carlson, Leeman, Holditch-Davis, & Soward, 2005).
- "We tested the hypothesis that children with acute lung injury treated with prone positioning would have more ventilator-free days than those treated with supine positioning" (Curley et al., 2005).

These study purpose statements illustrate the variety of ways used to set forth study aims.

Hypotheses   Study hypotheses are quite specific; they name the aspects of the issue that will be studied and state the nature of the relationship between the aspects they expect to find in the study. For example, "An increase in X will be associated with an increase in Y." This hypothesis does not cast either X or Y as causing the other. It says only that the two phenomena are related in some way. The hypothesis "Patients classified as high in PHE (positive health expectations) were expected to report higher QOL (quality of life) scores than patients with lower PHE scores" (Sears et al., 2004) is by itself an associative hypothesis. In context of the whole study, however, it is clear that the researchers believe that health expectations determine quality of life, not vice versa.

Other hypotheses are explicitly directional, such as "Patients will find it more comfortable to be transferred on and off beds and stretchers using a mechanical lateral transfer device when compared to 'manual' lateral transfer methods" (Pellino, Owen, Knapp, & Noack, 2006). This statement is actually a causal hypothesis because it implies that one transfer method will cause less discomfort than the other.

Methods

In the Methods section, the author describes how the study was conducted, including information about the following:

1. The overall arrangements and mechanics of the study
2. The setting or settings in which the study was conducted
3. The **institutional review board** (**IRB**) that gave ethical approval to the study
4. How the sample was obtained
5. The number of people in the sample
6. How data was collected
7. Any measurement **instruments** that were used (i.e., scales, questionnaires, physiologic measurements)
8. How the data was analyzed

The information about the sample should be sufficient to inform the reader about the likelihood that the sample is a good representation of the **target population** or provide enough profile information about the sample to let readers decide to whom the results would likely apply.

The information about how the data was obtained also includes a statement about the organization that gave ethical approval to the study, procedures used to collect data, and descriptions of the measurement instruments used. For now, you should come away from reading the Methods section of the reports with an understanding of the characteristics of the people who were included in the study, the sequence of steps in the study, and the data collected.

Results/Findings

In this section, the results of the data analysis are reported. Results are the outcomes of the analyses. In quantitative studies, results are tables, graphs, percentages, frequencies, and statistics. There should be results related to each of the research questions, hypotheses, or aims. To illustrate, consider the following hypothetical statement that might be found in the Results section of a quantitative study: "The t-test comparing the functional status scores of those in intervention group A and intervention group B indicated a significant difference (mean A = 8.4; mean B = 6.1; p = .038)." This is a result statement; it reports the results of the statistical analysis.

The interpretation of a result is called a **finding**. A finding for the result statement just given would be stated something like, "The group who received nursing intervention A had a significantly higher functional level than did the group who received intervention B." Note how the findings statement interprets the statistical result but does not claim anything more than the statistical result indicated. Findings statements are usually found in the Conclusions or Discussion section of quantitative study reports.

To illustrate further, consider the results and findings of a hypothetical quantitative study comparing the effects of a new method for osteoporosis prevention education to standard education. A t-test was used to compare the scores of the two groups on an osteoporosis prevention questionnaire; the result of that test was t = 1.99, p = .025. This result indicates that the statistical calculation comparing the scores of the two groups resulted in a t-value of 1.99, which is statistically significant at the p = .025 level (I'll explain p-values in a later chapter). The finding was this: The new educational method on average produced higher osteoporosis knowledge levels than standard education did, and there is a very low chance that this claim is wrong.

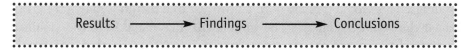

In qualitative research reports, data (results) and findings (e.g., themes) are often intermingled. Generally, qualitative study reports do not have a Results section, rather they have a Findings section in which themes, narrative descriptions, or theoretical statements are presented along with the data that led to them. Chapter 4 provides more explanation of the analytical processes used by qualitative researchers.

When you first begin reading research articles, you may have a tendency to skip over the tables and figures. This is not advisable because the real meat of the results is often in them. Most authors highlight or summarize in the text what is in the tables, but others assume the reader will get the information from the tables, thus they don't restate that information. In examining tables and figures, it is important to carefully read their titles so you know exactly what you are looking at. Also, within tables, the column and row labels are critical to understanding the data provided. Reading tables is a bit like dancing with a new partner—with a bit of practice, you will quickly get good at it.

Discussion or Conclusions

In the Discussion section, the researcher ties together several aspects of the study and offers possible applications of the findings. The researcher will usually open this section by stating the most important findings and placing them in the context of what other studies on the topic or question have found. In discussing the findings, many researchers describe what they think are the clinical implications of the findings. Here, they are allowed some latitude in saying what they think the findings mean. In the osteoporosis education for high school students example just given, the researcher might say, "The findings indicate that a short educational session is effective in increasing high school students' knowledge regarding osteoporosis prevention." This conclusion statement is close to the findings. On the other hand, if the researcher said, "Short educational sessions are an effective way of increasing osteoporosis prevention behaviors in high school students," the findings statement would be out beyond the results. Since the study only measured the outcome of knowledge, not behaviors, the author is adding an assumption to the results, namely, that knowledge produces behavior change—and that is a big assumption.

Authors are also expected to consider alternative explanations for their findings. This would include noting how research methods may have influenced the results, such as "The sample size may have been too small to detect a difference in the treatment groups" or "The fact that a high proportion of patients in the intervention group didn't return for follow-up may have made the outcomes of the intervention group look better than they would have been if post-data had been available from everyone in that group." At the end of this section, the authors usually comment on what they view as the limitations of the study and the implications of the findings for future research.

References

The reference list should include complete data for all citations made in the text. You might find it useful to circle in the text and in the reference list any articles that you want to obtain and read for greater understanding or because they studied a population of interest to you, for example, elderly persons living independently in the inner city. Perusal of the reference list also reveals how current other work on the issue is, who has done research on the issue, and which journals have published research articles about the issue.

Reading Approach

When you first read research reports, they may seem difficult to read. It's really like any new undertaking—at first it is confusing. However, the fog lifts rather quickly, the whole picture comes into focus, and the relationships between the parts become clear. For now, you should set three simples goals for yourself. You should come away from your reading of a research report knowing:

Why? How? What?

- **Why was the study done—to what purpose?**
  Found in Introduction and its subsections: background, literature review, theoretical framework, purpose, and hypotheses
- **How was the study done?**
  Found in Methods and its subsections: design, setting, sample, data collection, measuring instruments, data analysis
- **What was found?**
  Found in Results, Discussion, Conclusions.

Importantly, even seasoned readers of research reports find it necessary to read a research report at least twice. The first time you may only get a general sense of why the study was done, how it was done, and what was found. During the second reading, the why, how, and what should become clear to you.

During the second read, you also may begin to notice issues that make you wonder, such as the following:

- Why did the researchers exclude persons with heart disease?
- Did they take into account patients' balance when evaluating capacity for self-care?
- Did the fact that a study was going on put the nurse participants on best behavior?

These are important observations and questions; they will become important later when you are also required to appraise the **credibility** of study findings. For now, your aim is to get a grasp of the WHY, HOW, and WHAT of the study.

Wading In

Having considered how research reports are organized and noted some difference between the formats of qualitative and quantitative study reports, it is now time to delve into reading one of them; two are suggested at the end of this chapter. Your instructor may pick one for everyone in the class to read or assign one that is not on the list.

The research reports reprinted in full in subsequent chapters are considered exemplars in that they are typical or representative of a particular type of healthcare research. Most of the exemplar studies were also very well conducted, but they were not chosen because they are perfect models—all studies have warts. Rather, they were chosen because they used a research design that is widely used in healthcare research. Hopefully, you will actually "wade around" in these studies enough to acquire a thorough understanding of them.

References

Alsén, P., Brink, E., & Persson, L. O. (2008). Living with incomprehensible fatigue after recent myocardial infarction. *Journal of Advanced Nursing, 64*(5), 459–468.

Beitz, J. M., & Goldberg, E. (2005). The lived experience of having a chronic wound: A phenomenologic study. *MEDSURG Nursing, 14*(1), 51–82.

Crane, P. B. (2005). Fatigue and physical activity in older women after myocardial infarction. *Heart & Lung, 34*(1), 30–38.

Curley, M. A. Q., Hibberd, P. L., Fineman, L. D., Wypij, D., Shih, M., Thompson, J. E., et al. (2005). Effects of prone positioning on clinical outcomes in children with acute lung injury. *JAMA, 294*(2), 229–237.

Pellino, T. A., Owen, B., Knapp, L., & Noack, J. (2006). The evaluation of mechanical devices for lateral transfers on perceived exertion and patient comfort. *Orthopaedic Nursing, 25*(1), 4–12.

Persily, C. A., & Hildebrandt, E. (2008). The theory of community empowerment. In M. J. Smith & P. R. Liehr (Eds.), *Middle range theory for nursing* (2nd ed., pp. 131–144). New York, NY: Springer.

Sears, S. F., Serber, E. R., Lewis, T. S., Walker, R. L., Connors, N., Lee, J. T., Curtis, A. B., et al. (2004). Do positive health expectation and optimism relate to quality-of-life outcomes for the patient with an implantable cardioverter-defibrillator? *Journal of Cardiopulmonary Rehabilitation, 24*, 324–331.

Skelly, A. H., Carlson, J. R., Leeman, J., Holditch-Davis, D., & Soward, A. C. M. (2005). Symptom-focused management for African-American women with type 2 diabetes: A pilot study. *Applied Nursing Research, 18*, 213–220.

SUGGESTED READING

Fink, R. M., Hjort, E., Wenger, B., Cook, P. F., Cunningham, M., Orf, A., et al. (2009). The impact of dry versus moist heat on peripheral IV catheter insertion in a hematology-oncology outpatient population. *Oncology Nursing Forum, 36*(4), E198–E204.

Pellino, T. A., Owen, B., Knapp, L., & Noack, J. (2006). The evaluation of mechanical devices for lateral transfers on perceived exertion and patient comfort. *Orthopaedic Nursing, 25*(1), 4–12.

CHAPTER FOUR
Qualitative Research

Research methods that delve deeply into experiences, social processes, and subcultures are referred to as qualitative research. As a group, qualitative research methods:

- Recognize that every individual is situated in an unfolding life context, that is, a set of circumstances, values, and influences
- Respect the meanings each individual assigns to what happens to and around him or her
- Recognize that cultures and subcultures are diverse and have considerable effect on individuals

Qualitative researchers feel strongly that a person's experiences, perceptions, and social interactions are not reducible to numbers and categories—they are much too complex and situated in the context of a person's life. They believe that the researcher attempting to understand experiences, perception, and social interaction must enter into a person's life-world and let the participant's words and accounts lead the researcher to understandings that would remain hidden without deep and open-minded exploration (Munhall, 2007). Thus, qualitative researchers go into their exploration with as few assumptions as possible.

Data Collection and Analysis

The data collection techniques used to understand subjective realities include:

- Nonintrusive, often prolonged, observation
- Conversational interviews
  - ✓ Open-ended questions
  - ✓ Careful listening
  - ✓ Follow-up questions
  - ✓ Helping persons to be reflective about their experiences
  - ✓ Requesting elaboration
- Validation (when making an interpretation of observations or what was said, ask the informant if the interpretation is accurate)

Often, detailed notes are kept or interviews are recorded and subsequently transcribed. The researcher spends considerable time going back and forth through the notes to identify important connections. As the researcher gains greater insight into the issue, the questions asked of subsequent study participants may change (Swanson, 2001). The researcher works inductively, that is: moving from details to a slightly more general encompassing phrase or concept, and finally to a set of themes or patterns that portrays important aspects of the experience, social process, or culture.

The term *qualitative research* actually refers to methodological traditions and methods with diverse aims, data collection techniques, and analysis techniques. The methodological traditions were developed in disciplines such as sociology and anthropology—and nursing has adopted them (see Table 4–1).

The **phenomenological research** tradition is useful in gaining insight into human experiences, whereas the grounded theory tradition enables researchers to understand the fundamental social processes involved in healthcare situations, say, the workings of emergency care transports or how families make the decision for a child to have an organ transplant. The **ethnographic research** tradition creates descriptions of healthcare subcultures, such as chronic renal dialysis units or Alzheimer support groups—from the insider perspective. Two other qualitative research traditions are discourse analysis and historical analysis. Discourse analysis is used to analyze the dynamics and structure of conversations, such as patient–provider dialogue. Historical research examines past events and trends, usually through records, documents, articles, and personal diaries from the past.

Table 4–1 QUALITATIVE RESEARCH TRADITIONS

TRADITION	COMMON AIM IN NURSING STUDIES	DATA COLLECTION TECHNIQUES	DATA ANALYSIS TECHNIQUES
Phenomenologic research	To produce understanding of the lived experience of persons with a particular health condition or situation	1. Select persons who are living or have lived the experience. 2. Set aside preconceived ideas. 3. Engage in dialogue with each participant. 4. Explore the person's life-world. 5. Assist person to be reflective about his or her experiences and what they mean to him or her. 6. Stay in the setting until no new insights are emerging and all issues are understood.	1. Transcribe interviews. 2. Look for segments in the account. 3. Identify significant phrases. 4. Group phrases with common thoughts into themes. 5. Confirm themes with the participants.
Ethnographic research	To produce a rich portrayal of the norms, values, language, roles, and social rules of a health or healthcare culture or subculture	1. Immerse self in the culture/setting, typically for long periods of time. 2. Observe social interactions. 3. Seek out and informally question good informants. 4. Analyze documents. 5. Take detailed notes.	1. Identification of social rules and understandings. 2. Analysis of social networks. 3. Confirmation of interpretations. 4. Produce a coherent account of the culture. 5. Check out description with key informants.

(continued)

Table 4–1 (CONTINUED)

TRADITION	COMMON AIM IN NURSING STUDIES	DATA COLLECTION TECHNIQUES	DATA ANALYSIS TECHNIQUES
Grounded theory research	To produce a theory (i.e., a tentative, coherent explanation) about how a social process works	1. Gain access to the social setting. 2. Observe social interactions. 3. Conduct informal interviews. 4. Keep field notes. 5. Identify useful written materials. 6. Stay in the setting until no new insights are emerging and all issues are well understood.	1. Intermix data collection and analysis. 2. Name what is happening in the data with codes. 3. Analyze the use of language. 4. Proceed from concrete codes to theoretical ones. 5. Constantly compare new data with previously acquired data. 6. Generate hypotheses and check them out with participants.

Each of these traditions requires techniques for collecting and analyzing data appropriate to its purposes. After looking across the rows of Table 4–1, which will give you a sense for each tradition, look down the columns and note how the purposes and methods of these traditions differ.

Qualitative Description

Not all questions in nursing and healthcare can be investigated in a clinically useful way using the methods of one of the traditions just described. As a result another method that draws on features from the traditional approaches has evolved. This somewhat eclectic approach is called *qualitative description* (Neergaard, Olesen, Andersen, & Sondegaard, 2009; Sandelowski, 2000, 2010; Thorne, Kirkham, & MacDonald-Emes, 1997). The goal of qualitative description is to produce a straightforward description of participants' experiences in words as similar to what the participants said as possible. Most often, but not always, the participants are patients. Commonly used methods of qualitative description include, but are not limited to the following:

1. Sampling for diversity
2. Data collection by interviews of individual or focus groups
3. Data analysis by qualitative content analysis
4. Generation of themes or patterns that capture what has been said

Even quantitative data collection and analysis techniques can be incorporated into a study using the qualitative description method.

Understanding how *qualitative content analysis* is done is key to understanding this qualitative research method. If you think about it, you will realize that qualitative data collection produces an abundance of data— pages and pages of transcripts of interviews and dialogue or of written material. To extract meaning from all this raw data, researchers identify sections of data that convey an idea and assign it a word or phrase code that conveys its essence. The code should be data-derived, i.e., generated from the data itself (Sandelowski, 2000). In assigning a code to a section of transcribed narrative or a section of a diary, the researcher is always aware that she is making an interpretation and therefore must be careful that the code does not change the original meaning of what was said.

Content analysis is not a linear, constantly forward-moving process. Rather, it is dynamic and reflexive. If none of the previously used codes captures the meaning of a section of text, the researcher will create a new code.

The new code may or may not lead the researcher to revise the coding of already coded text.

A list of codes can be informative, but it may be more useful if coding is taken a step further. That step involves identifying similarities in the codes; it may be possible to group similar codes without losing the meaning of the first round of codes. This broader grouping may be a category, a chronological order, or a theme. Again, the researcher is on guard to not lose the meaning of the original data and codes.

> Original quote → Code
> Several similar codes → Theme

Importantly, even though qualitative description is somewhat eclectic in the methods used, researchers who use it remain committed to rigor of method by using methodological principles widely recognized by other qualitative researchers. In summary, qualitative description is a very pragmatic approach to doing qualitative research. It is characterized by using a combination of methods that will produce a useful description of the experience, perceptions, or events of interest. Any interpretation produced should not be far removed in meaning from the data provided by the study participants.

Uniqueness of Qualitative Studies

Some findings from qualitative research are useful in their own right, whereas others produce hypotheses that require further study using quantitative methods. Certainly, in-depth descriptions of patients' experiences of illness and health care are directly useful to nurses in understanding what their patients are experiencing and in communicating helpfully with them. They may also be useful in developing nursing assessment guides and teaching plans.

Other findings from qualitative research are hypotheses about associations and causal relationships at work in the situation of interest. These hypotheses require further study using quantitative methods—to acquire knowledge regarding the degree to which the identified associations are true across different segments of the population or to test possible causal relationships identified by the qualitative study.

At first, qualitative research methods may seem "unscientific" to you. Although it is true that they are very different from what most people view as "scientific," the reality is that these methods have been developed to acquire insights into subjective experiences and social processes—complex human realities that cannot be broken apart, manipulated, and examined the way physical realities can be. The rich and nuanced understandings of human experiences and social interaction produced by qualitative methods cannot be achieved using methods that reduce human characteristics to numbers and the context of human lives to the status of "variables."

Qualitative studies are sometimes criticized for having small sample sizes or for not being objective. These criticisms are based on a lack of understanding of what qualitative studies aim to produce and how their methods produce unique and valuable forms of knowledge for the clinical professions. Both qualitative and quantitative research methods have a place in the scientific toolbox of the clinical professions. Just as a house cannot be built with only one type of tool, e.g., saws, so it is that producing the full range of knowledge required for clinical practice requires the use of both qualitative and quantitative research methods.

Exemplar

📖 *Reading Tips*

I want to call your attention to the structure of this chapter. I do so because the same structure will be used in the rest of the chapters in Part I of the book. Each chapter is made up of three sections:

1. Introductory information about the featured method in an opening section such as you have just read about qualitative methods
2. A reprinted Exemplar article of an actual study using the featured method
3. A Profile & Commentary on the exemplar article

The Jacobson et al. (2008) article uses qualitative description methods; do pay attention to the full-page box called *More on Methods and Analysis* in the article. The Profile & Commentary that follows the article will refer quite a bit to the information provided in that box.

Patients' Perspectives on Total Knee Replacement

Ann F. Jacobson, Rodney P. Myerscough, Kirsten DeLambo, Eileen Fleming, Amy M. Huddleston, Natalie Bright, and Joseph D. Varley

American Journal of Nursing (2008), 108(5), 54–63.

Abstract

Objective: Because patients' perspectives on total knee replacement (TKR) surgery have rarely been the topic of research, this study sought to describe their pre- and postoperative experiences. *Methods:* Using a qualitative descriptive design, researchers collected data from a convenience sample of 27 patients who were about to undergo or had recently undergone TKR. Preoperative data were obtained in focus group sessions (n = 17); postoperative data were obtained in individual interviews (n = 10). All data-collection sessions were tape-recorded and transcribed, and transcripts were analyzed. The researchers isolated themes by identifying recurrent words and phrases and then sorted the data into thematic categories. *Results:* Four main themes emerged. First, many participants delayed surgery for months to years, despite increasing pain and limitation. Second, once participants decided to proceed with surgery, they entered a period of waiting and worrying about what would happen during and after surgery. Third, both pre- and postoperative participants struggled with the need for independence, as well as with learning to accept the new knee. And fourth, patients experienced postoperative pain associated with surgery and rehabilitation, yet reported having hope that they'd regain function. *Conclusions:* These findings suggest that patients need to be better educated and supported before and after TKR surgery. More research is needed to shed light on how patients' experiences influence their decisions about the surgery and its outcomes.

Key Words

total knee replacement, total knee arthroplastym, patient response to surgery, pain, functional ability, patient education

Total knee replacement (TKR) is one of the most common orthopedic operations in the United States,[1, 2] but few researchers have examined patients' experience of the procedure. The operation, performed to improve function and relieve pain in people with osteoarthritis or rheumatoid arthritis, involves resurfacing damaged bone and cartilage and replacing them with plastic or metal parts.[2] Yet numerous studies of total joint replacement (of the hip or knee) indicate that eligible patients delay or decline the procedure for reasons that aren't well understood.[3, 4] One recent literature review reported that a significant proportion of people who were eligible for joint replacement were unwilling to consider surgery.[4] It concluded that patients' expectations of outcomes are significantly influenced by factors such as sex, race, ethnicity, and socioeconomic status and that patient education materials "may not address the concerns of many individuals." (For more on total knee replacement, see *Facts About Total Knee Replacement Surgery*.)

Facts About Total Knee Replacement Surgery

- The first hinged knee prosthesis, made of ivory, was inserted in 1891 by German surgeon Themistocles Gluck to replace a tubercular joint.[1]
- According to the Agency for Healthcare Research and Quality's Healthcare Cost and Utilization Project (HCUP) (http://hcupnet. ahrq.gov), the number of total knee replacements (TKRs) performed in the United States almost doubled between 1995 (293,086) and 2005 (549,867).
- The proportion of patients ages 40 to 49 years and 50 to 59 years having TKRs increased by 95% and almost 54%, respectively, from 1990 through 2000.[2]
- Significantly fewer eligible black patients elect to have TKR than do eligible white patients.[3, 4]
- According to the HCUP, acute care discharge disposition for TKR in 2005 was 41% to another institution such as a rehabilitation center or nursing home, 32% to home health care, and 26% to home.
- Indications for TKR include "radiographic evidence of joint damage, moderate to severe persistent pain not adequately relieved by an extended course of nonsurgical management, and clinically significant functional limitation resulting in diminished quality of life."[3]
- Advances in implant composition and placement techniques have increased the popularity of TKR surgery. The longevity of the implant depends on individual factors such as the amount and type of postsurgical activity and the patient's weight, age, and sex.[5-8]

References

1. Shetty AA, et al. The evolution of total knee arthroplasty. Part II: the hinged knee replacement and the semi-constrained knee replacement. *Curr Orthop* 2003;17(5):403-7.
2. Jain NB, et al. Trends in epidemiology of knee arthroplasty in the United States, 1990-2000. *Arthritis Rheum* 2005;52(12):3928-33.

3. NIH Consensus Development Conference on Total Knee Replacement. NIH Consensus Statement on total knee replacement. *NIH Consens State Sci Statements* 2003;20(1):1-34. http://consensus.nih.gov/2003/2003 TotalKneeReplacement117main.htm.

4. Weng HH, Fitzgerald J. Current issues in joint replacement surgery. *Curr Opin Rheumatol* 2006;18(2):163-9.

5. Beadling L. TKA can be an option for the young active patient. *Orthop Today* 2003;23(10):43.

6. Dennis DA. Trends in total knee arthroplasty. *Orthopedics* 2006;29(9): S13-S16.

7. Jenabzadeh AR, Haddad FS. Novel strategies in joint replacement. *Br J Hosp Med Lond* 2006;67(6):294-8.

8. Vazquez-Vela Johnson G, et al. Patient demographics as a predictor of the ten-year survival rate in primary total knee replacement. *J Bone Joint Surg Br* 2003;85(1):52-6.

One orthopedic surgeon who has written on this topic, Peter Bonutti, put it this way: "Maybe we don't understand what our patients care about."[5] He cited two studies' findings that one-third of patients who'd had TKR were dissatisfied with it, and he identified the need to consider the procedure from the patient's, rather than the surgeon's, point of view. The difference in perspective was highlighted in another study of 108 patients who underwent 126 TKRs: patients' subjective and physicians' objective assessments of outcomes correlated poorly.[6] The researchers concluded that "surgeons are more satisfied than patients."

In 2003 the National Institutes of Health held the Consensus Development Conference on Total Knee Replacement, calling in particular for research into patients' decisions about surgery and the factors that affect outcomes.[7] Members of the expert panel also suggested that the use of qualitative rather than quantitative methods might reveal a fuller range of experiences. And a British review examining qualitative research concluded that it "has particular strengths in uncovering evidence that is discrepant with researchers' or practitioners' prior assumptions" and revealing "significant but unanticipated factors."[8]

Methods

In seeking to describe patients' experiences with TKR, we used a qualitative descriptive design, collecting data from 17 preoperative and 10 postoperative patients during focus group and individual interviews, respectively. The focus group session immediately followed the hospital's joint-replacement class. Because of the limitations imposed by postoperative recovery and the variety of care sites, we collected data on patients' postoperative experiences during individual interviews. Table 1 shows the demographic characteristics of the sample. (For additional details about the methods, see *More on Methods and Analysis*.)

Table 1   PARTICIPANT CHARACTERISTICS (N = 27)

DEMOGRAPHIC	MALE (N = 13)	FEMALE (N = 14)	TOTAL (N = 27)
Mean age, in years (SD)	66.5 (12.8)	65.6 (11.9)	66.03 (12.1)
Range in years of age	45–83	49–83	45–83
Race, n (%)			
African American	1 (7.7)	2 (14.3)	3 (11.1)
White	12 (92.3)	12 (85.7)	24 (89.9)
Marital status, n (%)			
Married	8 (61.5)	7 (50)	15 (55.6)
Widowed	3 (23.1)	2 (14.3)	5 (18.5)
Divorced	1 (7.7)	1 (7.1)	2 (7.4)
Single	1 (7.7)	4 (28.6)	5 (18.5)

SD = standard deviation
Note: Percentages in the middle columns are percentages of the column totals (n) rather than the total cohort (N). Demographic data are not categorized by pre- and postoperative samples because the study did not investigate the differences between these groups; rather, it sought to fully describe patients' experiences.

Results

We identified four overarching themes in patients' experiences of TKR, which we named "putting up and putting off," "waiting and worrying," "letting go and letting in," and "hurting and hoping." Our purpose was to describe overall experience; we did not compare and contrast the data from the pre- and postoperative samples.

Putting up and putting off characterized the period before the decision to have surgery was made. It typically lasted for years and involved "putting up" with knee pain and resulting limitations and "putting off" TKR by modifying activities, using adaptive equipment, and undergoing less drastic treatments.

Putting up: pain limits what you can do. Participants described a gradual increase in knee pain, which they usually characterized as constant and aggravated by walking and other movements. Sometimes the joint gave out unexpectedly when they were walking or climbing stairs. They frequently described the knee as "bone on bone" with "no cartilage." Some reported that the knee was bending to the side or "bowing out."

One participant said, "Pain limits what you can do," a sentiment echoed by many. Another said,

> I'm tired of it. . . . I am a very active person. My favorite comment is 'I can't.' I can't take the trash to the street. I can't cut the grass. . . . I am a car salesman. I feel like a flat tire, and in my business you can't have a flat tire.

Knee pain limited participants' ability to perform many daily activities, including dressing, cooking, cleaning their homes, shopping, using stairs, dancing, and playing golf. Many activities required careful planning, such as bringing crutches or a wheelchair, premedicating with analgesics, and planning routes.

> If I went to the store, I had to know exactly what I could get and just hold onto the shopping cart. . . . [Eventually] I could only go to the stores that had [electric shopping carts]. I really couldn't even walk. . . . [The physician] even encouraged me to get handicapped parking, which I did.

Outings often resulted in fatigue and prolonged or exacerbated pain. Some participants described crying because of the pain and becoming depressed and isolated. As the condition worsened, participants began to limit their activities to those that required little walking or could be accomplished with frequent rest breaks or the use of mobility aids. Some relied on others for transportation; some obtained handicapped parking permits. One participant took her cell phone everywhere, even inside her own home, so that she could "call someone in case I get stuck." Others described modifying the way they approached tasks—for example, placing pillows under the knees when kneeling, sitting or lying down instead of kneeling, and crawling instead of walking.

For some, knee pain and functional limitations changed how they viewed themselves or how they believed others viewed them. They considered themselves active people who had been forced into inactivity. They saw their knee problems as constricting, and even controlling, their lives.

Putting off: getting to the point. Most participants delayed surgery for as long as possible, and for many, that was years after the option was first presented.

> It was something I knew I had to do, but you just keep hoping that it will get better. . . . You get to the point where finally you figure, "I got to do something."

Some said that they'd put off surgery because they'd hoped that medical science would eventually offer a less drastic alternative or because they wanted to first try to strengthen their knees. Most participants said they wished they hadn't delayed surgery for as long as they had and would advise others not to wait so long. But that view was not universally shared. One postoperative participant "wanted to make sure that . . . there wasn't any doubt, that [surgery] was my only recourse."

During this period, participants often received treatments such as cortisone or hylan G-F 20 (Synvisc) injections. These gave transient relief to some; others said the treatments either weren't effective or worsened their condition. Participants referred to these treatments as "Band-Aids," "just temporary," or "a prelude to having [TKR] done."

Waiting and worrying. Once participants decided to proceed with TKR, they entered a period of waiting and worrying about what would happen during and after surgery.

Waiting: let's get it over with. As participants prepared for TKR, they became anxious to put the surgery behind them: "I put this off for years. I can't wait to get it over with." They described the waiting period as one filled with apprehension; one spoke of "anxiety that is cursing my life."

Many participants prepared by maintaining or increasing their activity level, believing that would aid recovery: "The better shape you are in, the better you get through surgery." Some worked to get "everything in as much order as [they] possibly can" to prepare for a postoperative period of limited functioning.

Worrying: 'something can go wrong.' Participants reported having concerns about anesthesia, surgery, and complications. Many viewed anesthesia as particularly risky. Participants were given the choice of a spinal or a general anesthetic. Most chose general, even if they felt it was riskier and would prolong recovery; they didn't want to be aware of any aspect of surgery.

I had general anesthesia, it was my choice. . . . [I'm] a nurse; I didn't want to wake up in the middle and hear things. . . . I've been scrubbed in for orthopedic surgeries so I kinda know the sounds and noises, and I didn't want to wake up and hear the jigsaw or anything.

Some expressed a generalized fear about surgery: "Any time you have surgery, anything can happen." Specific fears involved the risk of complications, such as a blood clot, infection, or death. Some had had complications with prior procedures or knew someone who had, which led to their current fear.

More on Methods and Analysis

Design. The qualitative descriptive method entails collecting data and presenting findings in everyday language, with minimal inference and interpretation by researchers, unlike other qualitative methods (such as grounded theory).[1] As Sandelowski states, this method is "especially amenable to obtaining straight and largely unadorned . . . answers to questions of special relevance to practitioners."[1]

The study was approved by the institutional review boards at the university where the first author (AFJ) worked and the hospital where the patients were scheduled for their operations, a large urban medical center with an active orthopedic surgery department. All participants were informed of the nature of the study and signed consent forms. At the end of data collection, each participant was paid $25.

Sample. Data were obtained from a convenience sample of 27 patients (see Table 1, page 49) who either were scheduled for total knee replacement (TKR) surgery within one month or had undergone the surgery within the previous two months. Preoperative data were obtained in four focus group sessions in which a total of 17 patients participated; postoperative data were obtained in individual interviews with 10 patients. Inclusion criteria were being able to speak English, being 21 years of age or older, having had no previous total joint replacement, and either being scheduled for (preoperative sample) or having undergone (postoperative sample) a single TKR within the periods specified. Exclusion criteria were having cognitive impairment, rheumatoid arthritis of the operative joint, or significant postoperative complications (such as surgical site infection or thrombophlebitis). In addition, participants in the preoperative sample could not be in the postoperative sample, to avoid the possibility that participation in a preoperative focus group might influence postoperative views. Participants were recruited into both samples until data saturation occurred (with the additional interviews yielding only redundant information).

Instrument. All data collection sessions were tape-recorded and transcribed, with the transcripts serving as the units of analysis.

Preoperative focus groups. Four different focus groups with patients scheduled to undergo their first TKR within one month were held. The focus groups were moderated by one of the authors (RPM), a clinical psychologist with extensive experience in facilitating group discussion. One or two other research team members, RNs with research experience (AFJ and EF), served as assistant moderators, organizing participant recruitment and consent, keeping track of time, observing and recording nonverbal cues, and making other field notes.

Focus group participants were recruited from among people attending a class on total joint replacement, which was held in a conference room of the hospital where they would have the surgery. The nurse leading the class (not a research team member) mentioned the study at the end of class and invited attendees scheduled for a single TKR to remain if they wanted more information. Those who were interested met with one of us (AFJ), who explained the study. Participants signed a consent form and remained for the focus group session, at which participants and moderators were seated around a conference table. The session started with the moderator explaining basic concepts and expectations (for example, that there are no right or wrong answers in descriptive research and that it's hoped that everyone will participate).

The moderator then facilitated the discussion. First, to discourage "group think" (a phenomenon marked by a failure to express views that differ from the perceived group consensus), participants were asked to write down their three main concerns for later discussion. Next, the moderator prompted discussion by asking questions that progressed from the general (such as "As you've been thinking about the surgery, what's been on your mind the most?") to the more specific (such as "What are some of your concerns?"). (The complete list of *Questions for Focus Group and Interview Sessions* is available at http://links.lww.com/A422.) Follow-up questions were based on the participants' responses and were asked as they arose during the sessions. Each focus group session lasted about one hour, after which the moderators held a debriefing session to review responses and note emerging themes.

Postoperative interviews. Potential participants—patients who had undergone TKR in the previous two months—were identified by the orthopedic unit's patient care coordinator, an RN, who notified them of the study and obtained their permission to be contacted by the research team. Those who were interested in participating signed a consent form and scheduled a date for the interview with the research team member (NB), an RN graduate assistant with perioperative experience. Interviews took place on the post-acute rehabilitation unit or the patient's home. The researcher interviewed the patient using open-ended questions. Interviews ranged from about 15 minutes to about 60 minutes in length.

Data analysis. Transcripts from the focus group, debriefing, and interview sessions were first read through. Next, each transcript was read and analyzed using principles of qualitative content analysis, an approach that's "oriented toward summarizing the informational contents of [the] data" with minimal inference and interpretation.[1] Using the study's stated purpose as a guide, the researchers selected relevant sections of the transcripts, defined themes by identifying recurrent words and phrases, sorted the data into the thematic categories, and drew conclusions. Two members of the research team (AFJ and KD) analyzed the data independently and met periodically to compare findings and resolve category coding discrepancies ("check coding"). Codes were repeatedly revised as similarities and differences were noted across categories, until the final categories were considered robust and complete with agreement between coders.

References
1. Sandelowski M. Whatever happened to qualitative description? *Res Nurs Health* 2000;23(4):334-40.

But some said they had no concerns. Many said they tried to maintain a positive attitude, believing a negative one would worsen their outcome.

> I sure don't want to be negative going into it. . . . I mean, it's either go [in] up, or go in down and out. And if you go in down and out, there's . . . a worst-case scenario, that you will have complications.

One factor contributing to worry was having too little information about the operation: "I have no idea how long it will take. . . . Everything is ambiguous. . . . Please tell me what you are going to do." Most wished they'd received more information from their surgeons preoperatively and had better understood what to expect during recovery. One postoperative participant said that understanding the "backward-and-forward" nature of recovery beforehand would have made it "less scary and less traumatic than afterwards thinking, 'Why, what's wrong?'" (For more, see *Questions Participants Had About Surgery*.)

Questions Participants Had About Surgery

- When can I take a shower?
- How can I get up and down stairs?
- Will they give me a temporary wheelchair card for my car?
- How much pain will I have?
- When can I drive?
- What will the incision look like?

Some participants reported feeling well prepared for surgery and recovery. Those who'd received detailed and graphic information from their physicians appreciated it: "He was very explicit about what . . . the surgery would entail. [The surgeon] was great. . . . He let me hold the [replacement] joint in my hand."

Letting go and letting in. Pre- and postoperatively, participants struggled with the need for independence and with allowing others to help, comfort, and support them. "Letting in" also involved learning to accept the knee implant as part of their bodies.

Letting go: accepting a loss of control. Participants described themselves as independent people who found it difficult to rely on others: "I had to accept the loss of control." Many said they'd needed increasing assistance in performing activities of daily living preoperatively. Participants worried about being dependent on others, usually family members, while recovering.

> When you're used to being the caregiver, that's hard, having somebody take care of you. . . . The first night I came home from the hospital . . . I went to the bathroom and I made a mess and I couldn't clean it up. . . . That night [my partner] was fine, he didn't mind cleaning up my mess or doing all that, but I asked him to just leave the room and just let the music play and shut out the lights. I put the pillow over my head and I cried.

Sometimes, participants resisted relinquishing control and exercised their independence, ignoring the advice of clinicians or family members. One participant planned to sip ginger ale after surgery during the period when fluids weren't allowed, believing that it would relieve postoperative nausea. Some planned to get out of bed on their own right after surgery: "I can't be tied down." One planned to bring his pajamas to the hospital, saying he couldn't sleep in anything else. A participant with diabetes planned to adhere to his usual diet after surgery, rather than the one prescribed.

Religion helped some participants; one spoke of God: "He will take care of this." Others articulated a philosophical acceptance: "Life is a road and you have to go down it, and this is something that I have to do."

We observed that letting go was accompanied by letting in—receiving encouragement from others, establishing trust with clinicians, and accepting the new knee.

Letting in: accepting encouragement. Many participants knew others who'd undergone TKR and found their accounts of successful outcomes encouraging: "It is wonderful . . . just thinking that I am going to come out the same way." Some of these acquaintances had spoken about wishing they'd had the procedure years earlier and being happy with the results; they told our participants that after TKR they'd "feel brand-new." But reports of negative outcomes (such as continuing pain or poor knee function) left participants feeling frustrated or fearful, and many said they tried to avoid hearing such stories: "I don't want any negativity around me right now. I want the positive stuff."

Several participants said that having more opportunities to talk with people who'd had the surgery or with providers would have increased their confidence going into surgery.

> Don't let me just read it in a book or in a pamphlet or whatever. That's all well and good, but I want to talk to somebody. I want to bounce things off of them. I want to put myself more at ease. I want to get rid of that stress.

They would also have appreciated a structured peer-support group: "[It helps] knowing that other people have the same discomforts that I have. . . . You know, misery loves company and I'm sure we can compare notes."

Letting in: trusting the team. Participants spoke favorably of physicians who took the time to explain the surgery and answer questions. They valued a direct approach: "He's the nuts-and-bolts type of doctor that I like"; "He's not into fooling around. He tells you what's happening." They related having "100% confidence" in their physicians and their recommendations. Many chose a surgeon based on the recommendations of friends and family; some had solicited opinions about surgeons from others who'd had TKR.

Participants also noted the caring and skills of nurses and other hospital workers, especially those who had helped with transferring and walking. They appreciated nurses who assessed their pain and suggested or administered analgesia. They felt cared for by nurses who "hovered over" them or helped with personal care.

Letting in: accepting the new knee. Participants referred to how "bad" their own knees were and asked questions about the new one. (For more, see *Questions Participants Had About the New Knee.*) Postoperative participants said their muscles needed to "learn" to work with the new knee, which they described as stable and strong.

> I just feel like it's part of my knee. I don't feel like there's anything metal in there, or there's anything different, and if you hold one of those joints in your hands, they're real heavy. But I don't feel it at all. . . . In fact, it feels more steady than [the other] leg, to stand on it.

Questions Participants Had About the New Knee

- What is it made of?
- How long will it last?
- What if the implant wears out?
- Is it heavy?
- Can I get through airport security?
- Do they use the original kneecap?
- Can I kneel on it?
- Will I sink if I go swimming?

Many wished they had seen an actual model. One preoperative participant had, but only after asking the surgeon to show it to her. Another asked his surgeon whether the operation would be videotaped so that he could watch it later.

Hurting and hoping. During the recovery period patients were in pain, and they hoped that regaining lost function would make it worthwhile.

Hurting: pain is the thing. Pain was a prevalent theme. Preoperatively, participants anticipated postsurgical pain; as one said, "The pain is the main thing with the knee." They expressed the hope that adequate analgesia would be given; some discussed pain management preoperatively with the surgeon or anesthesiologist. One quoted her anesthesiologist's advice to take pain medications at regular intervals rather than as needed, "because if you let that pain get ahold of you, it is really hard to get rid of." Another's physician had said, "Take pain medicine when I tell you to take it and you won't hurt."

Many preoperative participants said that postoperative pain was inevitable and that they would endure it.

> I don't care how much pain medicine you give—it's still going to hurt. The pain medicine's going to wear off. And I know I'm probably going to go through . . . about two weeks of just a lot of pain. And then once that passes, the healing begins, it gets better.

All who underwent surgery reported immediate postoperative pain that was intensified by movement of the leg and by physical therapy. For some, the pain level diminished daily. Several reported being pleasantly surprised to find that they were in less pain than they'd anticipated: "I thought it would be a lot more painful than what it was. . . . I thought it would be a different type of pain." Yet others described severe, continuous pain. One explained how she would prepare someone else considering TKR for post-surgical pain.

> Even if they give you morphine, the pain's still there. . . . I think that would be one thing I would tell a patient: that we can relieve the pain afterward, but you're gonna have pain. And the pain medications will ease it a little bit, but it will never take it away completely.

Pharmacology was the primary pain management strategy—nonpharmacologic measures such as meditation, walking, transcutaneous electrical nerve stimulation, and topical application of ice were less frequently reported. Some participants' care teams advised them about pharmacologic strategies preoperatively. Some noted that nurses' postoperative strategies helped. For example, a home health care nurse advised a participant to take smaller doses of oxycodone with acetaminophen (Percocet) more often, rather than larger doses at greater intervals, with good results: "That really worked for me." Another participant said, "I feel really good in the morning because they medicate me during the night. . . . They said they should give it to me before I start to hurting real bad." But another described losing sleep because of pain and repeatedly asking for analgesia.

> I . . . just cried this morning 'cause it hurt so bad I couldn't stand it. And I couldn't get no more pills. . . . Just wish I could get a doctor in here to . . . give me something a little stronger.

Some participants worried about potential problems with analgesics (such as constipation, nightmares, becoming addicted, breakthrough pain, and reduced mental acuity), and some reported adverse effects.

Hurting: rehabilitation is work. Preoperative participants viewed the rehabilitation period as necessary to returning to normal life, saying that they knew it would involve "slow, hard work." Postoperative participants described physical therapy regimens including exercise, walking, and other measures as a necessary stage: "You have to give it time." Adaptive devices such as canes, walkers, and dressing aids (a trouser pull, for example) were used. Regular supervision was important to ensure adherence to the physical therapy program.

> My second physical therapy session in outpatient was tough. . . . They put you on your stomach and they bend your knee. . . . They try to break up the scar tissue, and push on it until you scream. . . . I know they have to do it. I know I can't do it all on my own.

Some made steady progress: "I expected to be able to get up and walk right away, and I did." One found rehabilitation to be "not as bad as what I figured it would be," as did others. But many voiced frustration over a lack of progress. How long is it gonna take? 'Cause I haven't felt like anything has changed. Everybody says it looks like it has, but I can't see that and I don't feel that.

Hoping: eyes on the prize. Participants envisioned a timeline for recovery, although the duration of the timeline varied, and some patients were more specific than others. Many predicted that they'd be independent, able to return to work, or both within three weeks. Some predicted it would take several months to a year. They emphasized the need to stay motivated during recovery: "Gotta keep your eye on the prize." They talked about pushing themselves or being pushed by providers or family members.

Since I couldn't go outside much, [the physical therapist] told me, "Just walk." So I walk from one end of the house to the other. I try to keep walking.

Participants believed that if they didn't perform the prescribed rehabilitation exercises, their new knees would be "stiff" or painful or wouldn't bend. Some said they thought that if they didn't bend their knees as prescribed, the surgeon would "take you back to surgery and bend it for you."

So I'm telling myself, and I'll tell somebody else, "Don't give up until you get full mobility back." Because if you don't gain it in this window of time . . . you're not gonna. You can't decide a year from now, "I'm gonna rehabilitate my knee and get more mobility." It's gone.

Many identified having a positive attitude, before and after surgery, as being necessary. One referred to this as "mind management."

Hoping: back to normal. Participants articulated specific activities they hoped to be able to perform as a result of the surgery, especially those they had been capable of doing "without having to think about it" and without pain, such as housework, gardening, and walking the dog. (For more, go to http://links.lww.com/A423.) The phrase "normal human being" was often used.

I'm going to be back out hiking and biking and doing all those things I haven't been able to do. Get down on the floor with my grandkids. I have no fear that it's not going to be good; I know it's going to be good.

Discussion

Many of our 27 participants reported delaying the surgery for months to years, despite increasing pain and limitation. Similarly, prolonged "enduring" was identified in a qualitative study of nine people in New Zealand who had had TKR surgery.[9] While our study included only people who ultimately did have the operation, their comments suggest that possible reasons for delay include the hope that the knee would get better on its own or that surgical advances would offer less drastic alternatives to total joint replacement. The latter reason echoes findings from a 1997 study of 30 people with osteoarthritis of the hip or knee, in which women were more likely than men to delay surgery because they expected that technology would improve.[10]

Once participants decided to proceed with surgery, they typically anticipated it with anxiety and felt a desire to "get it over with." Common sources of anxiety were general fears about anesthesia, surgery, and complications. Another frequent concern was their lack of information about the implant and what surgery and recovery would entail. In contrast, two quantitative surveys of patients planning to undergo total joint replacement identified more specific concerns, the most prominent of which involved postsurgical pain and mobility and the ability to care for oneself.[11, 12] This discrepancy may result from the selection of items included in the quantitative surveys and the forced-choice responses they entailed. In our study, participants' responses were not so restricted.

Although we conducted the preoperative interviews after patients had met with their surgeons and attended the hospital's joint-replacement class, our findings strongly suggest that patients wanted more information. But does additional information improve outcomes? A recent review of nine studies involving a total of 782 patients about to undergo joint replacement suggests that it does not. The researchers concluded that "there is little evidence to support the use of preoperative education . . . to improve [most] postoperative outcomes," although they said that "there is evidence that preoperative education has a modest beneficial effect on preoperative anxiety."[13] Similarly, a Swedish study found that giving patients specific information about pain management before TKR lessened their anxiety.[14] Such educational programs are increasingly common, but because they don't report on the theoretical or empirical basis for their design, the mechanisms that might explain their effectiveness remain obscured, limiting their applicability.[15, 16] More research is needed. Approaches tailored to a patient's age, race, and sex may be most effective.[11, 12]

Many participants indicated that they would have liked to have talked with others who had had successful TKR; those who had done so reported feeling that it was helpful. Other qualitative studies of people considering total joint replacement have described similar findings.[10, 17] Further investigation into the efficacy of formal peer-support interventions—which have been effective in other patient populations (such as people with cancer[18] or diabetes[19])—for people preparing to undergo TKR is warranted.

The adequacy of participants' postoperative analgesia was inconsistent. For some, acceptable pain control was obtained with strategies such as routine dosing (rather than dosing as needed) and consultation with providers. Some comments reflected acceptance of postoperative pain, which was perceived as inevitable. Because preoperative expectations of postoperative pain and doubt about one's ability to manage it can increase pain levels,[20] effective pain management strategies should be developed and shared with patients before surgery.

Limitations. The study has several limitations. Participants were recruited by convenience sampling from one healthcare institution, and their experiences may not be representative of all patients in all geographic regions. Another limitation was a lack of control over variables (such as the surgeon, the surgical technique, and the analgesic regimen) that could influence participants' experiences. And although we attempted to encourage participants to respond candidly, the fact that we identified focus group moderators and interviewers as healthcare professionals may have altered some of the responses we received.

Further Considerations

Our study revealed four themes reflecting patients' experiences of anticipating and recovering from TKR, extending the findings of several other studies in this population.

Findings from this and similar studies suggest that patients need better education and support and highlight the role of the healthcare team, particularly nurses and physicians, in providing both. Patients aren't prepared to make the decision to undergo TKR, and they don't know what to expect in the postoperative period. Anxiety and pain, which were common before and after surgery, may adversely affect outcomes. Participants emphasized the benefits of peer support and of having competent and caring surgeons, anesthesiologists, and nurses. Descriptive and interventional studies should be conducted to evaluate strategies designed to eliminate or reduce the negative aspects of TKR (such as preoperative pain and anxiety) and promote positive influences (such as peer support). More research focusing on the patient's perspective is also needed to explore how patients' experiences influence their decisions about TKR surgery and affect their outcomes.

Ann F. Jacobson is an associate professor at Kent State University (KSU) College of Nursing in Kent, OH. Rodney P. Myerscough is a clinical psychologist at Summa Health System in Akron, OH; this study was conducted at St. Thomas Hospital, a Summa site. Kirsten DeLambo was a postdoctoral fellow at the Summa Health System-KSU Center for the Treatment and Study of Traumatic Stress in Akron at the time of the study and is now a psychologist with KSU Health Services. Eileen Fleming is the nursing research coordinator and Amy M. Huddleston is a clinical psychologist at Summa Health System. Natalie Bright was a master's-degree candidate at KSU College of Nursing at the time of the study and is now an organizational learning and performance specialist at Hillcrest Hospital in Mayfield Heights, OH. Joseph D. Varley is chairman of the Department of Psychiatry at Summa Health System.

The study was funded by the Summa Health System-KSU Center for the Treatment and Study of Traumatic Stress; the KSU Research Council; and Sigma Theta Tau, Delta Xi Chapter. The authors have disclosed no other significant ties, financial or otherwise, to any company that might have an interest in the publication of this educational activity. They thank Patty Costigan, MSN, RN, and LeAnn Speering, MS, CCRP, for assistance with data collection; Claire Draucker, PhD, RN, for guidance on qualitative methods and analysis; and Elizabeth H. Winslow, PhD, RN, FAAN, for her review of a previous version of this article. Contact author: Ann F. Jacobson, ajacobso@kent.edu.

References

1. Agency for Healthcare Research and Quality. *HCUPnet, healthcare cost and utilization project* [database online]. http://hcupnet.ahrq.gov.
2. Kane RL, et al. *Total knee replacement*. Rockville, MD: Agency for Healthcare Research and Quality; 2003 Dec. AHRQ publication no. 04-E006-2. Evidence report/technology assessment, no. 86. http://www.ncbi.nlm.nih.gov/books/bv.fcgi?rid=hstat1a.chapter.16930.
3. Ballantyne PJ, et al. A patient-centered perspective on surgery avoidance for hip or knee arthritis: lessons for the future. *Arthritis Rheum* 2007;57(1):27-34.
4. Hawker GA. Who, when, and why total joint replacement surgery? The patient's perspective. *Curr Opin Rheumatol* 2006;18(5):526-30.
5. Bonutti PM. *Improving patient satisfaction through technique: minimally invasive TKA*. Clinical counterpoints: new techniques in total knee arthroplasty and pain management; 2005 Feb 24; Washington, D.C.: Medscape and the Postgraduate Institute for Medicine; 2005. http://www.medscape.com/viewarticle/502313_9.

6. Bullens PH, et al. Patient satisfaction after total knee arthroplasty: a comparison between subjective and objective outcome assessments. *J Arthroplasty* 2001;16(6):740-7.

7. NIH Consensus Development Conference on Total Knee Replacement. NIH Consensus Statement on total knee replacement. *NIH Consens State Sci Statements* 2003;20(1):1-34. http://consensus.nih.gov/2003/2003 TotalKneeReplacement117main.htm.

8. Murphy E, et al. Qualitative research methods in health technology assessment: a review of the literature. *Health Technol Assess* 1998; 2(16):iii-ix, 1-274.

9. Marcinkowski K, et al. Getting back to the future: a grounded theory study of the patient perspective of total knee joint arthroplasty. *Orthop Nurs* 2005;24(3):202-9.

10. Karlson EW, et al. Gender differences in patient preferences may underlie differential utilization of elective surgery. *Am J Med* 1997;102(6):524-30.

11. Macario A, et al. What questions do patients undergoing lower extremity joint replacement surgery have? *BMC Health Serv Res* 2003;3(1):11.

12. Trousdale RT, et al. Patients' concerns prior to undergoing total hip and total knee arthroplasty. *Mayo Clin Proc* 1999;74(10):978-82.

13. McDonald S, et al. Pre-operative education for hip or knee replacement. *Cochrane Database Syst Rev* 2004(1):CD003526.

14. Sjoling M, et al. The impact of preoperative information on state anxiety, postoperative pain and satisfaction with pain management. *Patient Educ Couns* 2003;51(2):169-76.

15. Prouty A, et al. Multidisciplinary patient education for total joint replacement surgery patients. *Orthop Nurs* 2006;25(4):257-61.

16. Tribbey F. Total joint replacement program. *Med-Surg Matters* 2005;14(1):9.

17. Clark JP, et al. The moving target: a qualitative study of elderly patients' decision-making regarding total joint replacement surgery. *J Bone Joint Surg Am* 2004;86-A(7):1366-74.

18. Ussher J, et al. What do cancer support groups provide which other supportive relationships do not? The experience of peer support groups for people with cancer. *Soc Sci Med* 2006;62(10):2565-76.

19. McPherson SL, et al. The benefits of peer support with diabetes. *Nurs Forum* 2004;39(4):5-12.

20. Granot M, Ferber SG. The roles of pain catastrophizing and anxiety in the prediction of postoperative pain intensity: a prospective study. *Clin J Pain* 2005;21(5):439-45.

Profile & Commentary

WHY *Study Purpose*

In the introduction, the authors set forth the reasons *why* they conducted this study, namely that patients' subjective experiences of having a total knee replacement (TKR) are not well understood. The lack of understanding is reflected in the findings of several previously conducted studies. The authors cite several studies in which patients were found to delay having a TKR for a long time even though they were having considerable pain and functional limitations. Also, two studies found that after surgery a third of the patients were dissatisfied with their outcomes. The goal of the study was to describe patients' experiences before and after uncomplicated TKR. The restriction to patients with uncomplicated results is important as it limits the variation in the data; patients with complications undoubtedly have very different views than patients with smooth postoperative recoveries.

HOW *Methods*

How the study was done is described in a short section in the body of the report and in greater detail in the box called *More on Methods and Analysis*.

Ethics Review   The study was approved by the Institutional Review Boards at the university where the first author worked and the hospital where the patients were seen. An institutional review board (IRB) is a group of people appointed by a university, hospital, or other healthcare organization who are charged with the responsibility of ensuring that the rights of human subjects are protected when a study is conducted under their auspices. Federal law requires that IRBs be nationally registered.

A researcher must receive IRB approval prior to beginning a study and provide reports to the IRB about the ongoing status of the research. In reviewing proposals, IRBs consider the following information:

- How informed consent (knowledgeable choice to participate or not) will be ensured
- Whether pressure or coercion to participate in the study is completely absent
- How participants in the study will be informed about the purpose of the study, the basis of subject selection, the experimental treatments, assignment to treatment groups, and risks associated with each treatment

- How participants will be protected from discomfort and harm and treated with dignity
- How privacy, confidentiality, and anonymity will be ensured

Importantly, an informed consent document must be signed and dated by the participant or the participant's legal guardian. The informed consent document must include a statement giving the researcher access to the participant's protected health information, if that is needed to conduct the study.

Some studies, by their very nature, involve minimal risk of violating human rights, whereas others are very sensitive. Studies involving infants, children, reproductive issues, imposed pain or distress, and risks are considered sensitive, and thus the procedures of the study must be spelled out in great detail. Only individuals who are 18 years of age or older and legally competent can give their own informed consent. Parents or guardians must give consent for minors. The capacity of persons with cognitive and mental limitations to give consent is considered carefully by IRBs.

Recognizing the great diversity of studies, an IRB chairperson or committee designates a study as (1) exempt from review, (2) eligible for expedited review, or (3) requiring complete review (U.S. Department of Health and Human Services, 2005). The criteria for *exempt from review* status are spelled out in a U.S. Department of Health and Human Services policy. If the risk is minimal, an expedited review can be carried out by the IRB chairperson or by one or more experienced reviewers. A study that has greater than minimal risk must receive full review by the entire IRB. From the exemplar article, we don't know if this study underwent expedited review or full review; we do know that it was approved.

Design   In the text and the box we are told that the researchers used qualitative descriptive methods with the goal of conveying what patients said in everyday language.

Sample   Seventeen patients participated in preoperative focus groups, and 10 participated in postoperative individual interviews. Focus group participants were excluded from postoperative interviews to avoid having the preop focus group discussions influence what the patients said in the postoperative interviews. Note the inclusion and exclusion that were used to assure full participation in the focus groups and interviews and to control extraneous influences (e.g., postoperative complications). The sample size was not predetermined; rather, recruitment of new participants was closed when no new information was being contributed (i.e., **data saturation**). A brief demographic profile of the sample participants is provided in Table 1.

Data Collection   The preoperative focus group participants were recruited during classes on joint replacement held in the hospital; the focus groups were held immediately after the classes. The moderators, who were experienced in leading group discussions, used prompts that at first encouraged participants to say what was on their minds but subsequently asked participants to talk about more specific issues. Do look at the questions used for the focus group and the interview sessions that are provided at the online site given in the article. I would say that the questions are slightly more focused than what might be used by some other qualitative researchers. The postoperative interviews were held within 2 months of having undergone the TKR; they lasted 15 to 60 minutes. Transcripts of both the focus group dialogue and the interviews were produced to facilitate analysis.

Data Analysis   The researchers analyzed the data of transcripts using the principles of qualitative content analysis. They marked sections of the data relevant to understanding the patients' experiences and perceptions with word or phrase codes that conveyed the meaning of the section or comment. The codes were then grouped into themes based on similarity of the ideas expressed. Do note that the researchers took steps to control their own preconceptions during this interpretation process.

WHAT *Results*

Four overarching themes comprise *what* was found. Under the heading for each of these themes, the researchers provide general statements portraying participants' experiences. These statements expand on the abbreviated theme labels. Illustrative participants' quotes that led to the development of each theme are also provided. Notice how these quotes give life to the more abstract overall description. This is how it should be—the linkage between the themes and the quotes should ring true. The themes should not seem forced. The researchers provide these quotes to demonstrate to the reader that the themes did indeed arise out of the data and are close to it. Each reader then makes a judgment about the credibility of the themes.

Discussion

In the Discussion section, the researchers link their findings to findings from other studies. This is crucial to producing a coherent and broad body of knowledge about the issue. These authors (1) link their finding to similar finding in a New Zealand study; (2) contrast their findings to two qualitative surveys of patients planning to have total joint replacement; and (3) discuss the implications of participants' views that they would have liked more information preoperatively. To further place the findings in a larger knowledge context, the limitations of the study, as perceived by the researcher themselves, are set forth. Finally, clinical implications and issues needing further research are offered.

REFERENCES

Jacobson, A. F., Myerscough, R. P., DeLambo, K., Fleming, E., Huddleston, A. M., Bright, N., & Varley, J. D. (2008). Patients' perspectives on total knee replacement: A qualitative study sheds light on pre- and postoperative experiences. *American Journal of Nursing, 108*(5), 54–63.

Munhall, P. (2007). The landscape of qualitative research. In P. Munhall (Ed.), *Nursing research: A qualitative perspective* (4th ed., pp. 3–36). Sudbury, MA: Jones & Bartlett.

Neergaard, M. A., Olesen, F., Andersen, R. S., & Sondergaard, J. (2009). Qualitative description—the poor cousin of health research? *BMC Medical Research Methodology, 9,* 52–57. Advance online publication. http://www.biomedcentral.com/1471-2288/9/52/prepub

Sandelowski, M. (2000). Whatever happened to qualitative description? *Research in Nursing & Health, 23,* 334–340.

Sandelowski, M. (2010). What's in a name? Qualitative description revisited. *Research in Nursing & Health, 33,* 77–84.

Swanson, J. M. (2001). Questions in use. In J. M. Morse, J. M. Swanson, & A. J. Kuzel (Eds.), *The nature of qualitative evidence* (pp. 75–110). Thousand Oaks, CA: Sage.

Thorne, S., Kirkham, S. R., & MacDonald-Emes, J. (1997). Interpretive description: A noncategorical qualitative alternative for developing nursing knowledge. *Research in Nursing & Health, 20,* 169–177.

U.S. Department of Health and Human Services. (2005). *Code of Federal Regulations: Title 45, Part 46, Protection of Human Subjects.* Retrieved August 1, 2010 from http://www.hhs.gov/ohrp/humansubjects/guidance/45cfr46.htm

QUALITATIVE STUDIES USING VARIOUS METHODOLOGIES

Drew, D., & Hewitt, H. (2006). A qualitative approach to understanding patients' diagnosis of Lyme disease. *Public Health Nursing, 23*(1), 20–36. [Phenomenological study]

Eklund, P. G., & Sivberg, B. (2003). Adolescents lived experience of epilepsy. *Journal of Neuroscience Nursing, 35*(1), 40–49. [Content analysis]

Gullick, J., & Stainton, M. C. (2008). Living with chronic obstructive pulmonary disease: Developing conscious body management in a shrinking life-world. *Journal of Advanced Nursing, 64*(6), 605–614. [Phenomenological study]

Knott, A., & Kee, C. C. (2005). Nurses' beliefs about family presence during resuscitation. *Applied Nursing Research, 18*, 192–198. [Qualitative descriptive study]

Leenerts, M. H. (2003). From neglect to care: A theory to guide HIV-positive incarcerated women in self-care. *Journal of the Association of Nurses in AIDS Care, 14*(5), 25–38. [Grounded theory study]

Penney, W., & Wellard, S. J. (2007). Hearing what older consumers say about participation in their care. *International Journal of Nursing Practice, 13*(1), 61–68. [Ethnographic study]

Renaud, M. T. (2007). We are mothers too: Childbearing experiences of lesbian families. *Journal of Obstetric, Gynecologic, and Neonatal Nursing, 36*(2), 190–199. [Ethnographic study]

Roberts, C. A. (1999). Drug use among inner-city African American women: The process of managing loss. *Qualitative Health Research, 9*(5), 620–638. [Grounded theory study]

Spector, D., Mishel, M., Sugg Skinner, C., DeRoo, L. A., VanRiper, M., & Sandler, D. P. (2009). Breast cancer risk perception and lifestyle behaviors among white and black women with a family history of the disease. *Cancer Nursing, 32*(4), 299–308. [Qualitative description]

SUGGESTED READINGS ABOUT QUALITATIVE RESEARCH METHODS

Holloway, I., & Wheeler, S. (2002). *Qualitative research in nursing* (2nd ed.). Oxford, England: Blackwell.

Parse, R. R. (2001). *Qualitative inquiry: The path of sciencing.* Sudbury, MA: Jones and Bartlett.

Polit, D. F., & Beck, T. B. (2004). Qualitative research design and approaches. In D. F. Polit & T. B. Beck. *Nursing research: Principles and methods* (7th ed., pp. 245–272). Philadelphia, PA: Lippincott Williams & Wilkins.

CHAPTER FIVE
Descriptive Research

W hen building knowledge about patients' illness situations or caregiving situations, a useful early step is learning about the elements and features that comprise it. Quantitative descriptive studies create detailed descriptions of the features of phenomena by obtaining structured data—that is, categorical or numerical data—about them. Structured data includes:

- measurements of physiologic states that produce a number value;
- questionnaires with choice answers that can be scored; and
- observations and verbal responses that are categorized and/or counted.

Some quantitative data is obtained directly in numerical form (e.g., white blood cell count), whereas other quantitative data is produced by converting phenomenon from natural form to categories or numerical values (e.g., exercise behaviors described by patients are converted into defined levels of exercise by the data collector). An advantage of quantitative data is that it can be summarized to create a concise snapshot of an experience or situation.

Natural Conditions

In quantitative descriptive research (from now on just called descriptive research), data is obtained from participants under natural conditions, with no attempt to manipulate the situation in any way—no treatment or intervention is given. For this reason, descriptive studies are classified as nonexperimental or observational designs. The aim is to capture naturally occurring variations in the features being studied. After the data is collected from individuals, it is summarized to produce a rather detailed, composite picture of the feature or features of interest. The composite picture portrays the frequency with which the features are present and the different levels at which they are present.

To illustrate, a descriptive study (Lauver, Connolly-Nelson, & Vang, 2007) examined two questions: (1) What are the stressors women experience at the end of treatments for primary cancer? (2) What coping strategies do these women use to cope with their stressors? The researchers had the women complete a problems checklist and a coping questionnaire with a scale. Among the findings were that the most common stressors at four weeks after treatment were difficulty concentrating, attitudes about their bodies, and dealing with mortality, each of these was reported by about one third of the women. To deal with their stressors, 80% to 90% of the women used acceptance, emotional support, and distraction. All the findings together provide a composite picture of the stressors this group of women experience and how they deal with them.

Another descriptive study examined factors associated with hospital arrival time for stroke patients (Maze & Bakas, 2004). Among the features of interest were stroke warning signs that most commonly result in the decision to seek hospital care and hospital arrival time in relation to the onset of the first warning sign. Data was collected from 50 stroke survivors and/or their companions in face-to-face interviews using a structured interview guide. The data about warning signs was categorized by the interviewer from what the patient said, and then the cases in each category were counted. The data about time to arrival at the hospital was quantified as minutes by the interviewer based on the information provided by the patient or companion.

The findings included the following:

1. "The most common stroke warning sign resulting in the decision to seek medical care was sudden confusion and trouble speaking or understanding speech, followed [in frequency] by sudden numbness or weakness on one side of the body" (p. 1).

2. "Only 28.9% of patients arrived at the hospital within 3 hours of the first warning sign, with the mean arrival time for the group being 330.4 minutes (5.5 hours)" (p. 1).

In both the studies just described, the goal was to capture certain aspects of reality as they exist and create useful descriptions of them. The stressor and coping study examined a patient experience, whereas the stroke study examined a situation. Descriptive methods also create descriptions of patient conditions, and the exemplar you will read in this chapter examined a caregiving situation.

Study Variables

In descriptive research, the features, characteristics, or properties of persons, experiences, situations, or things that are studied are referred to as *variables*. By definition, a variable changes or varies from person to person, thing to thing, or situation to situation. In other words, it is not constant. In fact, most characteristics of human nature and of situations vary. Examples of variables are anxiety level, blood pressure, gender, weight, infection, pressure ulcer rate, length of breast feeding, attitudes toward birth control, family unity, frequency of hand washing—quite a diverse list. To expand on one of these: Not every person on the day of surgery has the same level of anxiety; moreover, a person's level of anxiety varies over time depending on what is happening to him or her. Thus, anxiety varies across time in a person and across persons—it is a variable. Gender is an example of a variable that usually has just two variations, that is, categories (female and male), whereas ethnic identification could have several categorical variations (Asian American, black or African American, Hispanic or Latino, white or Caucasian, and so on).

Measurement of Variables

The variables are categorized, counted, or measured, i.e., a numerical value is determined. A person's anxiety level at any point in time can be measured using a questionnaire with a scale that the responder uses to indicate to what degree each statement is true for him or her (see Figure 5–1). The scores for all the statements are then summed to produce a total score. Other variables are categorized rather than measured. For instance, each participant could be asked to indicate her or his ethnicity from a list of six or seven categories.

Measurement involves involves determining one or all of the following:

- Whether the variable is present
- At what level it is present
- The features of the variable that are present
- The strength of the features

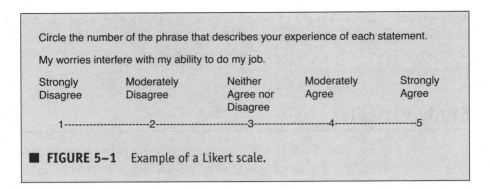

FIGURE 5–1   Example of a Likert scale.

Features of anxiety could include: frequency, degree of perceived threat, physiological sensations, interference with functioning, and duration of the experience. A subscore for each of these features, and a total anxiety score could be calculated. The devices used to measure variables are called tools or **instruments**. Commonly used nursing research instruments include rating scales, questionnaires, physiological measurement, and observational scoring.

In the clinical professions, healthcare providers are interested in the following information about variables of interest:

- Their level (average and range) in various populations.
  Example: How much knowledge do middle-age men have regarding the symptoms of heart attack?
- How they change over time.
  Example: How does hope fluctuate across time for women diagnosed with breast cancer?
- How they affect one another.
  Example: How does general health affect the exercise level of women in their 60s and 70s?

These interests stem from the nature of clinical practice, which uses information about expected levels, causative factors, and associated factors to diagnose the problems of individual patients and plan therapeutic and restorative care for them.

Good Data   In quantitative research, data is considered good when the measurement of variables is consistent and true. Consistent means the measurement method obtains values that are very close to actual values across time, persons, and settings. A measurement method that consistently yields values close to actual values is described in research terms as *reliable*.

A true measurement method captures the essence and attributes of what it is intended to measure. In other words, it really zeroes in on the variable of interest and captures it in its totality. When a measurement method captures to a high degree the totality of a variable of interest, researchers say the measure is *valid*. As you will learn, there are ways of testing a measurement method's reliability and validity, and the results of these tests are often provided in research reports.

Reliability Measurement is not as objective as one might think in that error and inconsistency can enter into measurement at many points. Consider the clinical situation in which two nurses obtain a blood pressure (BP) on a patient with a stable BP. Assume: (a) when the nurse meets the patient, he is standing at the doorway to the room; (b) the measurements are separated by a five minute interval; (c) the second nurse does not know the value the first nurse obtained. Most likely the two BP values obtained will not be exactly the same, even with digital machines. The difference is probably attributable to variations in their measurement methods more than it is to changes in the patient's BP. Differences in cuff size, improper application of the cuff, inconsistent patient body position, use of a different arm, arm position, failure to wait before repeating the measurement, and the calibration of the device used can contribute to variation in BP values.

To the extent that the BP measurements are obtained using the correct technique each time, they will have less error and will more consistently reflect actual BP. When a measurement method consistently captures the actual value, or close to it, the measuring method is considered reliable. To increase the **reliability** of blood pressure measurements in research studies, researchers spell out in great detail the procedure for obtaining and recording a blood pressure measurement to ensure that all persons collecting data do so in the same way.

Validity When measuring something across time and cases, low reliability is not the only problem. The measurement instrument or method may fail to fully capture the essence of the phenomena of interest. In other words, the measure does not truly measure what it is supposed to measure. Often this is because the variable is difficult to define. For instance, coping with a stressful situation is difficult to define—in contrast to blood pressure, which is much easier to define.

Conceptually, blood pressure is the pressure generated by the ejection of blood from the left ventricle into the aorta and dispersed throughout the arteries and capillaries. So, blood pressure is a combination of left ventricular ejection force, the elastic properties of the arterial system, and the location of the measurement relative to the level of the heart. The most direct measurement of blood pressure is achieved by placing a small catheter in a peripheral artery and connecting it to a transducer, which senses the pressure, converts it into a waveform, and eventually into a number value. Of course, blood pressure can also be measured indirectly by a blood pressure cuff and sphygmomanometer or nonmercury device. In most situations indirect BP measurement captures the totality that makes up blood pressure, which is to say that it is a valid measure of what is generally defined as "blood pressure."

In everyday usage, the word *valid* means "true." This is similar to the meaning of the word when used to describe a measurement instrument. It is a true (or valid) measure if there is data supporting that it accurately captures the concept it claims to represent. Over the years, a great deal of data supports the high validity of direct blood pressure measurement and the slightly lower validity of indirect BP measurement. The lower validity of indirect BP measurement is due to the fact that direct BP measurement produces accurate values under a wide range of conditions, including low cardiac output, high peripheral resistance, and patient obesity. However, indirect measurement is either difficult or inaccurate under these conditions. Thus, indirect BP measurement may be valid with some patient populations but have less validity with other populations.

The essence and features of coping are much more difficult to capture than BP. In part this is because coping is a complex, psychological, subjective response of a person over time. It has many features, contextual interactions, and manifestations, whereas blood pressure is made up of fewer, readily identified determinants that are very similar in everyone. Also, our understanding of coping is considerably less than is our understanding of BP. The result of the complexity, subjective nature, and limited knowledge of coping is that capturing its attributes and diverse manifestations is illusive.

Study participants can be asked to report their level of coping but the word itself means different things to different persons. Alternatively, the researcher could ask participants to complete a questionnaire asking them to rate various aspects of their daily functioning, emotions, thought processes, sleeping, and eating. A total coping score for each participant could then be produced to reflect various levels of coping. This measurement process sounds comprehensive and straightforward, but the reality is that the questionnaire would have to be developed carefully over time to be sure that it truly captures the many features and manifestations of coping. It would also have to be tested in various populations because it could be valid with some groups of people and not with others. It could be valid with persons with chronic pain but not with persons in a stressful marriage. In short, the measurement of coping is much more complex and much less objective than is the measurement of blood pressure. In general, obtaining valid measurements of psychological states is more difficult than obtaining valid measurements of physiological states.

> Reliability = Consistency of measurement
> Validity = Accurate capture of underlying concept

Psychosocial Variables   Measuring psychosocial variables is much trickier than measuring biophysical variables because psychosocial variables do not exist as physical realities. Rather, they exist in the minds, emotions, perceptions, experiences, and behaviors of individuals. They also exist conceptually as varying definitions that clinicians, researchers, and theorists assign to them. Thus, psychosocial variables are both subjective and intangible. Researchers develop questionnaires, scales, and observation scoring guides to get at the features specified by a particular definition of the concept. To make them reliable and valid, these instruments or tools need to be developed and refined over time, just as the indirect measurement of blood pressure was refined over the years.

To make a long story short, it takes conceptual clarity, testing, revision, and retesting to produce a valid psychosocial instrument. It is all too easy for a questionnaire to include features of another psychosocial phenomenon that is similar to but slightly different from the phenomenon it is intended to measure. For example self-confidence and optimism are concepts that have similarities to, even overlap with, coping. If the questionnaire items aren't chosen correctly and the balance of items about various features of coping isn't right, the questionnaire might capture self-confidence or optimism instead of coping.

Sometimes a physiological measure can be used as an indicator of a psychological state or behavior. Thus, instead of measuring a psychosocial variable by participant self-report, a physiological, trace indicator of that variable can be measured. For instance, salivary cortisol level is used as an indicator of stress (Galvin, Benson, Deckro, Fricchione, & Dusek, 2006), and serum glycosylated hemoglobin (HbA1c), which reflects average blood sugar over the past 1 to 3 months (but is heavily weighted to the past 2–4 weeks), is used as an indicator of patient self-management of diabetes (Whittemore, D'Eramo Melkus, & Grey, 2005).

Rather than explain here how researchers report validity and reliability of instruments, I explain it in the commentaries about the exemplar studies throughout Part I of the book. It is much easier to understand with specific numbers in front of you. However, you now have enough information to understand what the researcher is talking about when you read the exemplar report in this chapter.

> Appropriate choice of measurement instruments +
> Proven measurement instruments +
> Sound data collection procedures → Trustworthy data

Extraneous Variables

Before leaving the topic of variables, I want to point out that when designing a study the researcher decides which variables will be studied. Other variables may have influence in the situation but are not of interest in the particular study, and these are referred to as **extraneous variables**— *extraneous* meaning outside the interest of the study. Even though they are not of interest, if they influence the data being collected, they can lead to wrong conclusions. To prevent this, researchers try to anticipate these variables in advance of doing the study by eliminating or controlling them. Controlling means to isolate, eliminate, or hold steady their influence in the situation.

Let's say that a researcher is interested in studying whether women of different income levels have different levels of receptivity to TV spots about osteoporosis prevention. If the study involves collecting data from a random sample of women ages 15 to 50, age could be lurking as an extraneous variable. Thus, even though the data may be analyzed so as to answer the questions about how income influences receptivity to TV health messages, any differences found could actually be from a combination of income and age (women with lower incomes might be younger than women with higher incomes). Thus, age is an extraneous variable. It is not of interest in the study but it may be at work in the situation and could confound the findings—meaning that it confuses, or muddies, the interpretation of the results.

Recognizing this problem in advance would allow the researcher to conduct the data analysis in a way that takes the effect of age into account. To do that, the researcher could control the age variable by studying only women in a narrower age range, say, 35 to 50 years. The research question would still be about income level and responsiveness to the TV spots, but the influence of age differences would be greatly reduced. However, in the process the researcher will obtain less information; depending on the research question, this may be okay.

One extraneous factor that always must be kept in mind is that in most studies, the participants are aware of the fact that they are being studied or that their responses will be examined in detail by the researchers. This may make them think more about issues than they would ordinarily, thus they may report problems that persons who are not in the study are not consciously aware of. Another possibility is that the questions asked on a questionnaire influence the person's thinking and change how they answer subsequent questions. Researchers try to minimize the effect of participation in a study, sometimes referred to as the *Hawthorne effect*, by considering the order in which data is collected and/or by giving equal attention to all groups from whom data is collected.

Researchers design studies so as to gain control over extraneous variables and thereby produce findings regarding the variables that are of real interest. However, the world is complex and it is almost impossible to control all the extraneous variables that are operative in a situation. Therefore, researchers often point out in the Discussion section of the report any extraneous variables that were not well controlled in their study and may have influenced the findings. Moreover, as clinicians read study reports, they often identify extraneous variables that may have influenced the results—and which the researcher was not aware of.

Target Population and Sampling

Ultimately, the aim of research is to create knowledge about the levels at which variables of interest exist in a population of people, a population being a large group of persons with a characteristic in common (e.g., they all have chronic bone pain). However, data cannot be collected on all persons in the population—it is not possible for logistical and cost reasons. Instead, researchers collect data about the variables from a small group of people who are part of the larger population and who are more readily available to the researcher. This smaller group is the sample; the group to whom the researchers envision their findings being applicable is the **target population**.

Data is collected from the **sample**, and statistics are calculated. Thus, the levels at which the variables are present in the sample becomes known, and the known values become the basis for estimating the values in the target population. The population's values are inferred from the sample values. Said differently, the sample values are the best guess about the target population values (see Figure 5–2).

When a list of the entire membership of a defined target population exists, researchers randomly choose persons from the list to be in the study—after obtaining their consent, of course. These persons become the sample of the study. When a random selection process is followed, the sample is considered to be representative of the target population because all persons in the target population had a chance to be selected, and those who were selected were randomly chosen. The results from the sample are directly generalizable to the actual target population as per the top part of Figure 5–3.

If, however, obtaining a list of persons in the target population is not possible, the target population is specified differently. First, *available* persons who are presumed to be members of the assumed population are recruited. A sample created in this way is called a convenience sample.

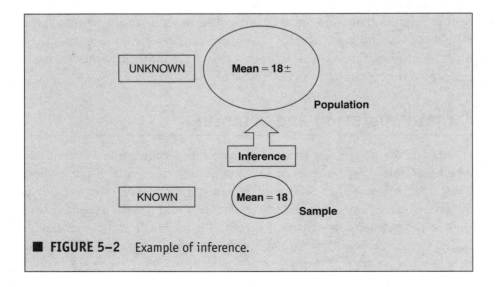

■ FIGURE 5–2   Example of inference.

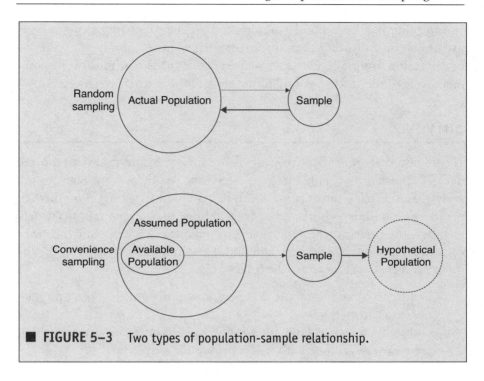

■ **FIGURE 5-3**   Two types of population-sample relationship.

Then a profile of the members of the sample is compiled. The sample may be profiled in terms of the setting in which they are receiving care, health status, disease, symptoms, age, or other demographic variable. The profile becomes the basis for specifying a hypothetical population (Huck, 2007). The hypothetical population is all persons who have a profile similar to that of the sample. The results from the sample are indirectly generalizable to persons who are similar to the sample profile (i.e., person in the hypothetical population). This is illustrated in the bottom part of Figure 5–3.

In healthcare research, complete lists of population members are quite rare, thus convenience samples and resulting hypothetical populations are quite common. Convenience samples also reduce the cost and effort of doing a study. Even when a list exists—of say, women who are having treatment for breast cancer, which could be obtained from cancer registries—it would be logistically very difficult to consistently collect data from a sample scattered across a state or nation. To make the study more feasible, the researchers might decide to recruit participants from one or two cancer centers and specify a hypothetical target population based on the profile of that sample.

Sampling is a broad and complex topic. The preceding explanations just touch on it. Rather than discuss it further here, I point out methods of obtaining samples and the consequences of those methods in the commentaries of the studies you read in this and the next three chapters.

Surveys

A common type of descriptive study is the survey. In surveys, self-reported data is collected by mail, Internet, telephone, or in person. Surveys are widely used because a lot of data can be collected from large numbers of people with minimal effort and expense. However, surveys are also widely misused—by persons who fail to recognize the various ways in which they can lead to erroneous results (Dillman, Smyth, & Christian, 2009). The main problems in surveys are the following:

- Failure to obtain a sample that is representative of the target population right from the start
- Difficulty in constructing questionnaires and interview questions that are clear to everyone who will complete the survey
- Low response rates, which make the respondents not representative of the target population (Dillman, Smyth, & Christian, 2009)

When conducted properly, surveys provide useful information, but when conducted by the inexperienced, they produce misleading information.

Results

Percentages

Descriptive studies report results in a variety of ways. Perhaps the most common way is percentages. In a study of Australian cardiac patients' knowledge and use of sublingual glyceryl trinitrate (commonly called sublingual nitroglycerin), results included the following: (1) 82% of participants carried the medication with them at all times, and (2) 24.4% knew that taking the drug to prevent chest pain was an appropriate use (Fan, Mitchell, & Cooke, 2007).

Center and Spread of the Scores

To convey the typical or representative score, the mean or median may be reported. Remember, the mean is the numerical average of the scores and is the best description of group average when the scores are evenly distributed around the mean. Means are reported when most of the scores are near the mean with gradual decreases in frequency of scores on both sides further from the mean. The median is more typical when the distribution of scores is skewed (i.e., there are a few scores strung out on *one side* toward the end of the score continuum—away from the majority).

In a study of why elderly people delay responding to heart failure symptoms (Jurgens, Hoke, Brynes, & Riegel, 2009), the median duration of various symptoms before hospital admission was reported. The median delay reported by patients experiencing dyspnea was 3 days. The authors reported the median because there were several persons who delayed for up to 90 days, and this skewed the data toward longer delay; those few cases elevated the mean so it was not representative of average or typical persons.

To convey the variability or spread in the data, researchers often report the range of scores (actual low score and high score) or the interquartile range, which indicates the spread of the middle 50% of scores (see Figure 5–4). Data with narrow ranges or interquartile ranges are less dispersed than are data with wide ranges. Sometimes data dispersion is of as much interest as is the average of the scores.

Case	1	2	3	4	5	6	7	8	9	10	11
Score	52	54	55	57	58	59	60	62	65	66	68
Quartile			Q1			Q2 Median			Q3		

[-------------------- IQR = 55–65 ----------------------]

■ **FIGURE 5–4** Example of interquartile range (IQR).

Percentages, means, medians, and ranges are widely used in reporting the results of descriptive studies. This, plus the natural conditions under which data is collected, makes descriptive studies generally easy to read and understand. Thus, a descriptive study serves as the first quantitative design to be considered.

Exemplar

📖 *Reading Tips*

If you don't know what an endotracheal tube is, you will get more from this research article if you take a few minutes to obtain some basic information about it from a medical–surgical text or medical dictionary.

An Observational Study on the Open-System Endotracheal Suctioning Practices of Critical Care Nurses

Sean Kelleher and Tom Andrews

Journal of Clinical Nursing (2008), 17(3), 360–369.

Aim and objectives. The purpose of this study was to investigate open-system endotracheal suctioning (ETS) practices of critical care nurses. Specific objectives were to examine nurses' practices prior to, during and post-ETS and to compare nurses' ETS practices with current research recommendations.

Background. ETS is a potentially harmful procedure that, if performed inappropriately or incorrectly, might result in life-threatening complications for patients. The literature suggests that critical care nurses vary in their suctioning practices; however, the evidence is predominantly based on retrospective studies that fail to address how ETS is practiced on a daily basis.

Design and method. In March 2005, a structured observational study was conducted using a piloted 20-item observational schedule on two adult intensive-care units to determine how critical care nurses ($n = 45$) perform ETS in their daily practice and to establish whether the current best practice recommendations for ETS are being adhered to.

Results. The findings indicate that participants varied in their ETS practices; did not adhere to best practice suctioning recommendations; and consequently provided lower-quality ETS treatment than expected. Significant discrepancies were observed in the participants' respiratory assessment techniques, hyperoxygenation and infection control practices, patient reassurance and the level of negative pressure used to clear secretions.

Conclusion. The findings suggest that critical care nurses do not adhere to best practice recommendations when performing ETS. The results of this study offer an Irish/European perspective on critical care nurses' daily suctioning practices.

Relevance to clinical practice. As a matter of urgency, institutional policies and guidelines, which are based on current best practice recommendations, need to be developed and/or reviewed and teaching interventions developed to improve nurses' ETS practices, particularly in regard to auscultation skills, hyperoxygenation practices, suctioning pressures and infection control measures.

Key Words

clinical significance, critical care, evidence-based practice, nursing practice, observation

Introduction

The ultimate goal of nursing is to provide evidence-based care that promotes quality outcomes for patients, families, health-care providers and the health-care system (Craig & Smyth 2002). While the literature has demonstrated that nurses are increasingly recognizing the role research has to play within modern health care (Hundley *et al.* 2000), it seems that many established nursing practices are not underpinned by sound evidence (Glacken & Chaney 2004). One area of nursing practice that has caused concern is the endotracheal suctioning (ETS) of intubated patients (Swartz *et al.* 1996, Thompson 2000, Sole *et al.* 2003). ETS is an important intervention in caring for patients with an artificial airway (Thompson 2000) and an essential aspect of effective airway management in the critically ill (Wood 1998b). It is an invasive, potentially harmful procedure, which when performed inappropriately or incorrectly can result in serious complications (Celik & Elbas 2000, Paul Allen & Ostrow 2000). It is important, therefore, that those carrying out such a procedure are aware of the potential risks and practice in a manner that ensures effectiveness and patient safety.

Literature Review

While ETS is an important intervention when caring for critically ill patients, the practice surrounding ETS can vary widely between institutions and practitioners (Swartz *et al.* 1996, Sole *et al.* 2003) with much of that practice based on anecdote and routine rather than research (Paul Allen & Ostrow 2000, Thompson 2000, Day *et al.* 2002b). This may partially have been influenced by a paucity of research evidence to guide practitioners in the care of a patient with an endotracheal tube (Thompson 2000). The last decade has seen a steady increase in the body of literature relating to how and when ETS should be performed (Glass & Grap 1995, Wainwright & Gould 1996, Wood 1998b, Thompson 2000, Day *et al.* 2002b, Moore 2003). Much of this evidence is in the form of succinct literature reviews (Wood 1998b, Day *et al.* 2002a) and systematic reviews (Thompson 2000) enabling practitioners quickly and easily to determine current research recommendations irrespective of their ability to interpret the research findings. Nonetheless, there is still some disparity in regard to what exactly constitutes the best ETS practice (Swartz *et al.* 1996) owing largely to a dearth of quality research on ETS techniques. While Thompson (2000), in a systematic review of the literature, isolated aspects of the ETS procedure that are generally accepted as being the most important, a lack of homogeneity and methodological flaws in some of the studies (Thompson 2000) resulted in 13 non-prescriptive recommendations for practice. Conversely, the more conventional literature reviews (Wood 1998a, Day *et al.* 2002a, Moore 2003), which are generally regarded as being less rigorous than systematic reviews (Dickson 2003), explicitly describe how ETS should be performed, but overlook the quality of the evidence from which they originate. Notwithstanding the lack of rigorous research concerning ETS practice, it is generally accepted that the ETS techniques, when used inappropriately or incorrectly can have deleterious effects on patients (Wood 1998b, Celik & Elbas 2000, Paul Allen & Ostrow 2000). It is important therefore to establish how critical care nurses perform ETS and establish how it compares with the current best practice recommendations.

Critical Care Nurses' ETS Practices

A study conducted by Swartz *et al.* (1996) used a quantitative, descriptive design using a survey method to examine 'national' suctioning practices on 80 paediatric intensive-care units (ICU) across the United States. The results indicated that suctioning techniques among critical care nurses varied and were based on a combination of nursing judgement and ward routine. Paul Allen and Ostrow (2000) report similar findings in a quantitative descriptive study which aimed to identify the closed-system ETS practices of 241 randomly selected critical care nurses. One hundred and twenty nurses (50%) responded to a mailed questionnaire. The findings indicated variations in nurses' suctioning techniques. While the results of both studies suggest that critical care nurses vary in their ETS practices, the '*ex-post facto*' focus of the studies may not necessarily be an accurate reflection of nurses' daily practice. Carter (1996), cited in Cormack and Benton (1996), suggests that the subjects' written responses to questionnaire items about how they carry out a procedure may bear little resemblance to how they actually perform it.

Day *et al.* (2002b) triangulated observation, interview and questionnaire methods to explore nurses' theoretical knowledge and practical competence in ETS. Using convenience sampling, 28 critical care nurses were recruited from three critical care wards in a large teaching hospital in the UK. The results indicated that many nurses failed to demonstrate an acceptable level of theoretical knowledge and competence in practice and that there was no significant relationship between nurses' theoretical knowledge and observed practice. Furthermore, many nurses were unaware of recommended practice and some demonstrated potentially unsafe practice. These findings are supported in the literature (Celik & Elbas 2000) and have considerable implications for the safety of critically ill patients.

The observational element of Day *et al*'s. (2002a) study ensures a more accurate reflection of what happens in practice than the descriptive retrospective studies discussed earlier (*Swartz et al.* 1996, Paul Allen & Ostrow 2000). This view is supported in the literature, which suggests that observational methods provide data on the realities of current practice from a firsthand perspective (Zeitz 2005). Day *et al*'s. (2002b) findings are, therefore, very significant as they support previous research that identified wide variations in nurses' ETS practices (*Swartz et al.* 1996, Paul Allen & Ostrow 2000) and that nurses are inclined to rely on personal experience and ward routine to inform practice over any other source (Sole *et al.* 2003).

Summary of the Literature

The literature search identified a paucity of empirical evidence relating to how well ETS is performed in the clinical area. The literature that does exist raises concerns about the standard of ETS practice among nurses (Paul Allen & Ostrow 2000, Day *et al.* 2002b). This evidence is predominantly American and based on descriptive, retrospective studies that focus on closed suctioning systems (Swartz *et al.* 1996, Paul Allen & Ostrow 2000, Sole *et al.* 2003). While such studies are important for describing and documenting the aspects of ETS practice, they have one primary limitation. Participants may have a tendency to misrepresent attitudes or traits by giving answers that are consistent with prevailing social views (Polit *et al.* 2001). A few observational studies addressing nurses' ETS practices are identifiable in the literature (Day *et al.* 2002b, McKillop 2004), with only one assessing how actual nursing practice is compared with the recommended practice (Day *et al.* 2002b).

The inconclusive literature relating to nurses' real ETS practices indicates the urgent need for more observational studies in this area. It is only by distinguishing between the real and perceived ETS practice that the degree of deviance, if any, from what the literature has established as being general best practice, can accurately be established.

Method
Aims
The purpose of the study was to investigate open-system ETS practices of critical care nurses. Specific objectives were to:

1. Examine critical care nurses' practices prior to, during and post ETS;
2. Compare nurses' ETS practices with current research recommendations.

Based on the evidence, it is hypothesized that critical care nurses do not adhere to the best practice recommendations when performing ETS.

Design
A non-participant structured observational design was used for this study to gain insight into what is happening in practice. Structured observational studies involve the collection of data that specify the behaviours or events selected for observation and are conducted in the participants' natural environments (Polit *et al.* 2001). Fitzpatrick *et al.* (1994) suggest that direct observation is potentially a more comprehensive method to ascertain how nurses perform in real situations and to identify differences, if any, in practice.

Sample and Setting
The study took place in March 2005 on two adult ICU in Ireland. At the time of the study, the general ICU (GICU) had nine beds with the facility to ventilate patients in all beds at any one time. The cardiac ICU (CICU) had six beds and could facilitate the mechanical ventilation of six patients. GICU employed 53 full-time equivalent nurses and CICU employed 34. The nurses were generally allocated to only one patient per shift. The targeted population of interest were critical-care nurses, as they

predominantly perform ETS, while the sampling unit was the ETS event itself. Event sampling was deemed the most appropriate method of observation because of the erratic nature of the ETS procedure. By means of quota sampling, a total of 45 individual ETS events was observed, whereby each nurse performed only one event. Quota sampling is procedurally similar to convenience sampling; however, the researcher can guide the selection of subjects so that the sample includes an appropriate number of cases from each stratum (Polit *et al.* 2001), the strata in this instance being GITU nurses and CICU nurses. The sample size ($n = 45$) (51%) to be a representative sample of a combined total of 87 nurses (GITU 53, CITU 34) working on both ICUs and compares favourably with previous observational studies addressing ETS, wherein sample sizes ranged from $n = 9$ (Blackwood 1998) to $n = 28$ (Day *et al.* 2002b) observations. Inclusion and exclusion criteria were maintained.

Inclusion Criteria

- Full-time ICU staff members;
- Nurses with a minimum of one-year ICU experience on the study ICU.

Participants were required to fulfil these inclusion criteria to be considered eligible for the study. This can be justified by the argument that an experienced ICU nurse from a different ICU, who has recently been appointed, may work from a different practice/knowledge base depending on the ICU he/she comes from. Equally, nurses who have minimal ICU experience may not have acquired/developed a satisfactory practice/knowledge base from which to work.

Data Collection

Data were collected using a 20-item structured observational schedule (Appendix) adapted from a previously validated survey tool (McKillop 2004), which was constructed to reflect the observable behaviours associated with best-practice suctioning of adults with an artificial airway (Thompson 2000). Aspects of ETS practice that were not specified in the observational schedule developed by McKillop (2004) but implied in a systematic review by Thompson (2000) and established elsewhere as best-practice recommendations (Day *et al.* 2002a, Wood 1998a) were added to the instrument on the recommendation of experts in critical care nursing. The observational schedule was piloted to identify practical or local problems that might potentially affect the research process. No changes were made to the instrument based on the pilot study.

All items on the observational schedule were weighted with the digits 0 and 1, or 0 and 2, respectively. The higher weighting (2) constituted adherence to the best ETS practice as recommended by Thompson (2000) following a systematic review of the literature. The lower weighting (1) represented adherence to what is marginally accepted as constituting best ETS practice as they emanate from traditional literature reviews (Day *et al.* 2002a, Moore 2003). The weighting of 0 represented non-adherence to either of the aforementioned. High observation scores represented closer adherence to recommended best practice.

Validity and Reliability

The observational schedule was distributed for appraisal to a range of experts in critical care nursing, including a university lecturer in critical care nursing, two senior nursing intensive care practitioners and the researcher who developed the original instrument. During the pilot study, the observational schedule was tested for interrater reliability using a second observer, and no significant discrepancies were identified.

Ethical Considerations

Ethical approval to conduct the study was obtained from the appropriate ethics committee, and all participants were informed that their participation was voluntary and that their right to withdraw from the study would be respected at all times. Measures to ensure confidentiality and anonymity were implemented.

Data Analysis

Descriptive statistics included frequency ratings and percentages for nominal-level data. A one-sample *t*-test was used to test the null hypothesis and compare participants' ETS practices to ideal ETS best-practice recommendations. Analysis was performed using the Statistical Package for the Social Scientists (SPSS, version 9.0) software.

Quality of Treatment

To assess how individual participants' performances and subsequently a group's performance compared with recommended best practice, a variable representing 'recommended best practice' had to be developed. This was developed by calculating the sum of the highest possible scores for each observation, which was established as being 35. Each of the 20 items on the schedule was weighted with 0 and 1, or 0 and 2 depending on the strength of supporting evidence for that particular aspect of ETS. The number 35 therefore represented perfect adherence to best-practice recommendations, or ideal treatment. The higher a participant's/group's observational score, the closer the participant/group adhered to best-practice recommendations. Similarly, the lower a participant's/group's score, the less likely was the adherence to best-practice recommendations. This additional variable was subsequently termed 'quality of treatment'. For analysis, the variable was further divided into four subscales to describe the different aspects of the quality of treatment: practices prior to suctioning, infection control practices, the suctioning event and postsuctioning practices.

Results

In accordance with the observational schedule, the results were divided into five sections: practices prior to suctioning, infection control practices, the suctioning event, postsuctioning practices and quality of treatment.

Practices Prior to Suctioning

When assessing the need for ETS, only two (12%) CICU and four (14%) GICU participants auscultated the patient's chest (Table 1). All CICU participants communicated in some form to patients about the imminent procedure; however, eight (28%) GICU participants failed to communicate in any form. Similarly, a greater number of CICU participants were observed to perform hyperoxygenation on patients prior to ETS ($n = 16$, 94%) compared with the GICU group ($n = 22$, 79%).

Infection Control Practices

In relation to wearing gloves and an apron during the ETS procedure, there was no difference between the two groups as both were fully compliant with practice recommendations (Table 2). Disparities in practices were noted, however, in relation to hand washing prior to the procedure, maintaining the sterility of the suction catheter until its insertion into the airway and wearing goggles. Only nine (31%) GICU participants washed their hands before performing ETS in contrast to 11 (65%) from CICU. Ten (59%) CICU and eight (29%) GICU participants failed to maintain the sterility of the suction catheter prior to its insertion into the patient's airway. Only two (12%) CICU, participants and one (3%) GICU participant wore goggles during the ETS procedure.

Table 1   PRACTICES PRIOR TO SUCTIONING

VARIABLE	CARDIAC ICU ($N = 17$)	GENERAL ICU ($N = 28$)
Patient assessment		
No	15 (88%)	24 (86%)
Yes	2 (12%)	4 (14%)
Patient preparation		
No	0	8 (28%)
Yes	17 (100%)	20 (72%)
Prehyperoxygenation/hyperinflation		
Not given	1 (6%)	6 (21%)
Given	16 (94%)	22 (79%)
NaCl (sodium chloride)		
No	17 (100%)	28 (100%)
Yes	0	0

ICU, Intensive-care unit; n = sample number.

Table 2   INFECTION CONTROL PRACTICES

VARIABLE	CARDIAC ICU ($N = 17$)	GENERAL ICU ($N = 28$)
Hand washing		
No	6 (35%)	19 (69%)
Yes	11 (65%)	9 (31%)
Gloves wearing		
No	0	0
Yes	17 (100%)	28 (100%)
Apron wearing		
No	0	0
Yes	17 (100%)	17 (100%)
Catheter sterility		
No	10 (59%)	8 (28%)
Yes	7 (41%)	20 (72%)
Goggles		
No	14 (88%)	27 (97%)
Yes	2 (12%)	1 (3%)

ICU, Intensive-care unit; n = sample number.

The Suctioning Event

Both groups complied fully with best-practice recommendations in relation to suctioning time and application of pressure; however, all participants in both groups exceeded the recommended suctioning pressure of 80 and 150 mmHg (Table 3). Seven (40%) of the CICU group and eight (28%) of the GICU group selected a catheter that was larger than the recommended size for suctioning, and six (21%) GICU participants required more than the maximum number of recommended suction passes.

Table 3 THE SUCTIONING EVENT

VARIABLE	CARDIAC ICU (N = 17)	GENERAL ICU (N = 28)
Catheter size		
> Half internal diameter of ETT	7 (40%)	8 (28%)
≤ Half internal diameter of ETT	10 (60%)	20 (72%)
Number of suctioning passes		
More than two	0	6 (21%)
Two or less	17 (100%)	22 (79%)
Suction time		
> 15 seconds	0	0
≤ 15 seconds	17 (100%)	28 (100%)
Suction pressure		
80–150 mmHg	0	0
> 150 mmHg	17 (100%)	28 (100%)
Suction applied during		
Withdrawal	17 (100%)	28 (100%)
Insertion	0	0

ETT, endotracheal tube; ICU, Intensive-care unit; n = sample number.

Postsuctioning Practices

Two (12%) participants from CICU and seven (24%) from GICU failed to provide post-ETS hyperoxygenation (Table 4). Only one (6%) CICU participant and two (7%) GICU participants auscultated the patients' chest to evaluate the effectiveness of the ETS procedure. The main differences between the groups were in relation to hand washing and providing reassurance, with four (23%) CICU participants failing to wash their hands after the ETS procedure in comparison to 11 (38%) GICU participants. Patients were reassured by 15 (88%) CICU participants in contrast to 11 (38%) from GICU.

Table 4   POSTSUCTIONING PRACTICES

Factor	Cardiac ICU (*n* = 17)	General ICU (*n* = 28)
Oxygen reconnection		
>10 seconds	0	1 (3%)
<10 seconds	17 (100%)	27 (97%)
Postsuctioning hyperoxygenation		
No	2 (12%)	7 (24%)
Yes	15 (88%)	21 (76%)
Post-ETS assessment		
No	16 (94%)	26 (93%)
Yes	1 (6%)	2 (7%)
Patient reassured		
No	2 (12%)	17 (62%)
Yes	15 (88%)	11 (38%)
Hand washing postsuctioning		
No	4 (23%)	11 (38%)
Yes	13 (77%)	17 (62%)
Safety		
No	0	0
Yes	17 (100%)	17 (100%)

ICU, Intensive-care unit; *n* = sample number.

Quality of Treatment

Using a frequency distribution, the average treatment quality across both groups was 22·62 (SD = 3·10) (Table 5). The quality of treatment scores ranged from 14–30. Within the subscales, the highest average score was found in postsuctioning practices (mean = 6·47, SD = 1·53) and the lowest average score was found in infection control measures (mean = 4·67, SD = 1·17). A symmetric distribution was identified in the variable 'treatment quality' and its subscales.

Testing the Null Hypothesis

To compare participants' ETS practices with best-practice recommendations, a one-sample *t*-test was conducted, which compared the treatment quality observed with the ideal treatment quality score (Table 6). The test identified significant differences between the quality of treatment and its subscales (representing the combined ETS practices on both units) and the perfect score (representing recommended best practice). In all categories, the quality of treatment observed was significantly lower than the quality of treatment required ($p = 0.01$). This indicates that our study's sample group only partially adhered to best-practice recommendations when performing ETS and hence rejects the null hypothesis.

Table 5   QUALITY OF TREATMENT

	Practices Prior to Suctioning	Infection Control Practices	Suctioning Event Practices	Post Suctioning	Quality of Treatment
N	45.00	45.00	45.00	45.00	45.00
Mea	5.56	4.67	5.93	6.47	22.62
Median	6.00	5.00	6.00	7.00	23.00
Mode	6.00	5.00	7.00	8.00	25.00
Standard Deviation (S·D)	1.27	1.17	1.12	1.53	3.10
Range	6.00	5.00	5.00	6.00	16.00
Minimum	2.00	3.00	2.00	3.00	14.00
Maximum	8.00	8.00	7.00	9.00	30.00

Table 6   A COMPARISON BETWEEN CURRENT PRACTICE AND BEST-PRACTICE RECOMMENDATIONS

Variable	Maximum Potential Score (representing best practice)	Mean (actual score)	SD	T	DF
Quality of treatment	35	22.62	3.10	−24.63*	44
Practices prior to suctioning	8	5.56	1.27	−12.90*	44
Infection control practices	9	4.67	1.17	−19.15*	44
The suctioning event	9	5.93	1.11	−18.43*	44
Postsuctioning practices	9	6.47	1.53	−11.10*	44

*$p < 0.01$.

Discussion

The findings from this study have raised some interesting issues relating to the current ETS practice of critical care nurses. Best-practice ETS recommendations suggest that, when performing a respiratory assessment, nurses should auscultate the patient's chest to verify the need for ETS (Thompson 2000, Day *et al.* 2002a, Wood 1998a). Our findings show that the participants generally failed to do this. Day *et al.* (2002b) reported similar findings in a study of acute and high-dependency ward nurses. Their findings showed that only two nurses were observed to have performed auscultation. Given that the majority of participants failed to auscultate lung sounds prior to ETS, it is possible that they were working from a combination of clinical signs that indicated the necessity for ETS, such as noisy breathing or visible secretions in the airway (Thompson 2000). A limitation of observational methods, however, meant that there was no way of establishing whether participants' decision to perform ETS was informed by such indicators or whether they were working from some other perspective, such as unit routine, as is suggested in the literature (Swartz *et al.* 1996, Day *et al.* 2002a).Despite abundant evidence on the negative consequences of suctioning induced hypoxemia (Wood 1998a, Thompson 2000, Day *et al.* 2002a) 17 participants still failed to provide hyperoxygenation/hyperinflation either before and/or after ETS. Day *et al.* (2002b)) reported similar findings, where only two out of 10 subjects in their study were observed to provide hyperoxygenation/hyperinflation in practice. Such findings are important as they have direct implications for patient safety and reflect poorly on a vital aspect of nursing care.

Nosocomial infections are among the most common complications affecting hospitalized patients (Burke 2003). Consequently, the importance of aseptic technique in suctioning practices and hand washing before and after such procedures is strongly emphasized in the literature (Thompson 2000, Wood 1998a, Day *et al.* 2002a). Twenty-five participants in our study were not observed to wash their hands prior to the ETS procedure. Boyce and Pittet (2003) suggest that nurses do not wash their hands as expected because of the time it takes out of a busy work schedule, particularly, in high-demand situations, such as critical care units, under busy working conditions and at times of overcrowding or understaffing. One study conducted in an ICU demonstrated that it took nurses an average of 62 seconds to leave a patient's bedside, walk to a sink, wash their hands and return to patient care (Boyce & Pittet 2003). Notably, however, all participants in our study were observed to wear gloves and an apron during ETS. This may suggest a perception among nurses that wearing gloves and using a 'non-touch' aseptic technique when inserting the suction catheter negates the need for frequent hand washing. However, the literature clearly suggests that gloves do not replace the need for hand washing (Pratt *et al.* 2001). These findings support earlier studies that report modest and even low levels of adherence to recommended hand-hygiene practices (Thompson 2000, Boyce & Pittet 2003).

Another area of particular concern is the suction pressure used when performing ETS. High negative pressure can cause mucosal trauma, which in turn predisposes the bronchial tree to a higher risk of infection (Wood 1998a). Using high negative pressures does not necessarily mean that more secretions will be aspirated; therefore, limiting pressures to between 80–150 mmHg is recommended (Wood 1998a, Thompson 2000, Day *et al.* 2002a). The results indicated that participants used suction pressures outside the recommend levels for safe practice with suction pressures ranging from 230 to 450 mmHg. Participants on GICU generally used lower suctioning pressures, ranging from 230–380 mmHg, which still exceeded the recommended pressures for safe practice. Again these findings support the study by Day *et al.* (2002b) which found nurses to be generally unaware of recommended best ETS practice.

Recommendations for Education, Practice and Research

- As a matter of urgency, institutional policies and guidelines, which are not based on current best-practice recommendations, need to be developed and/or reviewed.
- Teaching interventions to improve nurses' knowledge and competence in the care of patients requiring ETS is indicated particularly with regard to auscultation skills, hyperoxygenation practices, suctioning pressures and infection control measures.
- The orchestration and implementation of effective educational interventions to change practice may be time consuming. Therefore, in the interim, it is recommended that nurses become familiar with the clinical indicators for ETS and how to perform a simple respiratory assessment on ventilated patients.
- Infection control guidelines need to be reinforced and monitored to ensure compliance.
- A regular audit of ETS practice is recommended to ensure that patient safety is being assured.

This observational study was successful in achieving its objectives; however, further observational studies need to be conducted to substantiate the findings. Observation coupled with a form of 'think-aloud' methodology may uncover the reasons behind nurses' decisions (in 'think-aloud' techniques, subjects are questioned and asked to 'think aloud' in regard to a particular aspect of their ETS practice). Such methodologies are recognized as a useful source of data collection in observational studies (Yang 2003).

Limitations

Observation, like other methods has its own limitations and ethical implications (Parahoo 1997). One of the main problems is the effect of the 'observer' on the 'observed'. This is referred to as the Hawthorne effect and is an important threat to the validity of observational research, whereby participants' knowledge of being in a study may cause them to change their behaviour (Polit *et al.* 2001). In our study, the Hawthorne effect may have resulted in participants rehearsing ETS according to evidence-based recommendations prior to the observations. This being the case, it could be suggested that participants' practice is normally of a poorer quality than the results of our study suggests.

Given the observational nature of the study, there were several aspects of the ETS procedure that could not be assessed. It was not possible to determine participants' reasons for their practice, for example, the only observable aspect of patient assessment was the practice of auscultation, and even then, it was not possible to determine what participants heard and how it was interpreted. This may have resulted in an inaccurate interpretation of some of the data.

The sample size was not assessed for statistical significance. A power analysis would have established accurate sample size requirements for the study and consequently enhanced the representativeness of the findings (Polit *et al.* 2001). The evidence used to develop the observational tool for this study derived from what might be regarded as the best evidence available at the time of conducting the study; however, there is still some disparity in regard to what exactly constitutes best practice owing to the paucity of empirical research regarding ETS.

Finally, while the study was conducted on two different ICUs, they were both part of one institution. The findings therefore may not be representative of the general population of ICU nurses and threatens the external validity of the findings. This could have been enhanced by spreading observations over a range of sites, in different geographical locations.

Conclusion

This study supports the general finding in the literature that nurses adhere only partially to best-practice recommendations in relation to ETS (Celik & Elbas 2000, Paul Allen & Ostrow 2000, Day *et al.* 2002b). Under the code of professional practice, nurses are obliged to ensure patient safety and expected by the public and their employer to provide high-quality, efficient, well-executed and appropriate care of individuals (Huber 2000). By failing to adhere to what the literature has established as best ETS practice, nurses fall short of fulfilling any of the aforementioned expectations.

Despite an increased uptake in postregistration education among critical care nurses and a heightened interest in the expansion of their role, the literature indicates that they remain poor at many of the aspects of care that might be considered basic. Nurses need to assess and improve their current practices continually to guarantee that evidence-based practice recommendations are being adhered to and patient safety is being assured. This can only be achieved when nurses become more aware of their professional responsibilities and receive adequate support in practice.

Acknowledgement

We would like to acknowledge the advice of a statistician Itai Beerei, University College Cork.

Contributions

Study design: SK and manuscript preparation; SK, TA.

References

Blackwood B (1998) The practice and perception of intensive care staff using the closed suctioning system. *Journal of Advanced Nursing* 28, 1020–1029.

Boyce J & Pittet D (2003) Guideline for hand hygiene in health-care settings. Recommendations of the Healthcare Infection Control Practices Advisory Committee and the HICPAC/SHEA/ APIC/IDSA Hand Hygiene Task Force Morbidity and Mortality Weekly Report. *Centers for Disease Control and Prevention* 51(RR16), 1–44.

Burke J (2003) Infection control—a problem for patient safety. *The New England Journal of Medicine* 348, 651–656.

Celik S & Elbas N (2000) The standard of suction for patients undergoing endotracheal intubation. *Intensive and Critical Care Nursing* 16, 191–198.

Cormack D & Benton D (1996) (ed) *The Research Process in Nursing*, 3rd edn. Oxford Blackwell Science, pp. 357–372.

Craig J & Smyth R (2002) *The Evidence based Practice Manual for Nurses*. Churchill Livingstone, London.

Day T, Farnell S & Wilson-Barnett J (2002a) Suctioning: a review of current research recommendations. *Intensive and Critical Care Nursing* 18, 79–89.

Day T, Farnell S, Haynes S, Wainwright S & Wilson-Barnett J (2002b) Tracheal suctioning: an exploration of nurses' knowledge and competence in acute and high dependency ward areas. *Journal of Advanced Nursing* 39, 35–45.

Dickson R (2003) Systematic reviews. In *Achieving Evidence Based Practice. A Handbook for Practitioners* (Hamer S & Collinson G eds.). Balliere Tindall, London.

Fitzpatrick JM, While AE & Roberts JD (1994) The measurement of nurse performance and its differentiation by course of preparation. *Journal of Advanced Nursing* 20, 761–768.

Glacken M & Chaney D (2004) Perceived barriers and facilitators to implementing research findings in the Irish practice setting. *Journal of Clinical Nursing* 13, 731–740.

Glass CA & Grap MJ (1995) Ten tips for safer suctioning. *American Journal of Nursing* 5, 51–53.

Huber D (2000) *Leadership and Nursing Care Management*, 2nd edn. Saunders, Philadelphia.

Hundley V, Milne J, Leighton-Beck L, Graham W & Fitzmaurice A (2000) Raising research awareness among midwives and nurses: does it work? *Journal of Advanced Nursing* 31, 78–88.

McKillop A (2004) Evaluation of the implementation of a best practice information sheet: tracheal suctioning of adults with an artificial airway. *Joanna Briggs Institute Reports* 2, 293–308.

Moore T (2003) Suctioning techniques for the removal of respiratory secretions. *Nursing Standard* 18, 47–53.

Parahoo K (1997) *Nursing research, principles, process and issues*, Palgrave Macmillan: London.

Paul Allen J & Ostrow L (2000) Survey of nursing practices with closed system suctioning. *American Journal of Critical Care* 9, 9–17.

Polit D, Beck C & Hungler B (2001) *Essentials of Nursing Research. Methods, Appraisal and Utilization*, 5th edn. Lippincott, Williams and Wilkins, Philadelphia.

Pratt RJ, Pellowe C, Loveday HP, Robinson N & Smith GW (2001) The epic project: developing national evidence based guidelines for preventing health care associated infections. Phase 1: guidelines for preventing hospital acquired infections. *Journal of Hospital Infection* 47, S1–S82.

Sole M, Byers J, Ludy J, Zhang Y, Banta C & Brummel K (2003) A multisite survey of suctioning techniques and airway management practices. *American Journal of Critical Care* 12, 220–232.

Swartz K, Noonan D & Edwards-Beckett J (1996) A national survey of endotracheal suctioning techniques in the pediatric population. *Heart and Lung: The Journal of Acute and Critical Care* 25, 52–60.

Thompson L (2000) Suctioning adults with an artificial airway. A systematic review. *The Joanna Briggs Institute for Evidence Based Nursing and Midwifery*. Systematic Review No. 9.

Wainwright S & Gould D (1996) Endotracheal suctioning in adults with severe head injury: a literature review. *Intensive and Critical Care Nursing* **12**, 303–308.

Wood C (1998a) Can nurses safely assess the need for endotracheal suction in short term ventilated patients, instead of using routine techniques? *Intensive and Critical Care Nursing* **14**, 170–178.

Wood C (1998b) Endotracheal suctioning: a literature review. *Intensive and Critical Care Nursing* **14**, 124–136.

Yang SC (2003) Reconceptualizing think aloud methodology: refining the encoding and categorizing techniques via contextualized perspectives. *Computers in Human Behaviour* **19**, 95–115. Available at: http://www.elsevier.com/locate/comphumbeh (accessed 11 January 2005).

Zeitz, K. (2005) Nursing observations during the first 24 hours after a surgical procedure: what do we do? *Journal of Clinical Nursing* **14**, 334–343.

Appendix: Observational Schedule

Practices Prior to Suctioning

1: Patient assessment
Did the nurse auscultate the patient's chest before ETS?
0 = No
2 = Yes (Wood 1998a, Thompson 2000, Day *et al.* 2000)

2: Patient preparation
Did the nurse explain to/communicate with the patient about the procedure?
0 = No
2 = Yes (Wood 1998a, Thompson 2000, Day *et al.* 2000)

3: Presuctioning hyperoxygenation/hyperinflation
0 = Not given
2 = Given by means of manual resuscitation bag/given by ventilator (Thompson 2000, Day *et al.* 2000)

4: Sodium chloride instillation
0 = Yes
2 = No (Wood 1998a, Thompson 2000, Day *et al.* 2000)

Infection Control Practices

5: Hands are washed prior to suctioning
0 = No
2 = Yes (Wood 1998b, Thompson 2000, Day *et al.* 2000)

6: Gloves are worn
0 = No
2 = Yes (Wood 1998a, Thompson 2000, Day *et al.* 2000)

7: Apron is worn
   0 = No
   1 = Yes (Wood 1998a, Day *et al.* 2000)
8: Sterility of suction catheter maintained until inserted into airway
   0 = No
   2 = Yes (Wood 1998a, Thompson 2000, Day *et al.* 2000)
9: Goggles/face mask worn
   0 = No
   2 = Yes (Wood 1998a, Thompson 2000, Day *et al.* 2000)

The Suctioning Event

10: Size of suction catheter ....
Size of ETT ....
   0 = > Half of the internal diameter of ETT
   2 = ≤ Half of the internal diameter of ETT (Wood 1998a, Thompson 2000, Day *et al.* 1998)
11: Number of suction passes ....
   0 = > 2
   1 = < 2 (Thompson 2000)
12: Length of time suction applied to airway
   0 = More than 15 seconds
   2 = Less than 15 seconds (Wood 1998a, Thompson 2000, Day *et al.* 2000)
13: Level of suction pressure
   0 = < 80 mmHg/ > 150 mmHg
   2 = 80–150 mmHg (10·6–20 kPa) (Thompson 2000, Day *et al.* 2000)
14: Position of catheter when suction applied
   0 = suction applied during insertion
   2 = suction applied during withdrawal from airway only (Thompson 2000, Day *et al.* 2000)

Postsuctioning Practices

15: Patient reconnected to oxygen
   0 = > 10 seconds post suctioning
   1 = within 10 seconds post suctioning (Day et al. 2000)
16: Postsuctioning hyperoxygenation/hyperinflation
   0 = Not given
   2 = Given by means of manual resuscitation bag/ventilator (Wood 1998a, Thompson 2000, Day et al. 2000)

17: Post-ETS assessment
    Did the nurse auscultate the patient's chest?
    0 = No
    1 = Yes (Day et al. 2000)
18: Patient reassured
    0 = No
    1 = Yes (Day et al. 2000)
19: Hands washed postsuctioning
    0 = No
    2 = Yes (Wood 1998a, Thompson 2000, Day et al. 2000)
20: Used catheter and gloves are disposed of in a manner that prevents contamination from secretions
    0 = No
    2 = Yes (Thompson 2000)

Profile & Commentary

WHY *Study Purpose*

Two specific objectives are stated. The one that dominates the report is to compare open endotracheal suction (ETS) practices of critical care nurses with recent research recommendations. The researchers go a step further and hypothesize that critical care nurses do not adhere to a high level of best-practice recommendations for open ETS.

The adjective "open" is important because there are two different systems for suctioning the ET tubes of patients on mechanical ventilators: open and closed systems. Briefly, open systems require disconnecting the ET tube from the ventilator to allow suctioning, whereas closed systems allow the ET tube to stay connected to the ventilator during suctioning. Even now (as of 2010), neither system has been demonstrated to be superior to the other. There are clinical advantages and disadvantages to both systems. The exemplar study examined only open-system practices.

In the review of research that was done (studies prior to 2005), the authors note that most of the studies asked nurses about their ETS practices, as opposed to actually observing them perform ETS. The lack of reference to more recent studies is due in part to the lag in bringing this study to print. The data for this study was collected in 2005, the article was submitted in 2006, and the article was published in 2008. Unfortunately, lag is not uncommon. However, nurses practicing in critical care tell me that today's standards for ETS suctioning adults have not changed appreciably from those used in the study.

HOW *Design*

"A non-participant structured observational design was used . . ." Structured observation means they used a set of prespecified action statements to structure what they would observe; the actions either were or were not performed. The word *nonparticipant* indicates that the researcher did not participate in any of the nursing care actions, and did not intervene in any way (unless of course there was a distinct danger posed to the patient) but simply assumed the role of an onlooker (Kelleher, Sean, personal communication, February 25, 2010).

Sample

The hypothetical target population could be considered the suctioning practices of nurses working in general ICUs and cardiac ICUs who work full time and have a minimum of 1 year of experience in the ICU. More narrowly, it could be considered similar nurses working in the general ICU and cardiac ICU of this one hospital or of Irish hospitals.

The 45 nurses observed were selected using quota sampling, which is a form of convenience sampling that has as a goal of obtaining a sample with characteristics that are in proportion to how the characteristics exist in the population. Thus, the proportion of nurses observed from the two units was similar to their actual proportion in the setting. The characteristics of the setting are described, which helps envision the hypothetical population to whom the results could apply.

Measurement

The schedule, tool, or instrument used to observe and record observations was an adaptation of a previously validated survey tool. The adaptation involved adding several actions not in the original tool; the added actions were based on more recent research findings and best-practice recommendations. The observational tool was piloted, and **interrater reliability** was checked: "no significant discrepancies were identified." Presumably, this means that the level of agreement between two raters in scoring actions was at least 80%.

Looking at the tool itself (in the appendix of the article), you can see that the 20 specific actions observed were grouped in four sequentially-ordered categories. In observing an ETS event, the rater marked *Yes* or *No* for each action, thus indicating whether or not the action was performed. Note that the actual numerical value associated with a Yes or No answer varied; the authors provide a rationale for assigning numerical values to actions. In looking at the observational tool, it is not immediately obvious whether performance of the abbreviated action statement is best practice or whether its absence is best practice. However, you can tell by the scoring. I had to go through and mark the best-practice action for each action statement in Tables 1 through 4. Thus in Table 1, I put an asterisk beside:

- Assessment   Yes
- Preparation   Yes
- Prehyperoxygenation   Given
- NaCl   No

In addition to calculating scores for each of the four categories, an overall quality score was calculated by summing the scores from all the items.

Ethical Considerations

The study was reviewed and approved by the ethics committee at the hospital where the study was conducted. Written consents were most likely obtained from the participating nurses. This study could be viewed as sensitive as the nurses asked to participate might worry that their suctioning technique might be reported to their nurse manager; steps would have to be put in place to prevent this and assurances provided to the nurses asked to participate.

WHAT *Results*

Subcategory Results   The results for the four subcategories of actions are reported first in Tables 1 through 4; these tables are quite straightforward. They display how many of the possible actions occurred. Sizeable discrepancies between best practice and actual actions occurred for many actions, such as pre–hand washing, catheter sterility, catheter size, suction pressure, post-hyperoxygenation, post-assessment, post-reassurance, and post–hand washing.

Overall Quality   The mean total score was 22.6 out of an ideal of 35. Right off you know that the actual practice of the sample observed in this study fell considerably short of ideal practice. Looking at Table 5, you can see that the highest total score was 30 and the lowest was 14. The fact that the mean, median, and mode for overall quality are close to one another indicates that the scores were approximately normally distributed around the mean. Note that you have to be careful in comparing the mean scores for the four subcategory mean scores because prior to suctioning had eight possible points, whereas the other three subcategories had nine possible points.

The researchers went a step further than just noting the difference between the mean scores of the observed sample and the ideal score. They were interested in determining if the mean score attained (22.62) could just be the mean of this sample of 45 suction events, even though the target population mean is actually 35. A *t*-test was run to determine if the sample mean of 22.62 is just a sampling variation on a mean of 35; the result was $t = -24.63$, $p < .01$. The bottom line conclusion from this statistical result is that a mean of 22.62 is most likely not just a sampling variation on a population mean of 35, therefore a mean of 35 is highly unlikely in the target population.

p-Values   Since this is your first introduction to *p*-value results in this book, a few words of review might be helpful. Remember from your statistics course that when comparing the means of two samples drawn from the same population, it is not expected that the two means will be identical—some variation is expected. However, if the difference between the two means is large, it may be outside expected variation, indicating that the two means are not just variations on the same mean; rather, they are truly different. A true difference is one that is robust enough that it is likely to represent a true difference, not a chance one resulting from expected variation. Importantly, a true difference conveys that a difference is also likely in the population the sample represents.

To illustrate expected variation, if you selected two simple **random samples** (n = 50 in each group) from a list of 200 healthy 28- to 34-year-old soccer players, one sample might have a mean heart rate of 68.1, the other sample a mean heart rate of 67.4. The p-value of a t-test ($p > .05$) would lead to the conclusion that the difference is a chance difference due to expected variation, not a true difference between the two groups.

When comparing two means, the researcher compares the data-based p-value produced by the t-test with the level of significance he has predetermined. The level of significance is a decision-point p-level indicating the probability of making an error he would take on should he conclude that the difference found is a true difference. Clearly, the researcher wants to limit the probability of making such an error.

If a data-based p-value is equal to or less than the acceptable level of significance pre-selected by the researcher, e.g., $p \leq 0.05$, it indicates that the difference found has a low probability of being just a chance difference. Such a result is considered statistically significant and will lead the researcher to conclude that the two means are most likely truly different. In contrast, a high p-value (higher than the acceptable level of significance selected by the researcher, e.g., $p > 0.05$) indicates an unacceptably high probability that the difference found is a **chance variation**. This statistical result will lead the researcher to conclude that the difference found in the two means is just chance variation and does not represent a true difference.

> Data-based p-value = The probability that the difference found is a chance variation, not a true difference

The t-test in the study we are considering was run to determine if the sample score mean of 22.62 is just a chance variation and that the real mean, i.e., the mean in the population, could actually be 35 (the ideal). The p-value obtained is $< .01$. This indicates that there is a very low likelihood (less than 1%) that the difference between the sample mean of 22.62 and the ideal of 35 is just a chance result. Because the probability is so low, the difference is most likely a true difference. We call such a result "statistically significant" because the researcher can have confidence that the two means really are different (as opposed to being due to chance variation). For a graphical display of this explanation, see Figure 5–5.

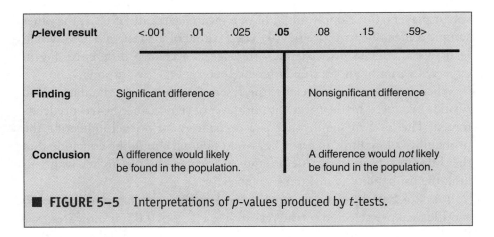

p-level result	<.001	.01	.025	**.05**	.08	.15	.59>

Finding   Significant difference   Nonsignificant difference

Conclusion   A difference would likely   A difference would *not* likely
                    be found in the population.   be found in the population.

■ **FIGURE 5-5**   Interpretations of *p*-values produced by *t*-tests.

Discussion

In this section, the researchers discuss the shortcomings in practice that are likely to have serious ramifications for patients' well-being. Recommendations based on the findings are also offered. Among the limitations of the study is the fact that the nurses knew they were being observed, so they may have used their best technique (i.e., Hawthorne effect); this led the researchers to the inference that unobserved technique may be of even lower quality.

Another limitation is that the 45 observed events of ETS practice were made in one hospital and therefore may not represent practice in other settings. This limitation is called limited generalizability. It reflects that one cannot be confident that the findings can be viewed as representing settings that are dissimilar from the one in which the study was done. However, other studies in other countries have also found only partial adherence to best-practice recommendations for ETS. Thus, although these findings are from one particular setting, they contribute to a larger body of knowledge about ETS practice.

Further Learning

To read another descriptive study article and commentary, see the posting on the companion website for this book, which can be accessed at ⌐ *go.jblearning.com/brown*.

REFERENCES

Dillman, D. A., Smyth, J. D., & Christian, L. M. (2009). *Internet, mail, and mixed-mode surveys: The tailored design method* (3rd ed.). New York, NY: John Wiley.

Fan, M. I., Mitchell, M., & Cooke, M. (2007). Cardiac patients' knowledge and use of sublingual glyceryl trinitrate (SLGTN). *Australian Journal of Advanced Nursing, 26*(3), 32–38.

Galvin, J. A., Benson, H., Deckro, G. R., Fricchione, G. L., & Dusek, J. A. (2006). The relaxation response: Reducing stress and improving cognition in healthy aging adults. *Complimentary Therapies in Clinical Practice, 12*(3), 186–191.

Huck, S. W. (2007). *Reading statistics and research* (5th ed.). Boston, MA: Allyn & Bacon.

Jurgens, C. Y., Hoke, L., Brynes, J., & Riegel, B. (2009). Why do elders delay responding to heart failure symptoms? *Nursing Research, 58*(4), 274–282.

Kelleher, S., & Andrews, T. (2008). An observational study on the open-system endotracheal suctioning practices of critical care nurses. *Journal of Clinical Nursing, 17(3)*, 360–369.

Lauver, D. R., Connolly-Nelson, K., & Vang, P. (2007). Stressors and coping strategies among female cancer survivors after treatments. *Cancer Nursing, 30*(2), 101–111.

Maze, L. M., & Bakas, T. (2004). Factors associated with hospital arrival time for stroke patients. *Journal of Neuroscience Nursing, 36*(3), 136–141.

Whittemore, R., D'Eramo Melkus, G., & Grey, M. (2005). Metabolic control, self-management and psychosocial adjustment in women with type 2 diabetes. *Journal of Clinical Nursing, 14*(2), 195–203.

OTHER DESCRIPTIVE STUDIES

Dibble, S. L., Casey, K., Nuseey, B., Israel, J., & Luce, J. (2004). Chemotherapy-induced vomiting in women treated for breast cancer. *Oncology Nursing Forum, 31*(1), E1–E8.

Dracup, K., Moser, D. K., McKinley, S., Ball, C., Yamaski, K., Kim, C., Doering, L. V., et al. (2003). An international perspective on the time to treatment for acute myocardial infarction. *Journal of Nursing Scholarship, 35*(4), 317–323.

England, M., Mysyk, A., & Gallegos, J. A. A. (2007). An examination of *nervios* among Mexican seasonal farm workers. *Nursing Inquiry, 14*(30), 189–201.

Johnson, J. J., & Stern, E. B. (2004). Readability of patient education material: A comparison of rural and urban cardiac rehabilitation sites in Minnesota. *Journal of Cardiovascular Rehabilitation, 24*, 121–127. [Posted with a Profile & Commentary at the companion website for this book, *go.jblearning.com/brown.*]

CHAPTER SIX
Correlational Research

Once qualitative and descriptive studies have provided knowledge about the variables at work in a health situation, researchers and clinicians naturally start asking questions about how the variables work together or influence one another. Questions such as: Is there a relationship between size of a family's social support network and their teenagers' emotional and social development? Is spousal or partner support associated with diabetics' self-care practices and blood sugar control? Are hearing loss and osteoporosis related? Do lung capacity scores predict exercise capacity? In general terms, these questions ask, "Are variable X and variable Y related?" These questions go beyond description of each variable separately to examine the relationship between them. They are the kinds of questions that can be answered by correlational research.

Relationship

Just what does this word *relationship* mean in the research context? In simplest terms, relationship describes a connection between variables—two variables are connected when a change in one is associated with a change in the other. The change has two dimensions: direction and strength. The direction of change can be in the same direction or in opposite directions. In a positive relationship, as one variable's values increase, the other's values also increase. In a negative relationship, as one variable's values increase, the other's values decrease.

A relationship can also be characterized as strong, moderate, or weak, indicating the strength of the relationship between the two variables. A relationship is strong when (1) persons who score high on variable A also score high on variable B, (2) persons who score low on variable A also score low on variable B, and (3) those who score intermediate on variable A also score intermediate on variable B. By contrast a weak relationship exists when (1) persons who score high on variable A have assorted scores (high, medium, and low) on variable B, and (2) persons who score low on variable A have assorted scores on variable B. In other words, there is very little connection between scores on A and scores on B. The opposite of relationship is *independence*, meaning that there is no connection between scores on the two variables.

Measuring Relationship

The direction and strength of a relationship between two variables are quantified using one of several statistical tests. The actual statistic used depends on the scale that was used to quantify the variables. When both variables were measured on an interval level scale, the Pearson *r* coefficient is used; it is the most widely used correlation statistic (Burns & Grove, 2005). An interval level scale is a measurement scale with a range of numerical values having equal distance between them, such as degrees on a thermometer, pounds on a weight scale. If either or both of the variables are measured using an ordered set of categories, for example, low, medium, high, the Pearson *r* coefficient is not used; rather another correlation coefficient would be used. There are several, but they all are interpreted similarly to how the Pearson *r* is interpreted.

The value of the Pearson *r* statistic varies from –1 to +1, which means that it can be –1, a minus decimal, zero, a plus decimal, or +1. The sign indicates whether the two variables have a positive or negative relationship; if positive, they move in the same direction (as one goes up, the other goes up); if negative, they move in opposite directions (as one goes up, the other goes down). The closer the value is to –1 or +1, the stronger the relationship between the two variables. Zero means the two variables are completely independent of one another, and a value close to zero indicates a very weak relationship.

Interpretation of *r*							
r Value	– 1	–0.8	–0.5	0	+0.6	+0.8	+1
Relationship	perfect negative	strong neg	moderate neg	none	moderate positive	strong pos	perfect pos

Graph Perspectives on Relationship   To illustrate relationship in the concrete, a hypothetical study (Box 6–1) and five possible datasets for the study are presented in the following figures (Figures 6–1 through 6–5). Each dataset is accompanied by a scatterplot for the data, the Pearson *r* coefficient for the data, and explanations about what these two analytical tools tell us. The samples in the datasets were limited to five to make it easier to see the relationship between the two variables, although a real study would not have as few as five cases. I would add that if you aren't up to speed regarding scatterplots, also called scatter diagrams, you should go back and read about them in your statistics reference text. You won't see many scatterplots in journal reports because they take up too much room, but they are helpful in acquiring an understanding of what Pearson *r* correlation coefficients mean.

Box 6–1   HYPOTHETICAL CORRELATIONAL STUDY

Study purpose: To examine the relationship between hope and adaptation in persons who have had multiple sclerosis for at least 3 years.

Measurement: Hope is measured on a 1 to 5 scale, 1 = barely present hope, 5 = an abundance of hope. Adaptation is measured on a 1 to 10 scale, 1 = not adapting, 10 = adapting without problems. Note that both variables are scored on continuous scales; this is a key requirement for using the Pearson *r* correlation coefficient to portray the relationship between the two variables. If one variable is a categorical variable (e.g., gender) and the other is a continuous variable (e.g., adaptation), the Pearson *r* statistic could not be used.

Sample: 5 persons

Results: Several possible sets of scores are presented in Figures 6–1 through 6–5. To make the relationship between the variables stand out, the Hope scores are the same from dataset to dataset, but the Adaptation scores are different.

Dataset 1	Person	Hope Score	Adaptation Score
	1	1	2
	2	2	4
	3	3	6
	4	4	8
	5	5	10

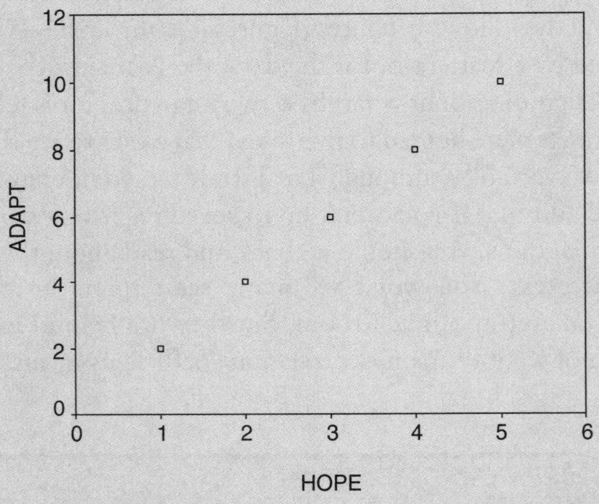

Note that for each increase of 1 point in Hope scores, there is a 2-point increase in the Adaptation scores. If you know a person's Hope score, you can accurately predict that person's Adaptation score; similarly if you know the person's Adaptation score, you can accurately predict his or her Hope score. When two variables change in lockstep with one another, we say that they have a perfect positive correlation. There is nothing magical about the 1-point Hope score to 2-point Adaptation score relationship. It could just as easily be that a 1-point change in Hope is related to a 4-point change in Adaptation.

Note that scatterplots provide the same information as the dataset table. Each point on the scatterplot represents one score. For example, the person who scored 1 on Hope scored 2 on Adaptation and has a point on the scatterplot as does the person who scored 4 on Hope and 8 on Adaptation. Because the relationship between the two variables is in lockstep, a line drawn between all the data points is a straight line.

The Pearson r statistic for this dataset is $r = +1$, which indicates a perfect positive relationship. The two variables move in lockstep with one another with high scores on one being paired with high scores on the other and low scores on one being paired with low scores on the other. The Pearson r statistic has possible values between +1 and −1.

■ **FIGURE 6-1**   Hypothetical dataset 1.

Dataset 2	Person	Hope Score	Adaptation Score
	1	1	10
	2	2	8
	3	3	6
	4	4	4
	5	5	2

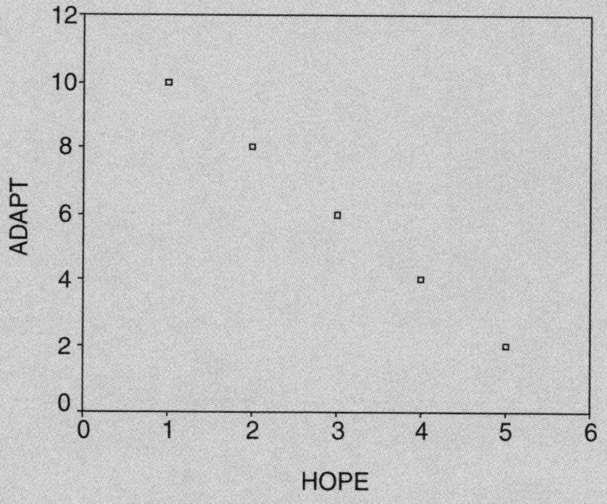

Note that for each increase of 1 point in Hope score there is a 2-point decrease in Adaptation score. Just as in dataset 1, if you know a person's Hope score, you can accurately predict that person's Adaptation score; similarly if you know the person's Adaptation score, you can accurately predict his or her Hope score. However, instead of moving in the same direction as they did in dataset #1, they move in the opposite direction. The variables in this dataset have a perfect negative relationship: As one variable goes up, the other goes down in lockstep a specific amount. Again, a line drawn between all the data points is a straight line. The Pearson *r* value for this dataset is $r = -1$, indicating a perfect negative relationship.

■ **FIGURE 6–2**   Hypothetical dataset 2.

Perfect correlations are, of course, a rare happening in the real world where variation and multiple influences are characteristic of reality, especially in the social, psychological, and behavioral realms. Instead, weak, moderate, and moderately strong correlations occur more often. These kinds of relationships are illustrated in the next three hypothetical datasets (Figures 6–3, 6–4, and 6–5).

Dataset 3	Person	Hope Score	Adaptation Score
	1	1	2
	2	2	3
	3	3	6
	4	4	9
	5	5	8

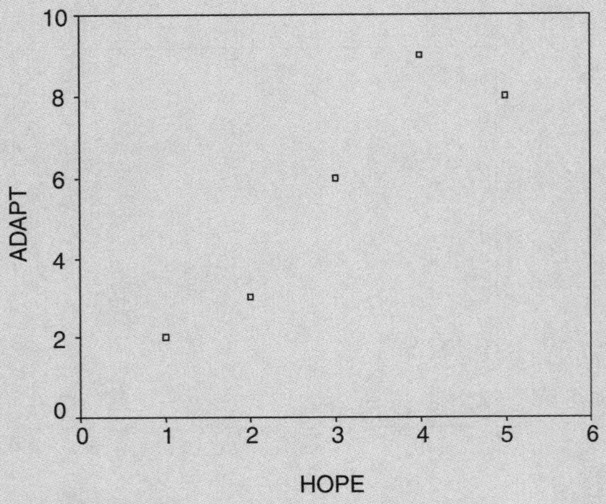

Note that an increase in Hope is roughly related to an increase in Adaptation. The two variables are strongly but not perfectly correlated. If you know a person's score on one variable, you can make a pretty good estimate of the person's score on the other variable.

A trend in the data is quite obvious, but all the data points are not in a straight line. If a straight line were drawn through the middle of the data, three data points would be on or very close to that line and two would be a bit farther away. The line is called the *trend line* and represents the middle of the data. Take a straight edge and add a trend line to this graph.

The Pearson *r* for this dataset is + .93, a strong, positive correlation.

■ **FIGURE 6–3**   Hypothetical dataset 3.

Dataset 4	Person	Hope Score	Adaptation Score
	1	1	2
	2	2	10
	3	3	6
	4	4	4
	5	5	8

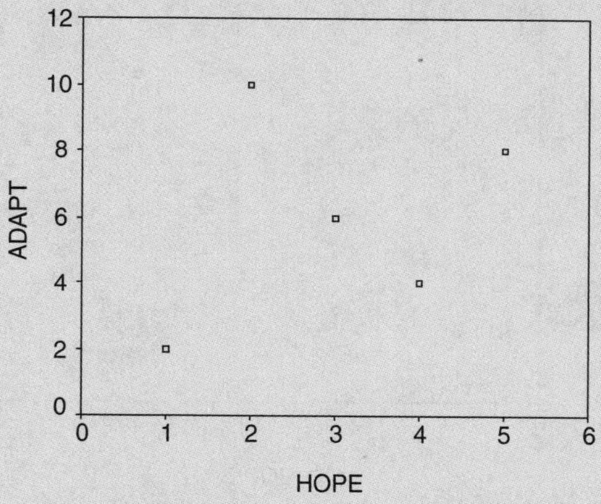

There is a bit of a linear trend in the relationship between Hope and Adaptation; as Hope scores go up, there is a bit of a trend for the Adaptation score to go up, but the relationship is weak. Any effort to base one score on the other score would have a low likelihood of being accurate.

A trend line drawn through the middle of the data would show that three data points are on or close to the trend line, but two are quite far from it. Thus, there is trend, but a weak one. The Pearson *r* for this dataset is +.30, indicating a weak positive correlation.

■ **FIGURE 6–4**   Hypothetical dataset 4.

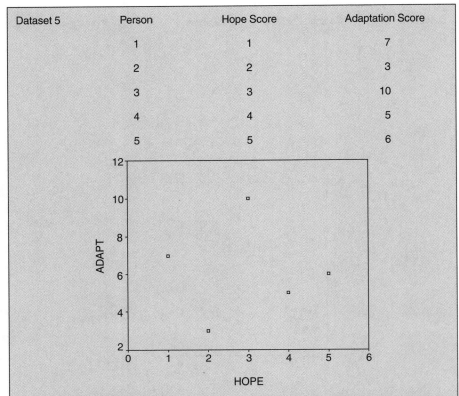

Dataset 5	Person	Hope Score	Adaptation Score
	1	1	7
	2	2	3
	3	3	10
	4	4	5
	5	5	6

In this dataset, there is no relationship between the Hope score and the Adaptation score; the two scores are independent of one another. Knowing one score will not enable you to predict the other one.

All data points are quite far from a trend line drawn through the data. The Pearson *r* for this dataset is 0, indicating no relationship between the two variables.

■ **FIGURE 6–5** Hypothetical dataset 5.

In summary, a correlation coefficient indicates the direction (positive or negative) and strength (perfect, strong, moderate, weak, or none) of a relationship.

Caveat Importantly, a strong relationship between two variables says nothing about the underlying dynamic that produces the relationship. Even a very high correlation (near –1 or +1) does not mean there is a cause and effect relationship between the variables. High correlation only conveys that there is a pattern in the relationship between the two variables. The relationship between the two variables could be much more complex than straightforward cause and effect.

For instance, look at Figure 6–3 again. On first blush, the scatterplot and the Pearson *r* of .93 *may seem to suggest that* level of hope determines level of adaptation. However, identical data could be found if the reverse were true, that is, successful adaptation generates hope. Another possibility is that the relationship between the two variables is not a direct one. There could be another lurking variable in the background that has a strong effect on both hope and adaptation and causes them to move in concert with one another; that lurking variable could be something like prognosis or response to treatment. In any of these three dynamics, the data could be the same as in Figure 6–3. The point is this: Correlation sheds no light on the dynamic underlying the relationship—even when one precedes the other in time. Correlation only detects a relationship. The dynamics of that relationship need to be ferreted out by further research using other research designs or justified by other knowledge about the two phenomena.

Correlation ≠ Cause
(Huck, 2004)

When the relationship between ratings of perceived exertion and heart rates of young African-Americans was studied in treadmill tests (Karavatas & Tavakol, 2005), the overall Pearson *r* was .58. The authors interpreted this result as a moderately strong relationship in which heart rate influences perceived exertion. This directional interpretation is justified by physiological knowledge, not by the statistical result itself.

Outliers   When looking at scatterplots, the researcher looks for **outliers,** which are cases which have very atypical pairings. An outlier's data point will lie very far from the trend line. Importantly, with small sample sizes, a single outlier can lower the Pearson *r* considerably. Consider the scatterplot in Figure 6–6. Note that most of the scores lie close to the positive correlation trend line, except for the person who scored 4 on hope and 1 on adaptation. This person's data is an outlier because it is very different from the other scores. The Pearson *r* for this dataset is .50, which is a modest correlation. However, when this outlier is removed, reanalysis produces a Pearson *r* of .99 for the other four scores. The Pearson *r* calculated with the outlier in is greatly influenced because the sample size is so small; still, studies with larger sample sizes can be moderately influenced by a single outlier.

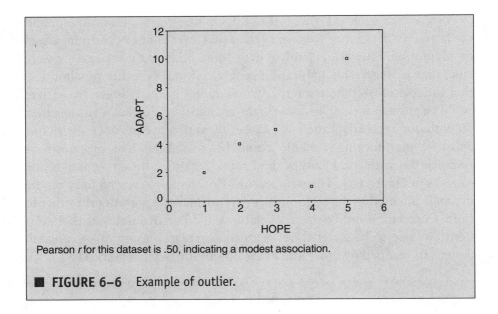

Pearson *r* for this dataset is .50, indicating a modest association.

■ **FIGURE 6–6**   Example of outlier.

An outlier can either understate or exaggerate the strength of the relationship between the two variables, depending on the values that make up the outlier. Removing an outlier, or even several in a dataset, can uncover a trend that would be less clear if the outliers were left in. When researchers remove data for an analysis, they should do so with good rationale and they should acknowledge that they did so. Removing data could be a form of bias, particularly when the study has a small sample size. Sometimes, a researcher will examine outlier cases in great depth because doing so can yield valuable insights that set the agenda for future research.

Practical Perspectives on r

Even though an *r* of 1.00 indicates a perfect positive relationship between hope and adaptation in which the variables move in lock step with one another, an *r* of .70 *does not mean* that 70% of the values of hope move in lock step with adaptation; rather the *r*-value indicates the relative strength of the relationship on a scale from −1 to +1.

Huck (2007) points out that *r* exaggerates how strong the relationship really is between two variables. A more realistic and practical perspective is gained by squaring the value of *r* to produce r^2, which is called the **coefficient of determination**. The r^2 value indicates the proportion of variation in hope that is related to adaptation and the proportion of variation in adaptation

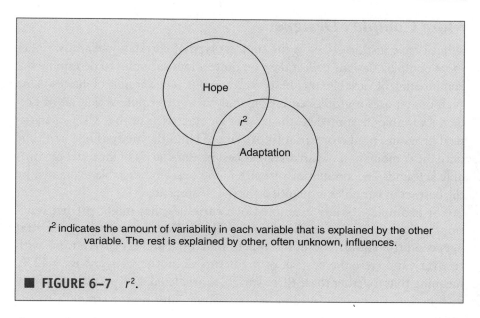

r^2 indicates the amount of variability in each variable that is explained by the other variable. The rest is explained by other, often unknown, influences.

■ **FIGURE 6–7** r^2.

that is related to hope. When an r of .70 is squared yielding an r^2 of .49, this tells us that about half the variation in hope is related to adaptation, and half of the variation in adaptation is related to hope (see Figure 6–7). The other 51% of both variables is attributable to other influences. In short, r^2 provides a more practical sense of the strength of the relationship between the two variables than r itself does.

Correlational Design

Purposes

The most straightforward correlational design is when the relationship between several variables is studied in a single group of people. The researcher measures the participants on each of the variables of interest using instruments that have been established as reliable and valid with the population under study (Brink & Wood, 1997), but no attempt is made to control or manipulate the situation. Analysis of the data consists of running correlational tests to determine if and how the variables are related. The analysis consists of measuring the correlation between various combinations of two variables, which is called *bivariate correlational analysis*. If there are three variables in the study, A, B, and C, bivariate analysis could be run on the relationship between A and B, A and C, and B and C, thus producing three correlation coefficients.

More Complex Designs

What I have just described is the simplest type of correlational study. Other more complex designs collect data on quite a few variables to determine the combination of variables that best *predict* an outcome variable of interest. One such design uses multiple regression analysis to determine which *set* of predictor variables best predicts the level of an outcome variable. Using a statistical program, predictor variables are entered into the analysis one at a time until the combination of variables that best predicts levels of the outcome variable is found. The amount of variance in the outcome variable explained by the best set of variables is quantified as the R^2 statistic.

For example, a study examined five variables that might predict functional recovery after a stroke (Hinkle, 2006). The major finding was that age, cognitive status, and initial function had the highest correlations with recovery and were the best set of predictors of motor recovery. $R^2 = 42\%$, meaning that together these three variables predicted 42% of the variability in functional recovery. Adding lesion volume and motor strength to the analysis did not increase the R^2.

Other studies involve using predictor variables to predict group membership (e.g., quit smoking/didn't quit smoking); this statistical technique is called discriminate analysis. Both multiple regression analysis and discriminate analysis are advanced forms of correlation in which the relationships among sets of predictor variables and an outcome variable are examined. The exemplar you will read examines bivariate correlations and includes a multiple regression analysis, so you will become familiar with the two most frequently used types of correlation firsthand.

Exemplar

Reading Tips

The only aspects of this research report that could be difficult are the physiological variables that comprise cardiac function. To make the reading easier, the following list defines those variables. Still, there are references to medications with which you may be unfamiliar; I leave it to you to look those up.

- Ejection fraction: Using one of several imaging techniques (cardiac catheterization, MRI, or CT scan), the percentage of blood that is pumped out of the left ventricle with each heartbeat is measured; a normal ejection fraction is 55 to 70 percent.

- Peak VO_2 (also called maximal oxygen uptake): During cardiopulmonary exercise testing (bicycle or treadmill), breathing exchange is measured. Peak VO_2 is the oxygen consumption per minute when the patient is exercising at a maximum level. An expected level is predicted based on age and gender. Generally, a value below 14 mL/kg/minute indicates a poor prognosis.
- Maximal workload: During exercise testing, the heart's work output at the safe target heart rate or when the test has to be stopped because of symptoms, exhaustion, or EKG changes is the maximal workload; it is expressed in watts per minute.
- Systolic heart failure: Inadequate pumping of blood from the left ventricle during contraction due to weakness of the ventricle walls results in systolic heart failure.

Correlates of Fatigue in Patients with Heart Failure

Lorraine S. Evangelista, Debra K. Moser, Cheryl Westlake, Nancy Pike, Alvina Ter-Galstanyan, and Kathleen Dracup

Progress in Cardiovascular Nursing (2008), 23(1), 12–17.

This study was conducted to determine the prevalence of fatigue and identify its demographic, clinical, and psychological correlates in 150 heart failure (HF) patients (73% men, 66% Caucasian, mean age 55.0 years, mean ejection fraction 26.7% ± 11%), from a single HF center, using the Profile of Mood States-Fatigue Subscale, the Minnesota Living With Heart Failure Questionnaire, and the Beck Depression Inventory. Sociodemographic and clinical data were obtained through self-report and chart abstraction. High levels of fatigue were reported in 50.4% of men and 51.2% of women. In a multivariate model, maximal workload, physical health, emotional health, and depression explained 51% of the variance in fatigue (P < .001). Fatigue in patients with HF is associated with both clinical and psychosocial variables, offering a number of targets for intervention. These findings suggest the need for multiple risk factor intervention strategies that improve physical and emotional health to decrease fatigue. Patients with depression warrant particular scrutiny. Prog Cardiovasc Nurs. 2008;23:12–17. ©2008 Le Jacq

Fatigue accompanies many illnesses and can be an incapacitating symptom that interferes with return to work, activities of daily living, and social or family responsibilities.[1] Factors underlying fatigue have been examined extensively in patients with cancer[2] and multiple sclerosis,[3] and findings strongly support an association between fatigue, depression, and quality of life (QOL). Fatigue in these conditions is multifactorial and involves complex pathophysiologic and psychological processes that reflect both disease conditions. Interest in the impact of fatigue in cancer patients has led to the development of a treatment algorithm in which patients are evaluated regularly for fatigue, and treatment is targeted to their fatigue level.[2] In addition, treatment strategies including exercise programs, cooling, dietary changes, and energy conservation have also been developed to ameliorate fatigue in these patient populations.[2,3]

Fatigue is one of the 2 most common symptoms (along with dyspnea) reported by patients with heart failure (HF).[4-7] Also commonly referred to as activity intolerance, fatigue in patients with HF is defined as persistent tiredness and the perception of difficulty performing daily activities because of this persistent tiredness. Fatigue is often one of the first symptoms of HF and is commonly overlooked because it is viewed by both lay people and health care providers as a vague complaint. Indeed, as many as one-third of patients with HF view fatigue as an unimportant symptom and up to 50% report having difficulty recognizing it as a symptom of worsening HF.[8] The origins of fatigue in HF are unclear and are likely to be multifactorial. Probable pathophysiologic causes of fatigue in HF include low cardiac output and poor tissue perfusion, muscle metabolic abnormalities, autonomic nervous system abnormalities, deconditioning effects, and endothelial dysfunction.

Investigators have examined the relative contribution of psychological factors and physical symptoms to the variance in fatigue in older women with HF and demonstrated that fatigue was related more to physical symptoms than to psychological factors.[4] In another study, both men and women with HF were examined during hospitalization to assess relationships among physical symptoms, functional limitations, and depression.[5] Depression was strongly related to physical symptoms but not functional limitations. Ekman and Ehrenberg[9] explored sex differences in experiences of fatigue and found that there was an agreement in fatigue prevalence between men and women with HF, but the rating for fatigue severity differed by sex. When describing the character and intensity of fatigue, women described their fatigue as severe, whereas men described their fatigue as mild.[9] Despite earlier studies examining the nature of fatigue in patients with HF, this symptom continues to be poorly understood by clinicians and researchers. The purpose of the current investigation was to examine the prevalence of fatigue and identify its demographic, clinical, and psychological correlates in patients with systolic HF. Knowledge of the patterns and mechanisms of fatigue experienced by HF patients may provide information about the type and nature of interventions needed to cope with this distressing symptom and the challenges related to living with the chronic illness of HF.

Table I. DEMOGRAPHIC AND CLINICAL CHARACTERISTICS OF HF PATIENTS WITH LOW OR HIGH FATIGUE LEVELS

	TOTAL (N=150)	LOW FATIGUE (N=74)	HIGH FATIGUE (N=76)
Age, y	55.0 ± 12.1	56.8 ± 2.2	54.7 ± 13.0
Years with HF	5.9 ± 6.1	5.8 ± 5.0	6.2 ± 7.1
Ejection fraction, %	26.7 ± 11.5	26.1 ± 11.7	27.3 ± 11.6
Maximal oxygen uptake (peak VO$_2$), mL/kg/min	15.8 ± 5.3	16.4 ± 5.3	13.2 ± 4.3[a]
Maximal workload, watts	96 ± 53	102 ± 52	72 ± 46[b]
Men, %	72.7	73.0	72.4
Race, %			
White	65.6	62.5	68.8
Black	26.9	28.8	25.0
Asians	7.5	8.7	6.2
Married, %	65.6	68.8	62.5
Education, %			
Some high school	12.5	12.5	12.5
High school graduate	21.9	25.0	18.8
Some college	37.5	25.0	50.0
College graduate	28.1	37.5	18.7
Not employed, %	78.0	72.0	75.0
Heart failure etiology, %			
Idiopathic	57.5	58.8	56.3
Ischemic	42.5	41.2	43.7
NYHA class, %			
II	44.8	46.3	43.3
III	42.7	41.2	44.2
IV	12.5	12.5	12.5
Medications, %			
ACE inhibitors	78.7	75.7	78.9
β-Blockers	73.3	68.9	68.4
Diuretics	96.0	93.2	93.4
Digoxin	57.3	58.1	48.7
Statins	64.0	63.5	68.4[a]

Abbreviations: ACE, angiotensin-converting enzyme; HF, heart failure; NYHA, New York Heart Association. Values are expressed as mean ± SD unless otherwise indicated. [a]$P < .05$. [b]$P < .001$.

Study Design and Patients

A cross-sectional, correlational design was used. A convenience sample of 150 patients with HF was recruited from a single outpatient HF clinic located within a tertiary, university-affiliated medical center on the US West Coast. Patients were included in the study if they were aged 18 years or older; able to read, write, and speak English; had a left ventricular ejection fraction < 40% documented by echocardiography or ventriculography; and had symptoms of HF for 6 months or longer.

Table II. QUALITY OF LIFE, PHYSICAL AND EMOTIONAL HEALTH, AND DEPRESSION SCORES (N = 150)

CHARACTERISTIC	MEAN	SD	RANGE[a]
Quality of life-total, sum score	42.2	26.7	0–100
Quality of life-physical health, sum score	18.0	12.0	0–40
Quality of life-emotional health, sum score	8.4	7.1	0–25
Depression, sum score	9.9	8.2	0–50

[a]These values reflect the actual range of scores for the sample.

Table III. CORRELATIONAL MATRIX FOR THE KEY VARIABLES (N = 150)

VARIABLE	1	2	3	4	5	6	7	8	9
Fatigue									
Age	−.067								
EF%	.095	.032							
Peak VO$_2$	−.227[a]	−.116	−.155						
Maximal workload	−.354[b]	−.178	.103	.203[a]					
Use of statins	.204[a]	−.230[b]	.010	.100	−.065				
QOL (total)	.596[b]	−.071	−.056	−.177[a]	−.318[b]	.182[a]			
Physical health	.595[b]	.002	−.039	−.167[a]	−.419[b]	.077	.945[b]		
Emotional health	.627[b]	−.069	−.056	−.172[a]	−.402[b]	.134	.807[b]	.638[b]	
Depression	.576[b]	−.166[a]	−.042	−.226[a]	−.249[b]	.239[b]	.511[b]	.367[b]	.684[b]

Abbreviations: EF, ejection fraction; QOL, quality of life; VO$_2$, maximal oxygen uptake. [a]$P < .05$. [b]$P < .001$.

Table IV. PREDICTORS OF FATIGUE (N = 150)			
VARIABLE	ADJUSTED R^2	F	P VALUE
Maximal workload, watts	.114	14.66	< .0001
Emotional health	.415	38.53	< .0001
Physical health	.466	31.8	< .0001
Depression	.506	28.13	< .0001

Procedures

Institutional Review Board approval was received before study initiation. Patients who expressed an interest in participating in the study signed an informed consent during their routine clinic visit and received a battery of paper and pencil instruments to complete. Sociodemographic (ie, sex, age, race, income, education, marital status, and employment status) and clinical data (ie, etiology of HF, left ventricular ejection fraction, current medications, maximal oxygen uptake [peak VO$_2$], and maximal workload) were obtained from patient self-reports and verified through most current (within 3 months of study participation) diagnostic tests obtained during medical records abstraction.

Instruments

The questionnaires took 10 to 15 minutes to complete and included the following:

Profile of Mood States-Fatigue (POMS-F).   The POMS-F, used to measure fatigue, is a 7-item subscale obtained from the 65-item Profile of Mood States instrument that was developed to assess transient distinct mood states specific to fatigue-inertia.[10] Participants were asked to rate their feelings related to being "worn out," "listless," "fatigued," "exhausted," "sluggish," "weary," and "bushed" on a 0 (not at all) to 4 (extremely) scale. Summative scores range from 0 to 28, with a higher score denoting greater fatigue. The standardized POMS-F scores were established in a sample of adult patients (N=400) between the ages of 18 and 94 years with a mean age of 44 ± 18.4 years. Sixty-four percent of the patients in the normative sample were married, 48% were men, and the average years of education was 14.3 ± 2.7 years. The mean scores for men and women in the sample were 7.3 ± 5.7 and 8.7 ± 6.1, respectively.[11] These mean values were used in the current study to determine the presence of low (ie, below norm) and high (ie, above norm) levels of fatigue. The POMS Total Mood Disturbance score correlated highly ($r = 0.79$) with a Visual Analog Composite score.[2] Reliability of the POMS-F was 0.91 in a sample of 428 cancer patients.[12] Internal consistency of the POMS-F was acceptable with a Cronbach's α of 0.88.

Quality of Life.   Quality of life was measured using the Minnesota Living With Heart Failure Questionnaire (LHFQ), a 21-item disease-specific tool that asks participants to indicate the extent to which various symptoms they have experienced in the previous month have prevented them from living as they wanted to. The items can be combined to form an overall QOL score as well as scores for physical health (8 items) and emotional health (5 items). The physical subscale contains items associated with the fatigue and dyspnea of HF. The emotional subscale consists of items such as being worried or feeling depressed. The remaining 8 items include questions about other areas of life affected by HF and are used to compute the overall QOL score.[13] Response options are presented as 6-point ordinal scales ranging from 0 (no) to 5 (very much), with a total maximum score of 105 (40 for physical and 25 for emotional health); a lower LHFQ score indicates better QOL.

Beck Depression Inventory (BDI).   Depression was measured using the BDI, which is widely used in chronically ill populations and is well validated.[14] The BDI is a self-reported inventory designed to measure severity of depressive mood or symptoms. The 21-item inventory consists of a Likert-type scale from 0 (absence of symptom) to 3 (severe or persistent presence of the symptom). Five of the BDI items pertain to somatic symptoms of depression (eg, loss of appetite and sleep disturbance) and 16 of the items reflect nonsomatic symptoms of depression (eg, hopelessness and social withdrawal). Scores on the BDI range from 0 to 63. Patients with BDI scores 0 to 9 are considered as having minimal symptoms of depression, scores 10 to 16 mild, scores 17 to 29 moderate, and scores 30 to 63 as having severe symptoms of depression.[15]

Data Analyses

Data were analyzed using SPSS for Windows (version 11.0; SPSS, Inc, Chicago, IL). Descriptive statistics were used to characterize the study population and analyze mean fatigue scores. Sex differences in fatigue scores were compared using the independent t test. Fatigue was dichotomized using validated cutoff points; a score > 7.3 for men and > 8.7 in women was indicative of moderate to high levels of fatigue.[11]

Univariate analyses were conducted to assess the impact of sociodemographic, clinical, and psychosocial factors on fatigue. Group comparisons of patients with low vs moderate to high fatigue levels were conducted using chi-square statistics or t test, depending on the level of measurement. Multivariate stepwise regression analyses were then used to identify which combination of variables provided the most predictive power for overall fatigue. Variables significant at an $\alpha < .10$ in the univariate analysis were included in the regression model.

To reflect the context variables, age and sex of patients were the first variables added to the model. Next, to depict the impact of clinical variables (peak VO_2, maximal workload, use of lipid-lowering medications [statins]) were added as a second set. Psychological factors including QOL, physical and emotional health, and depression were added last. Criteria for entry and removal of variables were based on the likelihood ratio test, with enter and remove limits set at $P \leq 05$ and $P \geq .10$, respectively.

Results

Mean age of the patients in the sample was 55.0 ± 12.1 years (range, 20–72 years). No significant differences were found in the sociodemographic characteristics and most clinical characteristics between patients who reported low vs high levels of fatigue (Table I). Ejection fraction was similar in both groups; however, peak VO_2 and maximal workload were significantly lower in patients who reported high levels of fatigue compared with those reporting lower levels of fatigue. This finding validates the measure of fatigue used in this study.

Fatigue scores for men and women were higher than the category scores for moderate-severe fatigue in a healthy adult population; men scored 9.5 (SD ± 7.5) and women scored 10.4 (SD ± 7.0). These scores reflect high levels of fatigue reported in 55 (50.4%) men and 21 (51.2%) women. The QOL, physical and emotional health, and depression scores are listed in Table II. No differences were found between men and women in the variables studied. Depression was detected in > 28% of the sample by the BDI questionnaire; 29 (19%) had mild depressive symptoms and 14 (9%) had moderate to severe depressive symptoms.

In a univariate analysis, age and sex were not correlated with fatigue; however, a strong correlation existed between fatigue, total QOL, physical and emotional health, and depression (Table III). Clinical and physiological variables associated with higher levels of fatigue were use of statins, lower peak VO_2, and lower maximal workload. Cardiac factors including HF etiology, New York Heart Association (NYHA) functional class, and left ventricular ejection fraction were not related to fatigue.

In a multiple regression model, lower maximal workload, physical and emotional health scores, and depression were found to be independent predictors of fatigue (Table IV). These 4 predictors accounted for 51% of variance in the fatigue scores of patients. There was evidence of a linear fit for each variable in the final model. Post hoc analysis, done to test for multicollinearity among variables, demonstrated that each of the predictors had unique effects on fatigue.

Discussion

Despite the pervasiveness of fatigue in patients with HF, little research has concentrated on this phenomenon. Given the importance of symptom status to patients and the value of symptom status as an indicator of the effectiveness of clinical therapies to clinicians, it is vital that research efforts are directed toward understanding fatigue. The current study is novel in that we used a multivariate model to determine correlates of fatigue and demonstrated the multifactorial nature of fatigue in this population. Both clinical and psychological variables were important correlates of fatigue: maximal workload, physical and emotional health scores, and depression were independent correlates of fatigue. In addition, we found that approximately one-half of the study participants experienced fatigue when compared with a healthy adult population utilizing the same measure.[11] Similar prevalence was also reported in a cohort of older women with HF in the United States[4] and in an elderly cohort of men and women with HF in Sweden.[16,17]

Lower peak VO_2 and maximal workload both correlated with higher fatigue; however, only lower maximal workload was found to independently predict higher fatigue in this sample. Peak VO_2 is traditionally used for risk stratification in HF; the impact it has on mortality is well supported in the literature.[18] Peak VO_2 has also been used to predict limitations (VO_2 ≤ 14 mL/kg/min) in daily activities as a result of poor exercise tolerance.[19]

Intuitively, patients with high levels of fatigue are less tolerant to increasing maximum workloads and experience decreased levels of peak VO_2. Although the mechanisms for these physiological responses are not well understood, our findings indicate that HF patients with lower maximal workload thresholds and peak VO_2 indices are at high risk for fatigue.

Higher fatigue correlated with poorer physical health. Our findings are consistent with previous study results that showed an association between fatigue and restrictions in physical activity and limitations in self-care.[7,16,17] Additionally, fatigue in older women with HF was related more to other concurrent physical symptoms than to psychological factors.[4] Investigators examined plausible explanations that link fatigue with higher functional limitations and identified impaired peripheral circulatory perfusion with reduced oxygen delivery and impaired muscle strength as potential confounders.[20] Fatigue and physical health warrant further investigation including what comes first, fatigue or physical health limitations. Our findings support the need to assess for ongoing physical symptoms (ie, dyspnea, edema) that may increase susceptibility to increased fatigue. At the current time, the best method of assessing for fatigue may be the most direct and simple, ie, asking patients about the presence of the symptom and helping patients to identify fatigue by specific questioning directed at uncovering fatigue in the context of daily activities. Patients who report a chronic physical symptom pattern should be screened for concomitant fatigue that may merit intervention. Finally, the need to consider interventions that focus on physical symptoms as a first step to managing fatigue in HF patients is vital.

Specific interventions to combat fatigue have not yet been tested in patients with HF, but data to date on the impact of exercise suggest that fatigue may be managed best by assisting patients to increase their activity levels. Given the relationship between depression and fatigue found in this and other studies, interventions to treat depression will likely have a beneficial impact on fatigue also. Exercise has a positive influence on depression. Assisting patients to increase their activity levels, which has been shown to be safe in the management of HF, can be recommended for the management of fatigue in patients with HF. It is also appropriate to teach HF patients energy conservation techniques for the management of fatigue, so their activity efforts are efficient and not exhausting.

The study supports previous reports that poor QOL and emotional health are common in patients with HF and that higher fatigue was related to poorer QOL.[17] Women who scored high on fatigue also scored high on stress related to illness and were less satisfied with life.[4] Our findings were similar and also showed that more than a fourth of the participants reported depressive symptoms, which is higher than depression rates reported among patients hospitalized with HF.[5] Both studies, however, consistently showed that higher depressive symptoms were associated with higher fatigue. The relationship between fatigue and depression has also been reported in women with breast cancer. Women reporting high levels of fatigue also reported greater symptom distress, lower activity, and poorer physical and social health status.[2] Hence, treatment strategies that help patients manage symptoms, relax, and obtain adequate sleep, especially patients experiencing greater emotional distress and depressive symptoms, may modify fatigue. Complementary therapies (eg, yoga, meditation, massage) and self-care strategies that promote sleep and exercise may also help patients cope with the emotional impact of fatigue.[5]

It may seem counterintuitive that we failed to find an association between fatigue and NYHA functional class or ejection fraction. However, given the nature of measurement of fatigue and the aspects of HF pathophysiology captured by NYHA functional class or ejection fraction, these findings are not unexpected. Given its subjective nature, fatigue is difficult to measure with precision. The NYHA classification also suffers from lack of precision in its measurement; at each of the 3 indicators at which symptoms are present (ie, classes II, III, and IV), the assessment seeks only whether any symptom is present, not specifically whether fatigue is present. Ejection fraction is likely not associated with fatigue because all patients with HF, regardless of ejection fraction, are expected to have symptoms such as fatigue, and symptom status has never correlated well with ejection fraction. This lack of correlation is one reason HF guidelines do not recommend using ejection fraction to reflect effectiveness of drug therapy, but they do recommend that symptom improvement be a major indicator.

Of interest, fatigue in HF was associated with the use of statins, which has been shown to increase the risk of myopathy, resulting in symptoms of fatigue, weakness, and pain. Although statin-related side effects were originally identified as affecting only 1% to 5% of patients,[21] some investigators have indicated that these effects may be common and often go unreported.[22] The risk of these adverse effects with statin use can be exacerbated by several factors, including compromised hepatic and renal function, hypothyroidism, diabetes, and use of concomitant medications, but the mechanisms causing statin-induced myopathy have not been elucidated and warrant further study.[23] Our finding, however, that statin use was not independently associated with fatigue suggests that discontinuation of statins to treat fatigue in patients with HF may not be warranted.

Some limitations must be considered when interpreting the results from our study. First, causation cannot be inferred; thus, we cannot say that low QOL, poor physical and emotional health, or depression leads to high levels of fatigue, nor can we comment on the direction of the hypothesized causality. The experience of severe fatigue may lead to low QOL, poor physical and emotional health, or depression. Our findings merely support the association between fatigue and several clinical and psychosocial variables. Next, the sample that was used for the study was fairly homogeneous; patients were all being seen at a single transplant referral center and their mean age was lower than the typical mean age for HF in the general community, thus limiting our ability to generalize to all patients with HF. Finally, the use of a convenience sample from a single center limits the utility of any estimate of prevalence of fatigue and could also introduce a bias in the ascertainment of correlates of fatigue.

Conclusions

Our data demonstrate that fatigue levels were moderately intense and highly prevalent in our sample of patients with systolic HF. We found that fatigue has predictable clinical dimensions and psychosocial correlates and is an important symptom to consider. Fatigue may influence patients' adherence to the medical regimen, their social relationships, and general QOL. Early identification of fatigue could facilitate the initiation of interventions to reduce the cost of associated health care.

Evaluation and treatment of fatigue in HF patients requires a multidisciplinary approach because the fatigue has many possible etiologies and several contributing factors. A comprehensive approach is required, especially for patients with moderate to severe fatigue, so that all possible contributing factors can be determined and an appropriate treatment plan created. The short- and long-term effects of various treatment strategies on the fatigue in HF patients should be assessed in future studies.

Disclosure: This research was partially supported by a grant from the American Heart Association Western Division (NCR, 133–09, PI, K. Dracup) and by a University of California School of Nursing Intramural Research Grant.

References

1. Solano JP, Gomes B, Higginson IJ. A comparison of symptom prevalence in far advanced cancer, AIDS, heart disease, chronic obstructive pulmonary disease and renal disease. *J Pain Symptom Manage.* 2006;31:58–69.

2. Payne J, Piper B, Rabinowitz I, et al. Biomarkers, fatigue, sleep, and depressive symptoms in women with breast cancer. *Oncol Nurs Forum.* 2006;33:775–783.

3. MacAllister WS, Krupp LB. Multiple sclerosis-related fatigue. *Phys Med Rehabil Clin N Am.* 2005;16:483–502.

4. Friedman MM, King KB. Correlates of fatigue in older women with heart failure. *Heart Lung.* 1995;24:512–518.

5. Friedman MM, Griffin JA. Relationship of physical symptoms and physical functioning to depression in patients with heart failure. *Heart Lung.* 2001;30:98–104.

6. Nordgren L, Sorensen S. Symptoms experienced in the last six months of life in patients with end-stage heart failure. *Eur J Cardiovasc Nurs.* 2003;2:213–217.

7. Mayou R, Blackwood R, Bryant B, et al. Cardiac failure: symptoms and functional status. *J Psychosom Res.* 1991;35:399–407.

8. Carlson B, Riegel B, Moser D. Self-care abilities of patients with heart failure. *Heart Lung.* 2001;30:351–359.

9. Ekman I, Ehrenberg A. Fatigue in chronic heart failure—does gender make a difference? *Eur J Cardiovasc Nurs.* 2002;1:77–82.

10. McNair D, Loir M, Droppleman L. *Profile of Mood States.* San Diego, CA: Educational and Testing Services; 1971.

11. Nyenhuis DL, Yamamoto C, Luchetta T, et al. Adult and geriatric normative data and validation of the profile of mood states. *J Clin Psychol.* 1999;55:79–86.

12. Baker F, Denniston M, Zabora J, et al. POMS short form for cancer patients: psychometric and structural evaluation. *Psychooncology.* 2002;11:273–281.

13. Rector TS, Johnson G, Dunkman WB. Evaluation by patients with heart failure of the effects of enalapril compared with hydralazine plus isosorbide dinitrate on quality of life. V-HeFT II. The V-HeFT VA Cooperative Studies Group. *Circulation.* 1993;87:VI71–VI77.

14. Beck AT. *Depression: Clinical, Experimental and Theoretical Aspects.* New York, NY: Hoeber; 1967.

15. Beck AT, Rial W, Rickels K. Short form of depression inventory: cross validation. *Psychol Rep.* 1974;34:1184–1186.

16. Falk K, Swedberg K, Gaston-Johansson F, et al. Fatigue is a prevalent and severe symptom associated with uncertainty and sense of coherence in patients with chronic heart failure. *Eur J Cardiovasc Nurs.* 2007;6:99–104.

17. Falk K, Swedberg K, Gaston-Johansson F, et al. Fatigue and anaemia in patients with chronic heart failure. *Eur J Heart Fail.* 2006;8:744–749.

18. Corra U, Mezzani A, Bosimini E, et al. Limited predictive value of cardiopulmonary exercise indices in patients with moderate chronic heart failure treated with carvedilol. *Am Heart J.* 2004;147:553–560.

19. Gitt AK, Wasserman K, Kilkowski C, et al. Exercise anaerobic threshold and ventilatory efficiency identify heart failure patients for high risk of early death. *Circulation.* 2002;106:3079–3084.

20. Drexler H, Coats AJS. Explaining fatigue in congestive heart failure. *Annu Rev Med.* 1996;47:241–256.

21. Dirks AJ, Jones KM. Statin-induced apoptosis and skeletal myopathy. *Am J Physiol Cell Physiol.* 2006;291:C1208–C1212.

22. Langsjoen PH, Langsjoen JO, Langsjoen AM, et al. Treatment of statin adverse effects with supplemental Coenzyme Q10 and statin drug discontinuation. *Biofactors.* 2005;25:147–152.

23. Thompson PD, Clarkson P, Karas RH. Statin-associated myopathy. *JAMA.* 2003;289:1681–1690.

Profile & Commentary

WHY *Study Purpose*

The stated purpose of this study is twofold: (1) to determine how prevalent fatigue is in patients with systolic heart failure (HF), and (2) to identify clinical and psychological states associated with HF. In the opening paragraphs, the researchers define fatigue and summarize research that has been done about the topic.

HOW *Study Design*

"A cross-sectional, correlational design was used." Cross-sectional means data was collected once from each participant; no effort was made to study change over time. The study used correlational design because data was collected about 10 variables, and the relationships among them were of interest.

Sample

The 150 patients that made up the sample were drawn from persons awaiting heart transplant who attended an outpatient clinic for HF patients at a referral medical center in the United States. A detailed profile of the patients in the sample is provided in Table I. This information provides a detailed portrayal of the hypothetical target population as a whole and of two subgroups (i.e., a low-fatigue subgroup and a high-fatigue subgroup). Notice how cutoff values were used to categorize sample patients into the subgroups.

Several pieces of information in this table are particularly noteworthy. First, the average age is quite young for persons with HF. I was puzzled by this until I read on the last page of the article that they were "being seen at a single transplant referral center." This explains the younger than expected age; very old people generally are not candidates for heart transplant. This means that the population to whom the results would apply are not the typical population of older persons with heart failure.

The researchers were interested is knowing whether persons in the high- and low-level groups had similar or different characteristics. The superscript *a* and *b* designations to the right of the right column help do this. They tell us about the results of the *t*-tests used to compare characteristics of the high- and low-level fatigue groups. Only the characteristics with an *a* or *b* beside them were different enough to be considered a real difference, meaning that it is likely that a different level of the characteristic would exist in high- and low-fatigue groups from the larger population of patients, not just in this sample. The *a* designation means that the difference in the two groups on that particular characteristic is large enough that there are only 5 chances in 100 that a difference that large would occur just by chance if the two groups in the population really had the same level of that characteristic. The *b* designation means that the difference between the two groups on that characteristic is large enough that it would occur just by chance 1 time out of 1,000—a rare occurrence indeed.

As the researchers tell us in the first paragraph under Results, the two groups were essentially similar on all variables except mean peak VO_2, mean maximal workload, and the proportion of participants who took statin drugs. This information suggests that people with high and low levels of fatigue do not have different clinical characteristics. This is perhaps counterintuitive.

Measurement

Three questionnaire-type instruments were used to measure fatigue, quality of life, and depression. The descriptions of these instruments are quite good, so I won't repeat that information other than to make a few points:

- The response scales of the three instruments are different (0–4, 0–5, and 0–3, respectively). Also note the direction of the scoring. A high number on the fatigue scale denotes greater fatigue (↑↑); a high number on the QOL scales indicates poorer quality of life (↑↓); and a high number on the depression scale denotes more severe depression (↑↑).
- "Normal" values for the POMS-F instrument have been established previously by having 400 healthy adults complete the instrument.
- All these measures and instruments are widely used. The report includes information about the reliability and validity of the POMS-F, and it provides references for the other two. You might want to look back to Chapter 5 to refresh your memory about reliability, validity, and the statistics used to represent them.

Data Analysis

Mean scores (with standard deviations and the range of scores) were calculated for the four psychological variables: quality of life–total, quality of life–physical, quality of life–emotional, and depression sum. Correlations statistics (Pearson r) were run on all different bivariate combinations of the 10 variables listed in Table III. And finally, a multiple regression statistical analysis was run to determine the best set of predictors of fatigue.

WHAT *Results*

The results in the first paragraph of the article are explained earlier in this commentary, where the sample was discussed.

Analyses of Fatigue   In the second paragraph, we learn that women, on average, reported more fatigue than men; women's mean level of fatigue was 10.4, whereas the mean for men was 9.5. Both levels are higher than the normative mean of 8.7 and 7.3, respectively. Thus both women and men have, on average, moderate to severe fatigue. Reported differently, about half the total sample had high levels of fatigue.

Analyses of Other Variables   Table II provides summary data for the total group scores of QOL total, physical health, emotional health, and depression. To put them in perspective, write the maximum possible score to the right of Table II. This makes clear that the mean level of depression (9.9) is rather low (based on a maximum of 63 possible) and in the mild depression range based on validated ranges. I consider this a bit of a surprise finding because I would have expected their depression to be higher, given the extent of their disease. However, looking at the range of depression scores reminds us that at least one person, and maybe more, did have a very high level of depression, even though the mean is rather modest.

Correlational Analyses   Now we get to the correlations. To make Table II more easily readable, I suggest that you put the variable numbers 1–10 down the left side of the table beside each variable. So variable 1 is fatigue, 2 is age, 3 is EF%, and so on to variable 10, depression. The column numbers across the top then correspond with those variables.

The numbers at each cross point of column and row are Pearson r correlation statistics for combinations of the column and row variables. For instance, the correlation between fatigue (column 1) and physical health (row 8) is .595. Note the small b beside this value, indicating that this is a **statistically significant** result, indicating that there is less than a 1 in 1,000 (0.001) probability that the correlation between these two variables is actu-

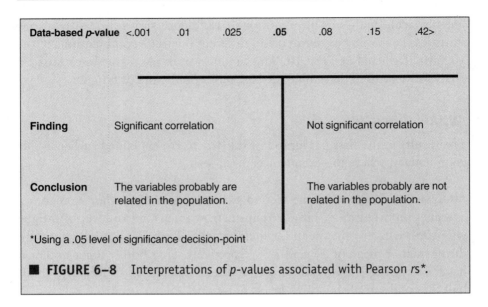

Data-based *p*-value	<.001	.01	.025	**.05**	.08	.15	.42>

Finding	Significant correlation	Not significant correlation
Conclusion	The variables probably are related in the population.	The variables probably are not related in the population.

*Using a .05 level of significance decision-point

■ **FIGURE 6–8** Interpretations of *p*-values associated with Pearson *r*s*.

ally zero in the target population. It may not be .595, but it is not zero (see Figure 6–8).

The most interesting findings are in column 1 because these indicate how the various factors correlate with fatigue. Here we learn that fatigue has a statistically significant correlation with all the other variables except age and ejection fraction. The highest correlations are between fatigue and emotional health, QOL, physical health, and depression.

To obtain perspective on the *r*-values, do as suggested in the introduction to this chapter, and square *r* to get r^2. In doing so, the *r* for emotional health and fatigue (*r* = .627) informs us that emotional health and fatigue have a moderately large overlap, 39% to be precise ($.627^2$ = .393). Therefore, when looking just at emotional health and fatigue, 39% of the variation in fatigue is explained by its relationship with emotional health, and 39% of the variation in emotional health is explained by relationship with fatigue— a moderate relationship. Clearly, other factors influence both fatigue and emotional health.

Other correlations in the table may also be of interest to you. For instance, physical health is correlated with QOL total (column 7) with a Pearson *r* of .945, a very strong relationship. You might be surprised to note that the correlations between ejection fraction (EF%) and the other variables are quite low. The authors address this counterintuitive finding in the Discussion section.

Multiple Tests of Significance   One final point needs to be made about correlation matrices, such as the one found in this report. Whenever a large number of statistical tests are conducted in a study, there is an increased chance that one or more of them will be statistically significant just by chance (Huck, 2007). To avoid accepting a correlation result resulting from multiple comparisons/tests, some experts advise that the level of significance required for each statistical test to be considered statistically significant should be raised. That is done using a procedure called Bonferroni correction. I will not go into how that is done here, but a more detailed explanation is provided on the companion website for this book, which can be accessed at ⊕ *go.jblearning.com/brown*. However, I will add that if the Bonferroni correction were applied to the results of this study, all of the correlations that were significant at the $p < .001$ level (those indicated by the [b] designation) will still qualify as statistically significant, albeit with less confidence that the relationship is not a chance result; the results that were significant at the $p < .05$ level would no longer be deemed statistically significant.

Multiple Regression Analysis   The multiple regression analysis uses a statistical program to find the set of predictor variables that best predict an outcome—in this case, fatigue. Looking at Table IV, we see that maximal workload was entered into the analysis first, and it predicted 11.4% of the variance in fatigue. When emotional health was also added, the two variables together predicted 41.5% of the variance in fatigue. Then physical health was added; it produced a 5% bump in explained variance to 46.6%. When depression was added, another 5% boost was achieved to arrive at the total variance in fatigue that was explained by the four variables of 50.6%. Adding other variables did not appreciably increase the amount of variance explained. The four best predictors are referred to as "the model." Predicting almost 51% of the variance in an outcome with just four predictor variables is a high level of prediction. (Note: The last two sentences in the Results section pertain to technical aspects of the analysis that relate to the confidence in the model—you can ignore them.)

Discussion

The discussion is long and a bit technical, but some of the takeaway points are as follows:

1. Fatigue is significantly associated with VO_2, maximal workload, use of statins, and with the psychological variables.

2. Approximately one-half of participants experienced fatigue when compared with what healthy adults experience, using the same measure of fatigue.
3. The discussion of peak VO_2 and maximal workload, and later ejection fraction, convey that only maximal workload was found to independently predict fatigue in the sample.
4. The best method of assessing fatigue is to directly ask the patient about it.
5. Interventions to control fatigue have not been tested, but based on the findings of this study, they could include help with getting good sleep, control of other sources of pain (e.g., arthritis), pacing activity to conserve energy, exercise to maintain conditioning, and relaxation therapies.
6. The authors issue a cautionary note about using the findings of this study in planning the care of other heart failure populations. The sample of this study is unique, not typical of the larger population of heart failure patients. Not only are they younger, they are at least being considered by a transplant program. They have some hope out in front of them. This makes them different from the typical population that will be managed by medications for the rest of their lives. In research language, I would say that the generalizability, or **external validity**, of the findings of this study is limited to heart failure patients being considered or awaiting heart transplant. The extent to which older persons with heart failure have the same experience profile as those in this study is not known.
7. The authors close with the mantra set forth in the introduction to this chapter: association/relationship does not confer causation. When you think about it, it makes sense that emotional health and fatigue are related, but which way is the direction of influence? Most likely it is a bidirectional relationship; the experience of fatigue influences emotional health while at the same time emotional health influences the experience of fatigue.

In summary, this correlation study provides insights regarding the complex nature of fatigue in heart failure patients. It reminds us that fatigue is not just a symptom of poor heart function; rather, it influences and is influenced by life perspectives.

REFERENCES

Brink, P. J., & Wood, M. J. (1997). Correlational designs. In P. J. Brink & M. J. Wood (Eds.), *Advanced designs in nursing research* (2nd ed., pp. 235–282). Newbury Park, CA: Sage.

Burns, N., & Grove, S. K. (2005). *Practice of nursing research: Conduct, critique, and utilization* (5th ed.). St. Louis, MO: Elsevier Saunders.

Evangelista, L. S., Moser, D. K., Westlake, C., Pike, N., Ter-Galstanyan, A., & Dracup, K. (2008). Correlates of fatigue in patients with heart failure. *Progress in Cardiovascular Nursing, 23*(1), 12–17.

Hinkle, J. L. (2006). Variables explaining functional recovery following motor stroke. *Journal of Neuroscience Nursing, 38*(1), 6–12.

Huck, S. W. (2007). *Reading statistics and research* (5th ed.). Boston, MA: Pearson.

Karavatas, S. G., & Tavakol, K. (2005). Concurrent validity of Borg's rating of perceived exertion in African-American young adults, employing heart rate as the standard. *Internet Journal of Allied Health Sciences and Practice, 3*(1). Retrieved from http://ijahsp.nova.edu/articles/vol3num1/karavatas.htm

OTHER CORRELATIONAL STUDIES

Dahlen, L., Zimmerman, L., & Barron, C. (2006). Pain perception and its relation of functional status post total knee arthroplasty: A pilot study. *Orthopaedic Nursing, 25*(4), 265–270.

Kara, M., & Mirici, A. (2004). Loneliness, depression, and social support of patients with chronic obstructive pulmonary disease and their spouses. *Journal of Nursing Scholarship, 36*(4), 331–336.

Kugler, C., Vlamick, H., Haverich, A., & Maes, B. (2005). Nonadherence with diets and fluid restrictions among adults having hemodialysis. *Journal of Nursing Scholarship, 37*(1), 25–29.

Mentes, J. C., Wakefied, B., & Culp, K. (2006). Use of a urine color chart to monitor hydration status in nursing home residents. *Biological Research for Nursing, 7*(3), 197–201. [Posted with a Profile & Commentary at the companion website for this book, *go.jblearning.com/brown*.]

CHAPTER SEVEN

Experimental Research

📖 Reading Tips

This is a very long chapter; therefore it is divided into two sections. The first section focuses on the methods used to conduct experimental studies testing the effectiveness of nursing interventions. The second section delves into the ways results of experimental studies are presented.

In the first section the methodological characteristics of experimental studies are considered, then the exemplar study is reprinted. At that point, you should read only the Introduction and Methods sections of the exemplar study, then the Profile & Commentary about its methods.

The second section of the chapter opens with an explanation of the results of experimental studies. After that you should read the Results section of the exemplar study and then the Profile & Commentary about its results. In other words, rather than have you ingest the whole research article at once, you will first consider the WHY and the HOW. Then you will delve into the WHAT. When you see the amount of information in this chapter, you will understand why it is divided into two portions.

The explanations in this chapter will be limited to the two-group experiment because most nursing intervention studies compare the effects of two interventions. Although in the future you will undoubtedly read three-group experimental studies, you should be able to understand them using what you know about two-group studies and reference to your statistics book.

Chapter Layout

Section 1
  Methods explained
  Exemplar study: Read Introduction and Methods sections only
  Profile & Commentary on methods

Section 2
  Results explained
  Exemplar study: Read Results and Discussion sections
  Profile & Commentary on results

Section 1: Understanding Experimental Methods

Determining the effectiveness of nursing interventions and treatments requires carefully designed studies. Assembling a group of willing participants and measuring them on a physiologic condition, psychological state, or knowledge level before and after receiving the intervention of interest is not sufficient (Kerlinger & Lee, 2000). It is insufficient because if an improvement is found, the researcher cannot claim with certainty that the intervention produced the improvement. Natural recovery, natural fluctuations in condition, or influences in the environment may have caused the observed improvements.

Key Features of Experimental Studies

When researchers want to test the effects of a nursing intervention on patient outcomes, the ideal research design is an experiment. A sample is drawn from a target population, and participants are randomly assigned to one of two groups. One group receives the test intervention and the other group receives no intervention or another intervention. At an appropriate time after the intervention, the researcher measures an outcome variable, or several, to determine whether one group did "better" than the other (see Figure 7–1). In designing an **experimental study**, the researcher tries to create conditions in which all influences on the outcome of interest, other than the effects of the different interventions, are the same for both groups. This sameness is necessary to be certain that any difference found in the outcomes of the two groups can be attributed to the fact that they received different interventions, not to some other influence.

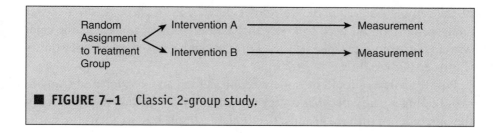

■ **FIGURE 7–1**   Classic 2-group study.

Good experimental studies have five key features:

- Adequate sample size
- Random assignment of participants to intervention and **comparison groups**
- Consistent delivery of interventions
- Control of extraneous influences and bias
- Low level of missing data

These features are key because they control error, bias, and unwanted influences, thereby bolstering confidence in the credibility of the findings.

Before explaining each of these key features, I want to say a word about the terminology used in reports of experimental studies: The new intervention (frequently the intervention of greatest interest) may be called the *experimental intervention* or *test intervention*; however, the term *experimental treatment* is also used. When referring to both interventions, the terms **independent variable**, *interventions*, or *treatment groups* may be used. The researcher's control over the design and delivery of the interventions may be referred to as *manipulation of the intervention*. I will use all these terms to help you get accustomed to them.

Adequate Sample Size

An experimental study's sample size must be large enough to detect a difference in the outcomes of the two groups if it actually occurs. Determining "large enough" requires taking into account several aspects of the expected results; these expectations are based on findings from similar previous studies. Foremost among the aspects taken into account are (1) the strength of the experimental intervention's impact vis-à-vis the impact of the comparison intervention, and (2) the desired level of significance (i.e., the *p* value that will be used as a decision-point for statistical significance). These values are entered into a calculation called a **power analysis**, which produces an estimate of the sample size required. You don't need to know how to do a power analysis, but you do need to know that doing a power analysis is the right way to determine sample size for correlational and experimental studies (Burns & Grove, 2009).

Power analysis should be done when designing an experimental study to avoid doing a study that has a very low capacity for finding a difference in the outcomes of the two groups. Insufficient sample size weakens the statistical calculations used to detect a significant difference in the outcomes of the two groups. It is like using a microscope with weak magnification—it just can't see everything that is there. Researchers use the terms *low statistical power* or *underpowered* to refer to a study with low capacity to detect a difference in the outcomes of the two groups. A common reason for low statistical power is small sample size.

When there is good reason to expect that the intervention will have a very strong impact on the study outcomes, the power analysis may indicate that a small sample size will be adequate. However, nursing interventions typically have modest impacts. The reality is that many nursing studies done with 30 persons in each group that find "no difference" in the outcomes of the two groups would find a significant difference had they been done with 100 persons in each group. If the purpose of a study is to determine if one intervention is more effective than another, doing a study with too small a sample is a waste of time, effort, and resources on everyone's part (Burns & Grove, 2009).

Random Assignment to Treatment Groups

Random assignment of enrolled participants to treatment groups is a defining feature of experimental studies. It is accomplished by assigning each person in the sample to either the **experimental group** or to the comparison group *based on chance determination*—not on the basis of patient preference for one treatment approach over the other, on physician request, or on the convenience of the research staff. Chance assignment requires that each participant have an equal chance of being assigned to either group. A flip of a coin is one way of randomly assigning each participant to one of the two study groups; computers can also generate a list of random numbers that can be used to determine each person's group assignment.

The contribution of random assignment to experimental design is that it controls differences in participant characteristics by distributing them evenly across both treatment groups, thus producing two groups that are similar at the start. Equivalent groups at the start are necessary in experiments because at the end of the study the researcher wants to be confident that the results were not influenced by different group compositions. When random assignment is not used, the possibility exists that some difference between the two groups that was present prior to delivering the interventions may have produced the difference found in the outcomes. This possibility creates lack of confidence in the study findings.

The larger the sample size the greater the chances are that random assignment will create treatment groups that are equivalent at baseline on important demographic and clinical variables (e.g., age, body mass index, disease severity). Nevertheless, even in large studies, researchers run comparison statistics on important demographic and clinical variables to make sure that random assignment worked effectively. A table profiling the two groups helps answer questions such as:

- Did the groups have similar mean ages?
- Did the groups have approximately equal proportions of men and women?
- Was the health status of the persons in both groups about the same?

In short, random assignment to treatment groups, sometimes referred to as *randomization*, is the most powerful way of ensuring that the two treatment groups are similar at the onset of the study; it works by evening out the presence of participant characteristics across both groups. Do note that random assignment is different from random sampling, which was discussed in Chapter 5. Briefly, random sampling is a way of obtaining a study sample that is representative of the target population, whereas random assignment is a way of determining the intervention each study participant will receive; what they share in common is the use of chance to control bias.

Inclusion and Exclusion Criteria   Although random assignment to treatment groups usually evens out the distribution of patient characteristics that could influence the outcome variable, their influence is still at work—albeit evenly in both groups. When it is known in advance that the influence of a patient characteristic on the outcome of interest is very strong, the researcher may decide to remove its influence completely. Removing it allows the effect of the treatment being tested to stand out. Removal of a very strong patient characteristic influence that is not of interest in the study is accomplished by including in the study only persons who do not have that characteristic.

To illustrate: If a study of persons with mild congestive heart failure examines the effects of two rehabilitation approaches on ability to walk for 6 minutes without stopping, the researcher might use exclusions to make the sample more homogeneous. This could be done without bias by excluding all persons with preexisting physical disabilities that affect mobility, such as stroke, severe arthritis, and neurological diseases. A homogeneous group would produce less scatter in the outcome data than a more diverse group would produce. Less scatter in the data would in turn increase the capacity of the statistical analysis to detect if one rehab approach was more effective than the other.

However, a long list of exclusion criteria can create problems in finding eligible participants for the study and problems with generalizing, or extending, the findings to patients found in real-world practice. If too many exclusions are used, the findings will only apply to a very narrow portion of the population clinicians are likely to see, and we would say the study has limited generalizability. Thus, researchers have to use exclusion criteria with awareness regarding how they will affect the clinical usefulness of the findings.

The important point here is that patient characteristics can influence the outcomes being studied and thereby complicate comparing the effects of the two treatments. Random assignment controls the influence of patient characteristics by ensuring that the patient characteristics are present to the same extent in both treatment groups. Judicious use of exclusion criteria ensures that very influential patient characteristics do not bury the effects of the treatment variable.

Having said that patient characteristics create problems in detecting treatment effectiveness, it also must be noted that there are study designs that analyze how patient characteristics affect response to the intervention. These designs (called factorial designs) make important contributions to clinical knowledge because they provide valuable information about persons with whom the intervention is very effective, moderately effective, or not effective. We won't go there because factorial designs are complex and describing them here would lead us astray.

Consistent Delivery of Interventions

Two-group experiments involve actively doing something to some of the participants and something else to the rest. In research language, one group receives the experimental intervention and the other group receives a comparison intervention. The experimental intervention is usually a somewhat "new" intervention in that its effectiveness has not been thoroughly evaluated; however, there should be good reason to believe that it will have a meaningful impact on the outcomes of interest. The comparison intervention can take one of five forms (Kerlinger & Lee, 2000):

- No intervention at all
- A placebo intervention
- A usual care intervention
- A different intervention
- Same intervention but of different dose (i.e., intensity, frequency, or timing)

A comment about placebo interventions: They are designed to look and feel similar to the intervention being tested but to not really have an effect on the outcomes being studied. At the very least, placebo interventions provide an "attention" activity for the comparison group to nullify the attention the intervention group receives. This is done because by itself the attention involved in delivering an intervention can have an impact on some outcomes. For this reason, studies of teaching or psychological support interventions often use a placebo group rather than a "no intervention" group.

Both the experimental and comparison interventions should be spelled out in considerable detail in advance of starting the study and consistently delivered throughout the study. If either intervention morphs during the course of the study, the contrast between them will be lost. This loss of contrast will invalidate the results because the comparison the researcher set out to make will no longer exist. Steps taken to ensure consistent delivery of the intervention include:

- specific study protocols,
- training of those who will be delivering the intervention, and
- checks on the delivery of the intervention to ensure compliance with study protocols.

Control of Extraneous Variables and Bias

Even when patient characteristics have been controlled, other sources of unwanted influence can affect the outcome data. Study activities and the settings in which the study is conducted can give rise to extraneous variables that influence the outcome variables directly. Steps must be taken to control them because they confound, that is, mix with, the situation and make it difficult to obtain a clear understanding of the relationship between the interventions and the outcomes. These influences can be persistent across the study setting or can influence one treatment group more than the other.

Sometimes "the setting" is the larger world of current events. For example, if during the time a study is being conducted to evaluate managing arthritis pain with the use of heat and cold, a new advertisement for a jazzy new whirlpool hits the TV waves big time, the advertisement could influence the results. Some persons in the heat group might be tempted to use the whirlpool instead of using heat according to the study protocol. In addition, some of those in the cold group might decide to abandon cold treatment all together. These changes in participant compliance with their assigned treatment method could result in persons in the treatment groups actually using different treatments than the study design indicates they are using. If the researcher is monitoring the study setting (immediate and more global), he may be able to detect such an extraneous influence and take steps to moderate it or check out its influence.

To control extraneous variables originating in the study activities, researchers develop very specific study procedures or protocols. In advance of starting the study, they specify:

- Characteristics of persons who are eligible for the study
- How participants are to be recruited
- How consent to participate in the study will be obtained
- How participants will be randomly assigned to treatment groups
- The activities that comprise each treatment
- The conditions under which the treatments will be delivered
- Training of data collectors
- How and when the outcomes will be measured

In studies where a research assistant observes and rates participants' responses, it is all too easy for well-intended data collectors to influence the **outcome measurement** even when they are trying to be neutral. "**Blinding**" the data collector controls this source of bias. Blinding is achieved by taking steps to ensure that the data collectors do not know which intervention the participant received. Obviously, blinding is not always possible. Consider a study comparing the effects of two positioning protocols on the comfort level of persons with fractured hips before they have surgery. It is almost impossible to blind data collectors as to which intervention the patient is receiving because the patient will be in a position associated with one or the other of the treatments when the data collectors obtain the comfort ratings.

Low Level of Missing Data

Missing data can be a problem in clinical studies. There are a variety of reasons for not having complete data on all participants who were entered into the study and were randomized to a treatment group, including:

- Some participants dropped out of the study (e.g., moved from the area, didn't want to continue in the study).
- The condition of some participants worsened so that they could not continue in the study (e.g., transfer to ICU, too sick to answer questions).
- Some participants were not available for measurement of the outcome variable at one or several data collection times (e.g., missed an appointment, couldn't contribute a specimen).
- The data collector failed to obtain some data (e.g., she was sick, she overlooked something).
- The burden of participating in the study was too great.

Generally, the reasons for missing data and the pattern of missing data are more important than the amount of missing data, although 20% missing data is clearly of more concern than 2% missing data. Also, random missing data is of less concern than is a pattern of missing data (Duffy & Jacobsen, 2001; Polit & Beck, 2004). Random missing data consists of values missing here and there throughout the data from both study groups. A pattern is present when more data is missing from one group than from the other, or when more data is missing from participants with a certain characteristic, such as the youngest or the oldest. Such a pattern can bias the findings.

In any case, the researcher is obligated to try and understand why the data is missing and decide how to analyze the results to prevent the missing data from distorting the statistical results. As a reader, you first suspect data is missing when you notice that the sample sizes of various analyses are different; there may be good reasons for this, but it could also be a result of problems in the way the study was conducted. Some researchers report and explain missing data, whereas others gloss over it.

Consider this description of missing data. If a randomized study evaluating the effectiveness of a smoking cessation method has a larger dropout rate in the test intervention group than in the comparison group, the results may be biased because only the people who found the test intervention agreeable would be included in the analysis. This would make the test intervention look better than it would have been had all the persons randomized to that group contributed outcome data. Also, the results are potentially biased because the even distribution of patient characteristics created by random assignment may have been destroyed; as a result the actual analysis may have been done on groups that do not have equivalent baseline characteristics. There are recognized ways of dealing with missing data—they will not be addressed here—but if there is considerable missing data, you should note if the researcher indicated how its influence was analyzed and managed.

Large numbers of dropouts and missing data also threaten the generalizability of the study's findings. For example, a randomized study of a new physical activity program for second- and third-grade inner-city children might find that the group who participated in the new program did better than those who received a placebo intervention. However, the study had a 26% dropout rate, which was evenly distributed across both treatment groups. Although the even distribution of dropouts may not have biased the study results, the benefit produced by the new program may not be realized if the program were given to all second- and third-grade inner-city kids. The high dropout rate could have produced a study sample that was not representative of the target population, and thus the generalizability of the study findings would be called into question.

Wrap-Up

In summary, an experimental study is usually sound when researchers do the following:

1. Determine sample size by doing a power analysis
2. Use random assignment to ensure that groups are equivalent at the start of the study
3. Ensure that interventions are delivered consistently
4. Control extraneous influences and potential bias
5. Take steps to ensure that participants stay in the study and contribute data at all collection times

Use of these research strategies ensures that any significant differences detected in the outcomes of the groups studied can with confidence be attributed to the difference in treatments the groups received. And if no differences are found, use of these research strategies ensures that the lack of difference can be attributed to the fact that the two treatments truly do not have different impacts.

Measurement of the Outcome Variables

As described in Chapter 5, an important standard for every quantitative study is good data. As this standard applies to experimental studies, the instruments used to measure the outcome variables should have high reliability and validity. This requires that even though an instrument or measure was found reliable and valid in earlier studies, the researcher should take some steps to evaluate its reliability and validity in the current application (Polit & Beck, 2004, p. 428). Checking validity is particularly important when the population of a study is unlike ones in which previously reported validity of the instruments was established. In short, reliability and validity of a measure are not established once and for all; they are established for each population studied. Having said this, this practice is not always followed, rather many authors report previously determined validity and reliability results from dissimilar groups and assume the measure performs similarly for their purposes. This assumption should be challenged more often than it is.

Limitations of Randomized Experiments

The randomized experiment is the gold standard study design for determining if a nursing intervention brings about desired outcomes. However, when clinicians read a study report of a randomized study, they often want to decide if they should use the intervention with their patients; in this regard randomized studies have limitations. One problem is that the findings of many studies are reported as average outcomes of the two treatment groups. However, clinicians treat unique individuals, not average individuals, and thus the clinician does not know if the particular patient will respond like the average patient in the more effective study group or in a different way. Even if 80% of patients in a group respond favorably to an intervention, the clinician does not know if the patient he is treating will respond like the 80% or like the other 20%.

A second limitation of randomized controlled experiments is that they may have weak generalizability resulting from the exclusion of patients with conditions other than the one of interest. Exclusions control extraneous variables and thereby afford more certainty about the effectiveness of the intervention. However, they pose a dilemma for clinicians in that the patients in the study may have fewer health problems (i.e., comorbidities) than do patients seen in everyday practice. As a result, the intervention itself may be difficult to use, or similar results may not be realized. For example, in studying the effectiveness of tai chi exercises on balance in the elderly, the research may have excluded persons who had a fall or dizziness during the last 6 months and those who have cardiovascular disease. From the point of view of establishing the effectiveness of tai chi, these exclusions make sense. However, many of the persons seen in a geriatric care setting have these problems, so the research findings would have limited application to a sizeable portion of them.

A third limitation of randomized controlled experiments is that the interventions are delivered in a controlled manner, whereas in everyday practice an intervention is delivered by a diverse group of people. Often it is not clear how much variation can be introduced into the delivery of an intervention and still retain its effectiveness.

These limitations do not mean that randomized controlled experiments are not useful; however, they do point to the need for multiple studies regarding an intervention—under different conditions and with diverse groups of people. The limitations also require that researchers explore deeply why some people responded very positively to an intervention, others responded in a moderately positive manner, and still others responded negatively or poorly.

Randomized Controlled Trials

You will see the term **randomized controlled trial** (often abbreviated as RCT) in the medical literature and less often in the nursing literature. RCTs in nursing are experimental studies in which study participants are randomly assigned to treatment groups and have large diverse samples (ideally in more than one setting); RCTs typically represent advanced testing of an intervention. Not all experimental studies are RCTs.

Quasi-Experimental Designs

Although experimental design is the gold standard for evaluating the cause–effect relationship between an intervention and an outcome, sometimes it is not possible to: (a) use random assignment to intervention groups; (b) to have tight control over the delivery of the intervention; or (c) to have a comparison group (Burns & Grove, 2009). In these situations, a quasi-experimental design is used to study the effectiveness of nursing interventions. These designs are enough like experiments to retain the word *experiment* in their description, but because they lack one of the important features of experiments, they leave open the door to uncontrolled extraneous variables and wrong conclusions to an extent that experimental designs do not.

To illustrate, if two methods for preventing heel pressure ulcers were studied on one unit of a long-term care facility, the staff might have difficulty keeping the two methods pure. So, the researchers might decide to use method A with at-risk patients on one unit and method B with at-risk patients on another similar unit. This would be a quasi-experimental study because individual participants are members of intact groups (patients on a particular unit) and that membership determines which intervention they receive, not random assignment. Even when the two groups seem similar, there is concern that they might be different in unidentified ways or that the levels of care on the two units are different. Any difference could act as an extraneous variable giving the impression of an intervention effect on the outcome. The researcher conducting such a study could take steps to identify, control, or take into account extraneous influences. These steps would include comparing the characteristics of the patients on the two units and comparing the two units on variables such as staffing pattern, years of experience of the staff, and their educational levels. Taking any differences into account in the analysis would build confidence in the study conclusions about the effectiveness of the two heel ulcer prevention interventions.

Another example of a quasi-experimental design is a study in which the first 100 participants receive treatment A and the second 100 receive treatment B. This would be a **consecutive series** method for assigning individuals to treatment groups; thus patient-participants are not randomly assigned to treatment groups. This design also raises concerns that the two treatment groups might not be equivalent at the start. Something may have changed in the environment during the time that lapsed between the beginning of one series and the beginning of the second series, such as a seasonal difference in patients, a change in staffing, or a change in work flow. Thus, an extraneous variable could be at work.

Generally, quasi-experimental study designs are considered weaker than randomized experimental design because there is lack of certainty that the two groups actually were equivalent at baseline or that they received exactly the same treatment. The reader of a report of a quasi-experimental study needs to be alert to nonequivalent groups, inconsistent treatment delivery, or the presence of extraneous variables because they could distort the findings and study conclusions.

Exemplar

📖 *Reading Tips*

One of the interventions evaluated in the exemplar study is the administration of promethazine, which is used to treat postoperative nausea and vomiting. If you are not familiar with this drug, you should look it up. Promethazine is widely used. Also, just to be clear: an alcohol prep pad is the little alcohol-impregnated piece of gauze used to cleanse skin prior to an injection or venipuncture.

At this point, read just the introductory and Methods sections (up to Results).

Comparison of Inhalation of Isopropyl Alcohol vs. Promethazine in the Treatment of Postoperative Nausea and Vomiting (PONV) in Patients Identified as at High Risk for Developing PONV.

Joseph Pellegrini, Jon DeLoge, John Bennett, and Joseph Kelly

AANA Journal (2009), 77(4), 293–299.

Frequently, patients identified as high risk for postoperative nausea and vomiting (PONV) are treated prophylactically with intravenous (IV) ondansetron and postoperatively with IV promethazine. The purpose of this study was to determine if using an aromatic therapy of 70% isopropyl alcohol (IPA) would be more effective than promethazine in resolution of breakthrough PONV symptoms in groups of high-risk patients administered prophylactic ondansetron.

All subjects enrolled were identified as high risk for PONV, administered general anesthesia and a prophylactic antiemetic of 4 mg of IV ondansetron, and randomized to receive IPA or promethazine for treatment of breakthrough PONV. Demographics, verbal numeric rating scale (VNRS) scores for nausea, time to 50% reduction in VNRS scores, and overall antiemetic and incidence of PONV were measured.

The data for 85 subjects were included in analysis; no differences in demographic variables or baseline measurements were noted between groups. The IPA group reported a faster time to 50% reduction in VNRS scores and decreased overall antiemetic requirements. A similar incidence in PONV was noted between groups.

Based on these findings, we recommend that inhalation of 70% IPA is an option for treatment of PONV in high-risk patients who have received prophylactic ondansetron.

Key Words

Isopropyl alcohol, postoperative nausea and vomiting (PONV), promethazine, risk factors for PONV

In the general surgical population, the risk of postoperative nausea and vomiting (PONV) is between 16% and 30%; however, this risk ratio is increased even further when certain factors are present that predispose a patient to PONV.[1-5] These risk factors include general anesthesia of more than 60 minutes' duration, female gender, nonsmoker, history of PONV, and history of motion sickness.[1-7] In fact, it has been noted that the incidence of PONV increases exponentially from 16% when no risk factors are present to as high as 87% when all risk factors are present.[1-9] Therefore, it has become routine in many anesthesia practices to screen patients preoperatively to identify the patients at high risk for PONV so that an aggressive management plan can be implemented to prevent or decrease the severity of PONV symptoms.

Most typically, this aggressive management plan involves the prophylactic administration of an antiemetic agent that works specifically on an area of the brain called the chemotaxic trigger zone (CTZ).[1-5] The CTZ, located in the area postrema of the brain, lacks a blood–brain barrier, thereby making it highly receptive to stimulation from specific neurotransmitters that have been shown to be integral in eliciting an emetic response.[1-5] These neurotransmitters include serotonin, dopamine, histamine, and acetylcholine.[1-5] Although a variety of agents can be administered prophylactically to prevent PONV, the agent most often used is the serotonin antagonist ondansetron, an antiemetic agent that has been shown to be highly effective in preventing PONV in a wide variety of patient populations, while still having a relatively low side-effect profile.[6-11]

Ondansetron, when used as a prophylactic agent, is routinely administered approximately 15 to 30 minutes before the conclusion of the surgical procedure. Studies have shown that the prophylactic administration of ondansetron results in a 50% to 80% reduction in PONV in groups of low-risk patients but only a 25% reduction in patients identified as high risk for PONV.[10–12] Because of this lack of effectiveness in preventing PONV in patients identified as high risk, the patients will often require a subsequent antiemetic for treatment, and one of the most common agents used to treat this breakthrough PONV is the antiemetic agent promethazine.[8,13]

Promethazine is a dopamine receptor blocking agent routinely administered because it has a rapid onset of action (within 3–5 minutes) and a relatively long duration of efficacy (approximately 2–6 hours).[8] However, unlike ondansetron, which has minimal side effects, promethazine is commonly associated with sedation, dry mouth, and, in rare cases, hypotension.[8,13] Despite these side effects, many practitioners prefer promethazine to other traditional antiemetic agents because it can be used in the inpatient and outpatient settings. Promethazine is routinely administered by the intravenous (IV) route to a patient while in the hospital but is also available in oral and suppository forms for outpatient administration.[8,13] However, some patients report hesitancy to taking an oral antiemetic when they are nauseous; therefore, many practitioners prescribe the suppository form to avoid oral administration and because it can be easily self-administered by a patient in the home setting. Despite this, many patients still report hesitancy toward self-administration of a promethazine suppository and often report that the side effects following administration are unacceptable.[9,14] Therefore, anesthesia practitioners are continually seeking alternative antiemetic treatments that are highly effective in treating PONV, can be easily self-administered in any setting, and have a low side-effect profile.

A PONV treatment that seems to meet all of these criteria is the aromatic treatment of 70% isopropyl alcohol (IPA) that is administered by simply using a single alcohol prep pad. Research has shown that inhalation of IPA from a simple alcohol prep pad is easy to administer in the inpatient and outpatient settings, is highly effective in treating PONV, and is associated with no side effects.[15–17] However, all of the studies to date using IPA have been done only with patients who are not classified as high risk for PONV, and IPA has never been used in a patient population that has been prophylactically treated with ondansetron. Therefore, the purpose of this study was to investigate the efficacy of IPA vs promethazine in treating breakthrough PONV in groups of high-risk patients who have received a perioperative prophylactic dose of ondansetron.

Methods

All patients scheduled for general anesthesia of more than 60 minutes' duration and having 2 of the 4 individual risk factors for PONV, (female gender, nonsmoker, history of PONV or motion sickness) were approached for possible inclusion in this institutional review board–approved prospective study. Patients were excluded from participation if they reported a recent upper respiratory infection; documented allergy to IPA, ondansetron, promethazine, or metoclopramide; antiemetic or psychoactive drug use within 24 hours; inability to breathe through the nose; pregnancy; history of inner ear pathology; and/or taking disulfiram, cefoperazone, or metronidazole. Patients with a body mass index greater than 35 kg/m² also were excluded from the study. In addition, following enrollment, the data were excluded from analysis for subjects who required inpatient hospitalization for reasons not related to PONV.

Once inclusionary criteria were met, informed consent was obtained and demographic data were collected, including age, height, weight, gender, ASA class, body mass index, race, and surgical procedure. All subjects were then randomly assigned using a computer-generated random numbers process into a control or an experimental group. The control group was assigned to receive 12.5 to 25 mg IV promethazine for complaints of PONV in the postanesthesia care unit (PACU) and same-day surgery unit (SDSU) and by promethazine suppository self-administration following discharge to home. The experimental group was assigned to receive treatment of PONV by administration of inhaled 70% IPA.

In the preoperative holding area, all subjects received instruction on treatments, study requirements, and the home data collection tool. A baseline level of nausea was obtained on all subjects following informed consent using a 0 to 10 verbal numeric rating scale (VNRS) in which a score of "0" indicated "no nausea" and a score of "10" indicated the "worst imaginable nausea." Before transport to the operative suite, preoperative medications for anxiolysis and sedation were administered based on individual requirements and anesthesia providers' discretion using 0 to 5 mg of midazolam and/or 0 to 3 µg/kg of fentanyl IV. All preoperative medications administered were recorded.

On arrival to the operative suite, blood pressure, electrocardiographic, and pulse oximetry monitors were applied and a baseline set of vital signs was obtained and recorded. Anesthesia induction was facilitated with propofol, 1.5 to 2 mg/kg IV; lidocaine, 0 to 1 mg/kg IV; fentanyl, 0 to 5 µg/kg IV; and a neuromuscular blocking agent of the anesthesia provider's choice. Following induction, all subjects were endotracheally intubated, and, based on surgical requirements, an orogastric tube was inserted and stomach contents were evacuated. All orogastric tubes were removed immediately before extubation, and the use of an orogastric tube was recorded. Maintenance of anesthesia was achieved with isoflurane, desflurane, or sevoflurane in combination with oxygen, 50% or 100%, and nitrous oxide, 0% or 50%. An opioid of provider choice was used for maintenance of analgesia. The doses of all opioids administered during the perioperative period were later converted to morphine equivalents for analysis.[18] Approximately 15 to 30 minutes before extubation, all subjects received ondansetron, 4 mg IV. Neuromuscular blockade was reversed, if necessary, using neostigmine, 0.05 mg/kg, and glycopyrrolate, 0.1 mg/kg IV. All medications administered intraoperatively were recorded on the data collection tool. Additional information collected and recorded included the type of surgery, use of laparoscopic technique, total estimated blood loss, total amount of IV fluids administered, estimated preoperative-postoperative fluid deficit, and anesthesia, surgical, and PACU times. All subjects were extubated before transfer to the PACU.

Following arrival to the PACU and SDSU, an admission VNRS for nausea was obtained and recorded. For the purposes of this study, *nausea* was defined as the subjective feeling of the urge to vomit, and *vomiting* was defined as the forceful expulsion of gastric contents. Each event had to be at least 60 seconds from any other event to be recorded as a separate event. In addition, VNRS scores were obtained and recorded at the first complaint of nausea, every 5 minutes following treatment for nausea for the first 30 minutes, and then every 15 minutes thereafter for 75 minutes after the event or until discharge from the PACU or SDSU. Nausea events were treated according to group assignment (IPA or promethazine).

Subjects in the control (promethazine) group received promethazine, 12.5 to 25 mg IV, at the first complaint of nausea in the PACU and SDSU; this dose could be repeated in 30 minutes for a maximum dose of 50 mg IV. For nausea that was refractory to promethazine, control subjects could receive metoclopramide, 10 mg IV every 15 minutes, not to exceed a total dose of 30 mg.

All subjects in the experimental (IPA) group received inhalation therapy using a commercially available 70% IPA pad (Webcol, Kendall Healthcare, Mansfield, Massachusetts). All subjects were instructed to remove the IPA pad from the protective covering, fold the IPA pad in half, hold the folded pad approximately 0.5 inches from their nares, and take 3 deep inhalations from the pad and discard it after use. This treatment could be administered by the PACU and SDSU nurses in the hospital setting or by the patient; however, subjects were instructed to self-administer their IPA treatments following discharge to home following the treatment regimen described above. The IPA treatments were ordered to be administered on an as-needed basis, up to a total of 3 separate applications (3 deep inhalations per application) every 15 minutes. For complaints of nausea refractory to IPA treatment (no resolution of PONV symptoms after 3 applications) or if a patient requested an antiemetic agent at any time, promethazine, 12.5 to 25 mg IV every 30 minutes was given, not to exceed a total dose of 50 mg IV, or metoclopramide, 10 mg IV every 15 minutes, not to exceed a total dose of 30 mg. These treatment protocols were the same in the PACU and SDSU settings. All pharmacologic treatments administered for nausea and VNRS score measurements were recorded.

Before discharge to home, all subjects were instructed to treat PONV symptoms based on their assigned group. The subjects in the promethazine group were instructed to treat any PONV using 25-mg promethazine suppositories every 6 hours on an as-needed basis. The subjects in the IPA group were instructed to use the folded IPA regimen as described in the hospital setting on an as-needed basis, up to a total of 3 separate applications. In addition, IPA subjects were also instructed that they could self-administer a 25-mg promethazine suppository for any PONV symptoms that were refractory to the IPA treatments or if they had exhausted the number of applications ordered and had not achieved resolution of PONV symptoms. All subjects were asked to record the time any antiemetic therapy was self-administered at home (IPA or promethazine), the number of nausea and emetic events, and the severity of nausea using the 0 to 10 VNRS scale before they self-administered any antiemetic therapy and every 15 minutes after initiation for a period of 30 minutes. Before discharge, all subjects were given a home data collection sheet to record these events and instructed that they would receive a telephone call by one of the investigators approximately 24 hours after surgery to obtain this information. In addition, during the telephone call, all subjects were asked to rate their level of satisfaction regarding their antiemetic therapy using the following scale: 1, totally dissatisfied; 2, somewhat dissatisfied; 3, somewhat satisfied; 4, satisfied; and 5, totally satisfied. All responses from the telephone interview were recorded on a data collection sheet.

Before initiation of this study, a power analysis was performed based on previous studies[15,16] that indicated that subjects in the IPA group would achieve a 50% reduction in their mean VNRS scores for nausea 15 minutes earlier than subjects randomized to receive promethazine treatment. By using an α of .05 and a β of .10, we determined that a sample size of 40 subjects per group would be required to determine if a difference between the groups existed. Factoring in a 20% attrition rate increased our sample size to 96 subjects (48 per group).

Statistical analysis was performed using SPSS software version 13.0 (SPSS Inc., Chicago, Illinois). Data analysis was accomplished using descriptive and inferential statistics. Demographic data and frequency data were analyzed using the χ^2 test and Pearson correlation. The VNRS scores and time to resolution were analyzed using a Student t test. Subject satisfaction scores, body mass index scores, and total promethazine requirements were analyzed using a Mann-Whitney U test. A P value of less than .05 was considered significant.

Results

A total of 96 subjects were enrolled, but 11 subjects were withdrawn, leaving a total of 85 subjects (IPA group, 42; promethazine group, 43) whose data would be included in the final analysis. Reasons for withdrawal included 4 subjects who received additional antiemetics intraoperatively (2 in each group), 1 subject inadvertently enrolled despite being scheduled for a nasal surgical procedure (IPA group), and 6 subjects who required postoperative inpatient hospitalization for reasons unrelated to PONV (3 in each group).

No differences were noted between the groups in relation to demographic variables, surgical times, anesthesia times, use of laparoscopy, orogastric tube use, time to first PONV event from PACU admission, history of motion sickness, primary volatile agent used, or the total number of PONV risk factors present. A noted difference was in the use of nitrous oxide between groups: 59% of the IPA group received 50% nitrous oxide compared with 37% in the promethazine group ($P = .049$). However when a separate analysis of nitrous oxide use and PONV was performed, no significance could be found to indicate that nitrous oxide administration increased the incidence of PONV. No differences in the amount of opioids administered during the perioperative period were noted between groups ($P > .05$) (Table 1). No differences in fluid deficit, estimated blood loss, type of surgical procedure performed, total amount of IV fluid administered, or total hours without oral intake were noted between groups.

Table 1. DESCRIPTION OF DEMOGRAPHIC DATA, PREOPERATIVE RISK
FACTORS, AND PERIOPERATIVE INFORMATION[a]

	ISOPROPYL ALCOHOL (N = 42)	PROMETHAZINE (N = 43)	P
Age (y)	33.98 ± 10.9	37.09 ± 11.0	.052
Weight (kg)	75.43 ± 17.4	74.84 ± 13.3	.939
Median (range) body mass index (kg/m²)	27 (22–34)	27 (21–33)	.947
Laparoscopy			
Total	21	20	.748
Gynecologic	14	11	.433
Gender			.763
Female	30	33	
Male	12	10	
Surgical time (min)	50.57 ± 34.32	57.63 ± 44.3	.416
Anesthesia time (min)	90.45 ± 39.5	101.1 ± 48.7	.272
PONV risk factors			.676
3 risk factors	24	26	
4 risk factors	12	9	
5 risk factors	6	8	
Time from PACU admission to PONV event (min)	90.9 ± 101.8	78.8 ± 76.7	.664
History of motion sickness			.723
Yes	26	25	
No	16	18	
Primary volatile agent used			.326
Desflurane	18	25	
Sevoflurane	22	16	
Isoflurane	2	2	
Opioid morphine equivalent			
Perioperative	24.05 ± 16.4	21.5 ± 9.1	.375
PACU	8.8 ± 5.7	9.3 ± 5.6	.775
SDSU	4.4 ± 2.5	4.1 ± 1.9	.736
Nitrous oxide use			.049[b]
Yes	25	16	
No	17	27	
Orogastric tube use			.668
Yes	16	19	
No	26	24	

PONV indicates postoperative nausea and vomiting; PACU, postanesthesia care unit;
SDSU, same-day surgical unit.
[a]Data are given as mean ± SD or number of cases unless otherwise indicated.
[b]Significant at $P < .05$.

Table 2. INCIDENCE OF NAUSEA EVENTS AND MEDIAN DOSES OF PROMETHAZINE REQUIRED PER GROUP PER SETTING

	ISOPROPYL ALCOHOL (N = 42)	PROMETHAZINE (N = 43)	P
No. (%) of nausea events			
PACU	7 (17)	10 (23)	.448
SDSU	17 (42)	10 (23)	.088
Home	19 (45)	10 (23)	.019[a]
Median (range) promethazine requirements (mg)			
PACU	0	12.5 (0–25)	.002[a]
SDSU	12.5 (0–25)	25.0 (0–50)	.033[a]
Home	12.5 (0–25)	12.5 (0–25)	.214

PACU indicates postanesthesia care unit; SDSU, same-day surgical unit.
[a]Significant at $P < .05$.

The overall incidence of postoperative nausea was similar between groups, with 76% (n = 32) of the IPA group reporting postoperative nausea compared with 60% (n = 26) of the promethazine group ($P = .119$). Analysis of the incidence of nausea based on setting revealed that a higher incidence of PONV occurred in the IPA group in all settings but achieved significance only following discharge to home ($P = .019$). Promethazine was administered as the primary antiemetic agent in the promethazine group and as a rescue agent in the IPA group. Not surprisingly, the median dose of promethazine was higher in the promethazine group in all settings, achieving significance in the PACU and SDSU (Table 2). Analysis of the need for promethazine suppositories following discharge revealed that 23% (n = 10) of the promethazine group self-administered a promethazine suppository compared with only 7% (n = 3) of the IPA group ($P = .039$). No subject in either group required metoclopramide as a rescue agent in any setting. No differences in the VNRS scores were noted between groups on initial complaint of nausea in any setting (Figure 1). However, when time to 50% reduction in VNRS scores for nausea was analyzed, we noted a significantly faster time to a 50% reduction in VNRS scores in the IPA group compared with the promethazine group in the PACU ($P = .045$), SDSU ($P = .032$), and the home ($P = .017$) settings (Figure 2).

Emetic events were similar between the groups in the PACU (none), SDSU (IPA group, 3; promethazine group, 2) and in the home (5 in each group). Satisfaction with nausea control was similar between groups: both groups reported a median of 4 (satisfied) with the level of nausea control for the respective treatment regimens ($P > .05$). No subject who received IPA treatments exclusively reported any untoward side effects, whereas

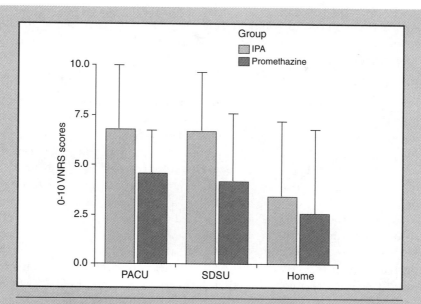

FIGURE 1. VNRS Scores on Initial Complaint Per Setting
VNRS indicates visual numeric rating scale; IPA, isopropyl alcohol; PACU, postanesthesia care unit; SDSU, same-day surgical unit.

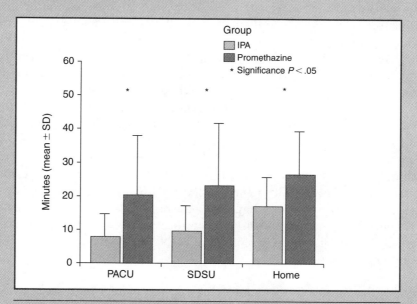

FIGURE 2. Time in Minutes to a 50% Reduction in VNRS Scores by Group Per Setting
VNRS indicates visual numeric rating scale; IPA, isopropyl alcohol; PACU, postanesthesia care unit; SDSU, same-day surgical unit.

subjects who received promethazine as a primary or rescue treatment reported mild to moderate degrees of sedation and dry mouth; however, no subject required treatment for side effects.

Discussion

Postoperative nausea and vomiting continue to be persistent problems following general anesthesia. In our study, we used the risk factors for PONV identified by Koivuranta et al.[1] that included the variables gender, smoking history, history of PONV, a history of motion sickness, and exposure to general anesthesia for more than 60 minutes to establish a risk of PONV. Koivuranta et al.[1] reported that the relative risk of PONV for someone with 3 risk factors is 54%, with 4 risk factors is 63%, and with all 5 risk factors is 87%.

Based on these findings, we anticipated the overall incidence of PONV to be approximately 60%, given that the number of risk factors ranged between 3 and 5 in both groups. We anticipated this number to be decreased by a ratio of 25% to 42% following ondansetron administration. We were surprised to find that the overall incidence of PONV ranged between 61% and 76%, thereby indicating that ondansetron prophylaxis was not as effective as we hypothesized. However, analysis of the incidence of nausea in the PACU and SDSU revealed that the overall incidence of nausea was approximately 45% in both groups, indicating that ondansetron is limited in providing prophylaxis for the first few hours after surgery. Because of this limited range of effectiveness, it is common for patients at high risk for PONV to require subsequent antiemetic agents for the treatment of breakthrough PONV, which can often result in some significant side effects such as sedation and hypotension.

Another problem with traditional antiemetic agents is that they often cannot be administered easily in the home setting. In addition, the potential for side effects may place postoperative patients at risk. We chose IPA aromatic therapy as an avenue for investigation because previous research showed that it is effective in treating the symptoms of nausea and can be easily administered in the home setting.[15,16] However, these earlier studies were not performed on a high-risk patient population or in groups of patients already given ondansetron. In this study, we showed that IPA is effective in alleviating the symptoms of PONV and works very well in concert with ondansetron.

There has been some research that found that IPA is no more effective than other aromatic therapies or having the patient take several deep breaths of ambient air. For example, Anderson and Gross[19] reported that no difference in nausea scores was found among groups of patients asked to inhale peppermint, IPA, or saline, and they concluded that it was the simple act of taking a deep inhalation of air that was the inducement to relieve PONV symptoms rather than any specific aromatic properties. However, it was noted that this study was done on a very small group of patients (33 subjects), and the researchers did not have control over subsequent antiemetics administered during the perioperative and postoperative periods; therefore, it is difficult to ascertain the specific agent that facilitated the relief of PONV symptoms in the study. The findings of Anderson and Gross are contradicted in an earlier study by Langevin and Brown,[17] who compared the inhalation of IPA with placebo (saline) in a double-blinded study (30 subjects; 15/group). These investigators reported that administration of IPA resulted in a complete resolution of PONV symptoms in 80% of patients treated with IPA and that deep inhalation from a saline-soaked pad was totally ineffective in resolution of PONV symptoms, indicating that simply performing deep inhalations through the nose is not effective in alleviating symptoms of PONV.

Our study had some limitations. The SDSU staff was required to record VNRS scores every 5 minutes on complaint of PONV; therefore, we were forced to limit our subject enrollment to 1 or 2 subjects per day to ensure quality data collection. Also, in the home setting, we found there was a social stigma associated with the insertion of suppositories, and some patients reported hesitancy to use the suppository. We specifically chose a suppository over oral medication because it has also been noted that many patients are also hesitant to orally ingest a medication when they are experiencing nausea. It is unknown what overall effect this hesitancy may have had on the number of subjects who reported that they did not use the promethazine suppository as a rescue medication in the home setting. In retrospect, perhaps a better choice of an antiemetic for use as a rescue agent following discharge to home may have been an agent that does not require oral ingestion or suppository insertion, for example, sublingual ondansetron.

Although this study was designed using a unimodal approach to PONV prophylaxis, many practitioners report that more clinical effectiveness is observed when a multimodal antiemetic approach is used. The multimodal approach is used in an effort to optimize coverage on different receptors in the CTZ. While using this approach has been shown to be more effective in preventing PONV than using a single modal approach, it usually results in an increase in side effects.[6-9] Because of this, we are planning a future study in which we plan to provide IPA prophylaxis immediately before induction of general anesthesia in addition to the standard ondansetron prophylaxis 15 to 30 minutes before the conclusion of the surgical procedure. It is unclear where IPA works in relation to blocking the receptors in the CTZ. We hypothesize that it may possibly work on several sites simultaneously in the CTZ; therefore, IPA pharmacokinetics may already use a multimodal approach. However, we note that the clinical duration of IPA is limited; therefore, we propose that in an effort to optimize this multimodal approach, it may be best tested by incorporating ondansetron prophylaxis into the design as well. To date, only 1 study has been performed in which IPA was administered prophylactically, and the investigators reported that the inhalation of IPA was no more effective than the administration of granisetron but was more effective than no prophylactic treatment.[20] This study indicated that IPA prophylaxis was effective in preventing PONV, but the study used a small sample and administered the IPA following extubation, a different method than the one we are planning.

We believe that we clearly showed that IPA is as effective in treating PONV as promethazine in patients who have been identified as high risk for PONV, but it works considerably faster, works well in concert with ondansetron, and can be easily administered in any setting. Therefore, we are confident in recommending that IPA be considered a viable option to conventional antiemetic therapy in treating breakthrough PONV in groups of patients identified as high risk for PONV who have received perioperative prophylactic ondansetron.

References

1. Koivuranta M, Läärää E, Snåre L, Alahuhta S. A survey of postoperative nausea and vomiting. *Anaesthesia.* 1997;52(5):443–449.

2. Eberhart LH, Högel J, Seeling W, Staack M, Geldner G, Georgieff M. Evaluation of the three risk scores to predict postoperative nausea and vomiting. *Acta Anaesthesiol Scand.* 2000;44(4):480–488.

3. Cohen MM, Duncan PG, DeBoer DP, Tweed WA. The postoperative interview: assessing risk factors for nausea and vomiting. *Anesth Analg.* 1994;78(1):7–16.

4. Haigh CG, Kaplan LA, Durham JM, Dupeyron JP, Harmer M, Kenny GN. Nausea and vomiting after gynaecological surgery: a meta-analysis of factors affecting their incidence. *Br J Anaesth.* 1993;71:517–522.

5. Kenny GN. Risk factors for postoperative nausea and vomiting. *Anaesthesia.* 1994;49(suppl):6–10.

6. Watcha MF, White PF. Postoperative nausea and vomiting: its etiology, treatment and prevention. *Anesthesiology.* 1992;77(1):162–184.

7. Apfel CC, Läärää E, Koivuranta M, Greim CA, Roewer N. A simplified risk score for predicting postoperative nausea and vomiting: conclusions from cross-validations between two centers. *Anesthesiology.* 1999;91(3):693–700.

8. Kovac AL. Prevention and treatment of postoperative nausea and vomiting. *Drugs.* 2000;59(2):213–243.

9. Tong G. Postoperative nausea and vomiting: can it be eliminated? *JAMA.* 2002;287(10):1233–1236.

10. Claybon L. Single dose intravenous ondansetron for the 24-hour treatment of postoperative nausea and vomiting. *Anaesthesia.* 1994;49 (suppl):24–29.

11. Kovac AL, O'Connor TA, Pearman MH, et al. Efficacy of repeat intravenous dosing of ondansetron in controlling postoperative nausea and vomiting: a randomized, double-blind, placebo-controlled multicenter trial. *J Clin Anesth.* 1999;11(6):453–459.

12. Jones S, Strobl R, Crosby D, Burkard JF, Maye J, Pellegrini JE. The effect of transdermal scopolamine on the incidence and severity of postoperative nausea and vomiting in a group of high-risk patients given prophylactic intravenous ondansetron. *AANA J.* 2006;74(2): 127–132.

13. Dillon GP Jr. Clinical evaluation of promethazine for prevention of postoperative vomiting. *Am Pract Dig Treat.* 1957;8(10):1571–1575.

14. Scuderi PE, James RL, Harris L, Mims GR III. Multimodal antiemetic management prevents early postoperative vomiting after outpatient laparoscopy. *Anesth Analg.* 2000;91(6):1408–1414.

15. Winston AW, Rinehart RS, Riley GP, Vacchiano CA, Pellegrini JE. Comparison of inhaled isopropyl alcohol and intravenous ondansetron for treatment of postoperative nausea. *AANA J.* 2003;71(2):127–132.

16. Cotton JW, Rowell LR, Hood RR, Pellegrini JE. A comparative analysis of isopropyl alcohol and ondansetron in the treatment of postoperative nausea and vomiting from the hospital setting to the home. *AANA J.* 2007;75(1):21–26.

17. Langevin P, Brown M. A simple, innocuous and inexpensive treatment for postoperative nausea and vomiting [abstract]. *Anesth Analg.* 1997; 84(suppl):S16.

18. Gordon DB, Stevenson KK, Griffie J, Muchka S, Rapp C, Ford-Roberts K. Opioid equianalgesic calculations. *J Palliat Med.* 1999;2(2):209–218.

19. Anderson LA, Gross JB. Aromatherapy with peppermint, isopropyl alcohol, or placebo is equally effective in relieving postoperative nausea. *J Perianesth Nurs.* 2004;19(1):29–35.

20. Teran L, Hawkins JK. The effectiveness of inhalation isopropyl alcohol vs granisetron for the prevention of postoperative nausea and vomiting. *AANA J.* 2007;75(6):417–422.

Authors

Joseph Pellegrini, CRNA, PhD, CAPT(ret), NC, USN, is the former director of research, Navy Nurse Corps Anesthesia Program, Bethesda, Maryland. He is currently an associate professor, Nurse Anesthesia Program, University of Maryland, Baltimore, Maryland. Email: Pellegrini@son.umaryland.edu.

LT Jon DeLoge, CRNA, MSN, NC, USNR, is a staff nurse anesthetist at Naval Medical Center, Portsmouth, Virginia.

LCDR John Bennett, CRNA, MSN, NC, USNR, is a staff nurse anesthetist at Naval Medical Center, San Diego, California.

Joseph Kelly, CRNA, MS, CDR(ret), NC, USN, is a staff nurse anesthetist at University of Florida, Shands Medical Center, Jacksonville, Florida.

Profile & Commentary: Introduction and Methods

WHY *Study Purpose*

The purpose of this study was to compare the effectiveness of the inhalation of isopropyl alcohol (IPA) from a 70% prep pad to the drug promethazine in the treatment of postoperative nausea and vomiting (PONV) in patients who are at high risk for PONV. The researchers note that prior research that found IPA to be effective was done with patients who were not classified as high risk for PONV, which is why this study is needed. Information about the high prevalence of PONV and the risk factors for it is presented in the first several paragraphs.

HOW *Study Design*

This is a two-group experimental study in which participants were randomly assigned to one of two treatment groups, and the researchers had good control over the conditions under which treatments were given and data was collected. It is cross-sectional because data were collected for just one episode of care. Collecting data at several times that are close to one another (i.e., hospital then home) does not make it a longitudinal design as the intent was not to examine change over time.

Sample

Although the target population from a narrow perspective is the patients who have surgery in the one hospital, from a broader perspective the target population is patients similar to those described in Table 1. The absence of information about the setting precludes including those features in the characterization of the target population.

Persons included in the sample were those who (1) were identified as at high risk for PONV, (2) met the inclusion criteria, and (3) agreed to participate in the study. These 96 persons were randomly assigned to receive one of the two interventions for PONV. Note that the list of reasons for exclusion is quite long; this was done to control extraneous influences that could alter the incidence of PONV and participants' responses to either of the interventions. Note also that the reasons for withdrawal from the study were given.

In the end data was available on 85 persons; 42 in the IPA group and 43 in the promethazine group. The sample size was determined by a power analysis that took into account the expected effect of the IPA over the promethazine and the statistical certainty they wanted, as indicated by the p-level decision point (α) and by the level of power they wanted (β); they also took into account that 20% of those enrolled might not complete the study.

The sample is profiled in Table 1. The two groups were compared on demographic characteristics, risk factors, and perioperative information. The p-value column informs us that the only significant difference in the two groups at the start of the study was the proportions who received nitrous oxide during the operation; the researchers did some analysis of this difference and decided it did not increase the incidence of PONV. All the other differences were just chance variations expected in obtaining two samples from a population. From this table, we can conclude that randomization was very effective in creating two groups with similar profiles. In other words, we don't have to worry that the two groups were different in some way right at the start; thus when we look at the results, we will be able to eliminate initial differences in group composition as an explanation for the results.

You might wonder about the effects of different kinds of surgery. This was controlled to some extent by including only persons who would have general anesthesia of at least 60 minutes duration. Also, the fact that the two groups were not different in terms of surgical time, anesthesia time, laparoscopy cases, use of orogastric tubes, and gynecological cases assures us that the distribution of types of surgical procedures was probably also evenly distributed across both groups.

Interventions

Many details about how the interventions were delivered are provided in the report. It is clear from this description that every effort was made to control the consistency with which the interventions were delivered, thus controlling another source of extraneous influences. Importantly, in hospital if IPA was not effective, patients in that group would be given IV promethazine, however we are not told how many patients in the IPA group ended up being given IV promethazine. After discharge, the patients were to continue using the intervention they had in the hospital although when promethazine was needed, it was to be taken via rectal suppositories (rather than given intravenously as in hospital).

Outcome Measures

The outcomes studied were

- Incidence of PONV
- Events of PONV
- Time to 50% reduction in the nausea
- Intensity of nausea
- Doses of promethazine required
- Satisfaction with nausea control

These outcomes were measured at various times.

The VNRS, which measured intensity of nausea, was obtained on admission to the PACU or SDCU, at the first complaint of nausea, and at defined intervals after the intervention was delivered. The VNRS is a 0 to 10 scale with 0 representing "no nausea" and 10 representing the "worst imaginable nausea." No information is provided about how well this scale captures gradations of nausea, but similar scales (visual analogue scales) are widely used in clinical practice and in symptom research. Reliability and validity of these scales are rarely discussed or provided.

At discharge, patients were given a home data collection sheet to record their events of nausea or vomiting and VNRS at intervals after an event. At the phone call 24 hours after discharge, patients were asked to rate their level of satisfaction with their treatment for nausea using a 5-point scale.

You should now have a sense of *how* this study was done. However, you may need to go back over it again to get some of the details fixed in your mind.

Section 2: Understanding Study Results

Was One Intervention More Effective Than the Other?

In most two-group experimental studies, the researcher's goal is to determine if one intervention is more effective than the other. Effectiveness is defined as impact or influence on the outcome variable, and more effectiveness is a greater degree of positive impact or influence.

There are two ways of thinking about effectiveness: from the clinical perspective and from the statistical perspective. At the center of both perspectives is a comparison of the amount of effect, or impact, each intervention had on the outcome variable. From the clinical perspective, the bottom line question is, "Is the difference in the outcomes of the two groups large enough to be clinically meaningful?" From the statistical perspective the bottom line question is, "Is the difference found a true difference or a chance difference?" When reading a report of an intervention study, too many people get hung up in the results of the statistical analysis (e.g., *p*-values, statistical significance). I suggest that you start by looking first at the results from a clinical perspective and then proceed to consider the meaning of the statistical tests of significance.

The Clinical Perspective

Generally speaking, the results of experimental studies are reported in one of two ways:

1. As the proportion of persons in each group who achieved a clinical outcome or milestone
2. As the mean scores of the two groups on the outcome variable

(The term *scores* refers to the numerical values obtained by all forms of measurement, be it physiological measurement, questionnaires, or rating scales.) When trying to get a read on the clinical significance of study results, proportions and mean scores require different analytical strategies.

Attainment of an Outcome   In some nursing studies and many medical studies, results are reported as the proportions of persons in the treatment groups who attained a certain outcome or milestone—say, not smoking for one year. When an outcome or milestone is reported as a "yes" or "no" outcome, it is called a dichotomous outcome. Other examples of **dichotomous variables** are these:

- Rated pain control as good or better–did not rate pain control as good or better
- Increased self-care knowledge–did not increase self-care knowledge
- Gained the ability to walk 50 feet without assistance–did not gain this ability
- Lived–died

In experimental studies with dichotomous outcomes, the proportion of persons in each group who attained the yes/no outcome is determined. When the outcome is a good event, the difference in these two proportions is called the absolute benefit increase (ABI). It is one of several measures of treatment effect used to portray the relative impact of the two treatments (Sackett, Straus, Richardson, Rosenberg, & Haynes, 2000). The other one explained in this chapter is number needed to treat (NNT).

Consider a fictional study in which a new program to encourage physical activity in second- and third-grade inner-city kids is evaluated. (Focus on the results, not the study design, and assume a low rate of dropout.) Two hundred children were randomly assigned to attend the new once-a-week after-school exercise program for three weeks or to receive a placebo treatment in which a study assistant played electronic, card, and board games with the kids in the comparison group once a week for three weeks. The milestone outcome being considered is actively exercising for 8 hours or more outside of school each week when measured three months after the program; this is a dichotomous outcome that is either achieved or not achieved. The results showed that 26% of the kids in the program attained the milestone outcome, whereas 12% of those in the placebo group attained it. So, the absolute difference between the proportion of those in the program who met the milestone and the proportion in the placebo group who met it is 14% (26%–12%); this is the **absolute benefit increase** (ABI) produced by the exercise intervention over the placebo intervention. The clinical ramifications of this measure of clinical significance should be considered: Is this a sizable enough difference to justify saying that the new program has a success rate that is clinically important?

The **number needed to treat** (NNT) provides another take on these results. It is the number of persons that would have to be given the more effective treatment rather than the less effective treatment for one additional person to achieve the milestone outcome—that is: one person more than the number that would have achieved the milestone outcome if the comparison treatment had been used. In our fictional study, the NNT is 8. This means that for every eight kids entered into the exercise program, rather than just getting attention, one additional kid will achieve the milestone exercise level than would have if all eight kids received just attention. This provides a practical sense of how much benefit the exercise program would produce, which is actually pretty impressive.

Note that the NNT is easily calculated from the ABI; it is the inverse (reciprocal) of the ABI. That is: 1/ABI rounded up to a whole number—we don't treat 0.1 of a person. The **treatment effect measures** of the exercise program are portrayed in Table 7–1.

NNT is useful in considering whether to implement a similar program because it estimates in concrete terms the benefit that is likely to be realized from the program. The NNT is useful for two reasons. First, it provides a clinical perspective on how many people are likely to benefit at a meaningful level from the program compared with no program. Second, the expected benefit can be considered in the context of the cost of the program, risks of exercise, and long-term risks of not developing an exercise habit.

Mean Level of an Outcome   When the outcome variable of a study is measured on an interval level scale, a score is obtained for every patient and group means are calculated. To make clinical sense of the results, you should first note the difference between the means of the two groups by subtracting one from the other—keeping in mind the range of the scale that was used to measure the variable. Then ask: Is this difference large enough to have clinical importance? For example:

- Is a 950-cc difference between the mean fluid intakes of two groups large enough to make a difference in patients' hydration status?

Table 7–1   TREATMENT EFFECT: EXERCISE PROGRAM FOR KIDS

MEASURES OF CLINICAL EFFECT (DICHOTOMOUS DATA)	
Milestone attained with program	26% (.26)
Milestone attained without program	12% (.12)
Absolute benefit increase (ABI)	14% (.14)
Number needed to treat (NNT)	1 ÷ .14 = 7.1 rounded up to 8

■ Is an 8-mm difference between mean diastolic blood pressure levels of the two groups large enough to represent better blood pressure control and lowered risk of complications?

Consideration of the size of the difference between the means provides some clinical sense of whether the difference in the impact of the two treatments is large, small, or somewhere in between.

The Statistical Perspective

When the outcome variable of a study is measured on an interval level scale and the results are reported as the means of each group, the statistical analysis provides information useful in answering the question: *Is the difference between the means of the two groups a true difference or a chance difference?* A true difference between the mean scores of the two groups is a difference that is robust enough that a difference is also likely to occur in the target population, not just in the study sample. Chance differences are caused by the normal variation in outcomes one would expect when measuring an outcome in two samples drawn from the same population.

In an experimental study, the two groups are treated differently; therefore a treatment effect is expected. A treatment effect is present when one treatment produces a larger effect on the outcome than the other treatment does. The larger the difference found between the outcome means of the two groups, the greater the chance that the difference is caused by one group receiving a treatment that was truly more effective than the other was. Moreover, the larger the difference in the means of the two groups, the greater the likelihood that a difference would be found if the whole population had been studied.

Note that even for the statistical question, your starting point is simple observation and common sense. Sometimes, just by looking at the mean outcome scores of the two groups and noting how different or close they are, you can get a first impression regarding whether the difference is caused by treatment effect or is just chance variation. If the difference is large, one treatment is most likely more effective than the other is and a benefit would probably be found beyond this one sample. If the difference in means is small, it is likely that it is just chance variation, which makes it unlikely that a benefit would be found in the target population. However, the definitive answer regarding whether the difference is a true difference or a chance difference is provided by inferential statistics, in particular the *p*-value result produced by a *t*-test.

t-Test and p-Value   The *t*-test is used to compare scores of two groups when the outcome variable is measured using an interval level scale; it cannot be used when the outcome variable is a dichotomous or categorical variable. The *t*-test analyzes the size of the difference between the means of two groups while taking into account the sample size and the spread of the scores across the possible range of scores (i.e., the standard deviation). It essentially asks: Even though a difference in means was found in this sample, what are the chances that in the larger population *no* difference would be found? The *t*-test produces a *p*-value indicating the probability that the difference found between the means is just a chance occurrence, not a true difference that would be found in the population.

This data-based probability *p*-value is then compared to a previously chosen level of significance probability *p*-level to determine if the probability that it is a chance result is acceptable or too high. If the data-based probability is acceptably low (i.e., lower than the level of significance decision-point probability), the difference is deemed statistically significant; if the data-based probability is too high (higher than the level of significance decision-point probability), the difference is deemed statistically not significant.

That last paragraph was a bit difficult—let's get more real-world. A hypothetical study tested the effects of two different methods of comforting babies during venipuncture (method A and method B); the infants' pain responses were measured 30 seconds after needle insertion using a scale with a value range of 0 to 10 (0 being no pain, 10 being a great deal of pain). Group A (n = 42) had a mean score of 3.6 and group B (n = 40) had a mean of 4.0, indicating that those in the method A group had on average less pain. A *t*-test was run on the difference between the means (0.4 points), and the result was $p = .02$. This is the data-based probability value; it indicates there are only 2 chances in 100 that a difference this large would occur because of chance variation. Said differently, if the researcher concluded that method A was more effective than method B, there would be 2 chances in 100 that his conclusion is wrong. When this data-based probability was compared to the decision-point level of significance probability ($p \leq .05$), the conclusion was that it is a true difference in outcome, because there is an acceptably low probability that the difference is just chance variation.

Consider a different result for this same study: Group A had a mean of 3.6, group B had a mean of 3.8, and $p = .10$. Now, the difference is just 0.2 point and there are 10 chances in 100 that the difference was a chance result.

With this result, *if* the researcher concluded that the difference is a true difference, there would be 10 chances in 100 that his conclusion would be wrong. Based on the researcher's chosen level of significance decision point ($p \leq .05$), this is too high a chance of being wrong so the researcher would conclude the two methods of comforting are essentially equivalent, i.e., a difference in effectiveness is doubtful, the difference found is not significant.

In summary, a difference in means associated with a low p-value (i.e., a data-based p-value that is below the decision-point p-level) is considered statistically significant; it is a true difference in treatment effectiveness, and a difference is likely to exist in the population as well. A difference with a high p-value (i.e., a data-based p-value that is above the decision-point p-level) is considered to be a not significant finding, meaning it very well may be a chance difference.

The level of significance at which a probability is considered low is often, but not always, set at $p \leq .05$. By setting the decision-point p-level at .05, a researcher is saying, "I am willing to accept up to 5 chances in 100 that I am wrong when I conclude that the difference found was not caused by chance." Said differently, by setting the decision-point for significance at the .05 level, the researcher is of the opinion that 5 or fewer chances in 100 of being wrong in calling the difference a true difference is an acceptable risk; more than 5 chances would make the risk of a wrong conclusion too great. This interpretation of p-values using a .05 decision-point for an acceptable level of significance is graphically displayed in Figure 7–2.

In study reports, the statistics just described are reported in a variety of ways. The absolute difference between the mean outcomes of the two groups may or may not be stated, but it can be easily calculated by subtracting the mean of one group from the mean of the other. The t-value may or may not be reported, but in-and-of itself it is not of importance to the clinical reader. However, the p-value associated with a t-test or an indication of whether the difference is statistically significant will almost always be provided in the text or in a table. The examples in Box 7–1 illustrate interpretations of p-values as they are expressed in research articles. The first example provides a p-value associated with a difference in means (i.e., a t-test), and the second provides a p-value associated with a difference in proportions (%s).

Borderline Results   So far, the decision regarding statistical significance has been portrayed as a cut-point decision. In reality, researchers some-

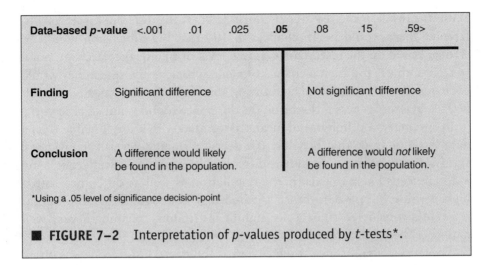

| Data-based *p*-value | <.001 | .01 | .025 | **.05** | .08 | .15 | .59> |

| **Finding** | Significant difference | | Not significant difference |

| **Conclusion** | A difference would likely be found in the population. | | A difference would *not* likely be found in the population. |

*Using a .05 level of significance decision-point

■ **FIGURE 7–2**   Interpretation of *p*-values produced by *t*-tests*.

Box 7–1   EXAMPLES OF *p*-VALUE INTERPRETATIONS

1. The effectiveness of a topical anesthetic in reducing the pain of subcutaneous measles–mumps–rubella vaccination in 1-year-old infants was studied in a double-blind, randomized, placebo-controlled trial (O'Brien, Taddio, Ipp, Goldbach, & Koren, 2004). The infants' pain levels were measured before the injection and after the injection; a high difference score from pre- to postinjection indicated more pain after the injection. Based on mean pre- to postinjection pain difference scores of 2.3 for the placebo group and 1.5 for the topical anesthesia group (*p* = .029), the researchers concluded that the topical anesthesia reduced the pain of vaccination. However, there is about a 3% chance that they are wrong in this conclusion, which is low enough that they are confident about their conclusion.

2. In a randomized controlled study evaluating the effects of a sliding-scale diuretic titration protocol for patients with heart failure in comparison to the usual method of set diuretic dosing, "There were significantly less ED visits in the diuretic titration group compared with the usual care group (3% vs 23%, *p* = .015)" (Prasun, Kocheril, Klass, Dunlap, & Piano, 2005). The researchers concluded that on average the diuretic titration protocol resulted in fewer ED visits because there is only between 1 and 2 chances in 100 that a 20% difference could have resulted from chance variation in sample groups. In other words, there is only a 1% to 2% chance that their conclusion that the titration method was more effective in reducing ED visits could be wrong.

times describe a result as being "highly significant" meaning that the data-based p-value was very small (e.g., $p = .001$). There is only one chance in a thousand that this is a chance difference and that the conclusion that there is a true difference is wrong. In contrast, when the data-based p-value is just slightly larger than the decision-point p-level (e.g., .06), researchers may say that the result was "marginally significant" or "approached significance" (Huck, 2007). This conveys that the difference was almost large enough to be considered a true difference result. Reporting marginal results is justified when the study is the first test of an intervention because it may indicate a promising intervention that warrants another study.

To recap issues pertaining to statistical significance, if the statistical result is significant (e.g., $p \leq .05$), researchers usually conclude that the cause of the difference is a result of the fact that one group received a more effective intervention than the other group did and that the effect is likely to hold up in the population as well. This conclusion is justified when all other factors that could have caused a difference were controlled in some way (i.e., in well-designed studies). If the data-based p-value is not significant ($p \geq .05$), researchers conclude that the difference between means is just chance variation, and the effect of the test intervention over the comparison intervention is so small that it is unlikely to represent a real effect that would exist in the population. They so conclude because there is a high probability that the difference found between them is just expected variation from one sample to another. This conclusion is justified when the study was well designed and the sample size was large enough to detect a difference.

Did I lose you in the last six to eight pages? If so, you need to go back to your statistics book and read about hypothesis testing and p-values. Even then, the concept may be less than clear to you—it is a tough topic. I offer the observation that the meaning of p-values will become clearer as you read more study reports. You will, however, have to pay attention to the p-values provided in reports and note how the researchers interpret them. This way, your understanding of them will increase over time. Understanding the meaning of p-values is crucial to understanding reports of quantitative studies. It is a concept that you must master.

Both Perspectives

Having explained both the clinical perspective and the statistical perspective on study results, I want to point out that statistical significance and clinical significance do not necessarily equate; rather, their relationship can take different forms:

1. The difference between the outcomes of the two treatment groups can be *clinically significant* and *statistically significant.* This would occur when the difference between means is large—of course, large is relative to the nature of the outcome being studied and to the scale used to measure it.

2. The difference can be *clinically not significant* and *statistically not significant.* This would occur when the difference between the means of the two groups is very small.

3. The difference between the two group means can be *clinically significant* but *statistically not significant.* This occurs most frequently in studies with small sample sizes, which are common in nursing. The clinician sees promise in the results, even though statistically they could be due to chance, and is of the opinion that the intervention needs to be studied with a larger sample.

4. The difference between two group means can be *clinically not significant* but *statistically significant*; that is, from a practical clinical perspective it is trivial or unimportant. Statistically significant but clinically not significant results occur most frequently in studies with very large sample sizes.

Possible Result Combinations

- Clinically Significant and Statistically Significant (CS-SS)
- Clinically Not Significant and Statistically Not Significant (cs-ss)
- Clinically Significant and Statistically Not Significant (CS-ss)
- Clinically Not Significant and Statistically Significant (cs-SS)

To illustrate some of the points made so far in this chapter, consider the results of a fictional randomized study comparing a new weight loss program to a program that has been around for a while (see Table 7–2).

First, note that the mean difference in weight lost by the two groups is not large (2.4 pounds). This difference is statistically significant, but is it

Table 7–2 WEIGHT LOSS EXAMPLE		
	NEW PROGRAM GROUP *n* = 50	OLD PROGRAM GROUP *n* = 50
Mean lb lost at 6 months	13 lbs (sd = 4.9)	10.6 lbs (5.3)
Difference in the two means = 2.4 lbs		
95% CI of the difference: 0.37 to 4.4 lbs *t*-test *p*-value: 0.02		
% achieved a 10 lb loss or more ABI = 20%	52%	30%
ABI = 22%		
NNT = 5 (1 ÷ .22 = 4.5 rounded up)		

clinically significant? The ABI and the NNT are more impressive than the mean difference. Based on the ABI and NNT for weight loss of 10 pounds or more, I am inclined to say that the new program achieves a weight loss that is clinically significant for more people than what the old program achieves. However, this is an opinion and others may look at the numbers and say that the effectiveness of the two programs is not different enough to make a meaningful change in weight over time. Ultimately, this call must be made with the details of the full report and within the context of participants' feelings about the demands and expense of the two programs.

In many nursing studies, consideration of the clinical significance of the difference between outcomes is as important, if not more important, than consideration of whether the results are statistically significant. Unfortunately, the size of the clinical impact of the test intervention is not always discussed in a useful way in reports of nursing intervention studies—even though it should be. Once again, I would advise you not to obsess over the statistical results in a report; rather, think about the size of the difference between the outcomes of the two groups from a clinical perspective before moving on to thinking about them from the statistical perspective.

Opinion Regarding Reporting of Outcomes

I would note that dichotomous clinical outcomes and their associated measures of effectiveness, ABI and NNT, are widely reported in the medical research literature but not as much in the nursing literature. Hopefully, reporting dichotomous clinical outcomes will increase in nursing research because they are often more relevant for clinicians than are mean scores on a test or scale. This is so because attainment of clinical outcomes and milestones are often important to patients—and memorable for clinicians. In contrast, mean scores on a scale or test are often indirect measures of outcomes important to patients and clinicians. I personally find that the reporting achievement of dichotomous patient outcomes adds clarity and clinical relevance to study reports.

Consider a fictional study in persons facing a risky medical procedure who were taught different ways of controlling anxiety in the days prior to the procedure; anxiety was measured on each of the three days before the procedure using a scale in which a low score indicated low anxiety and a high score indicated high anxiety. If the results reveal that the group taught method A had a mean anxiety score of 3 and group taught method B had a mean anxiety score of 7, we could say that clearly method A produced better anxiety prevention/relief, but we don't get a practical sense of how using method A actually improved patients' experiences of anxiety. In contrast, if the results were reported as 11% of the persons in group A reported enough anxiety that it interfered with their sleep during one of the three nights before surgery and 24% of those in group B reported sleep disturbance during those nights, the difference in treatment effectiveness has immediate clinical relevance.

Exemplar

You should now reread the Introduction and Methods sections in the exemplar (Pellegrini et al., 2009) and then carefully read the Results and the Discussion sections. The Profile & Commentary that follow will focus on the results.

Profile & Commentary: Results and Discussion

WHAT *Results*

The Results section starts with a description of the sample, which has already been discussed in the commentary on methods.

Incidence of PONV   In Table 2 we see that the in-hospital incidences of nausea in the IPA and promethazine groups (17% versus 23% in PACU and 42% versus 23% in SDSU) was not statistically different, whereas the at-home incidence of nausea events was higher in the IPA group (45% versus 23%). Note that this home difference was statistically different at the p = .019 level. The superscript a beside the p-value conveys this statistical significance by indicating that there are fewer than 5 chances in 100 that this difference is just due to chance.

Can you think of a reason why the incidence of nausea was higher at home in the IPA group than it was in the promethazine group? The reason that seems most likely to me is that IPA inhalation is shorter acting than is promethazine. Patients in the promethazine group may still have been getting benefits from the promethazine they received in the hospital.

In looking at Figure 1, focus on comparing the heights of the two bars in each setting. Doing so shows that in all three settings the VNRS scores at the time of the initial complaint of nausea were higher in the IPA group than the scores of the promethazine group. Although the bars make the differences look big, statistically they were not large enough to be considered a true difference, as stated in the text. In other words, these differences in all three settings are within what would be considered a normal variation around a mean common to both. (The lines with T endings are standard deviations; they provide a sense of how dispersed the scores were. We will not consider them.)

Comparative Effectiveness of the Treatments   In the text and from Figure 2, we learn that the time to a 50% reduction in the VNRS scores after the treatments was shorter for the IPA patients in all settings. For example, in the PACU a 50% reduction was achieved in approximately 8 minutes with IPA versus 20 minutes for the promethazine patients. You should think about whether or not you consider this a *clinically* significant difference. Would it be a benefit patients would value? Statistically, this difference was significant in all settings, as indicated by the p-values in the text and the asterisks in Figure 2; thus, the difference found in time to a 50% reduction in the VNRS is most likely not a chance result.

In the text we learn that vomiting (emetic events) were similar in both groups in all settings. So too were the median satisfaction with nausea control scores of the two groups. The report also informs us that no patients in the IPA group reported untoward side effects, whereas patients in the promethazine group did. Note how some results are found in both the tables and figures and the text, whereas other results are reported just in the text.

Dichotomous Outcome Although it is not addressed in the report, I was interested in knowing how effective IPA was in *avoiding* promethazine while in hospital; taking or not taking promethazine is a dichotomous outcome. To get at this I first needed to know the number of persons in each group who became nauseated and the number in each group who received promethazine. The number in each group who became nauseated is given in the article (32 in the IPA group and 26 in the promethazine group). I also knew that all the people in the promethazine group who became nauseated got the drug, according to the study protocol. The only missing piece was how many people in the IPA group who experienced nausea eventually had to be given promethazine. So I e-mailed the lead author, Pellegrini, who kindly responded with that information: 6 of the 32 persons in the IPA group who experienced nausea eventually required promethazine.

Now, to get at the outcome of interest (i.e., not requiring promethazine), I first determined the proportion in each group who experienced nausea but never had to take promethazine. That let me calculate the ABI and NNT for the benefit of IPA in achieving the outcome of not having to take promethazine at all. The calculation of the absolute benefit (AB) for both groups, the ABI achieved with IPA, and its NNT is as follows:

1. The number of persons in the IPA group who became nauseated and did *not* require promethazine was 26 (32 minus 6); in the promethazine group, the number who became nauseated and did *not* get the drug was 0 (26 minus 26).
2. 81% of the IPA group who experienced nausea did not get promethazine (26 ÷ 32), so the AB of IPA was .81. In contrast, 0% of the promethazine group who experienced nausea did not get the drug, therefore the AB of promethazine was 0 (0 ÷ 26).
3. The absolute benefit increase (ABI) for IPA over promethazine was 0.81 (0.81 minus 0).
4. The NNT for IPA inhalation for the benefit of not requiring promethazine is $1 \div 0.81 = 1.23$; this rounded up to an NNT of two persons.

This NNT means that just two persons would have to be treated with IPA as the first line of treatment in hospital for PONV instead of giving promethazine as the first line of treatment to achieve one patient not having to receive promethazine at all. Thus, IPA inhalation has a strong clinical benefit in avoiding another drug at a time when patients already have several medications active in their body. Do you think this is a clinically significant result?

It may take you a couple of times through this calculation to get your head around NNT, but it is not higher mathematics. It involves some reasoning and simple subtraction and division. I think the perspective on clinical effect that is gained from the calculation is worth the effort because NNT provides a real-world sense of the benefit of one treatment vis-à-vis another in terms of an actual clinical event occurring or not occurring.

Discussion

The section starts with a discussion about how the number of risk factors a person has increases their probability of PONV. They note that ondansetron, which is given in the operating room as the surgery is coming to a close to prevent postoperative nausea, is not as effective as expected with high-risk patients.

Limitations of the study are noted, particularly the reluctance of patients to self-administer a promethazine suppository at home. The researchers clearly have an interest in conducting future research to determine if IPA is effective in combination with ondansetron in preventing PONV. They conclude that the findings of the current study show that IPA inhalation is as effective as promethazine in treating breakthrough PONV in patients who are at high risk for PONV and have received ondansetron; they further note that it works faster and is easier to administer than promethazine.

The results of this study add to the knowledge about IPA effectiveness by focusing on patients who are at high risk for PONV. It is a good example of the methods of experimental design.

REFERENCES

Burns, N., & Grove, S. K. (2009). *Practice of nursing research: Conduct, critique, and utilization* (5th ed.). St. Louis, MO: Elsevier Saunders.

Conn, V. (2007). Personal communication. In H. A. DeVon, M. E. Block, P. Moyle-Wright, D. M. Ernst, S. J. Hayden, D. J. Lazzara, et al. (Eds.), A psychometric toolbox for testing validity and reliability. *Journal of Nursing Scholarship*, 39(2), 155–164.

Duffy, M. E., & Jacobsen, B. S. (2001). Univariate descriptive statistics. In B. Hazard Munro (Ed.), *Statistical methods for health care research* (4th ed., pp. 29–62). Philadelphia, PA: Lippincott.

Huck, S. W. (2007). *Reading statistics and research* (5th ed.). Boston, MA: Pearson.

Kerlinger, F. N., & Lee, H. B. (2000). *Foundations of behavioral research* (4th ed.). Fort Worth, TX: Harcourt College.

O'Brien, L., Taddio, A., Ipp, M., Goldbach, M., & Koren, G. (2004). Topical 4% amethocaine gel reduces the pain of subcutaneous measles-mumps-rubella vaccination. *Pediatrics, 114*(6), e720–e724.

Pellegrini, J., DeLoge, J., Bennett, J., & Kelly, J. (2009). Comparison of inhalation of isopropyl alcohol vs. promethazine in the treatment of postoperative nausea and vomiting (PONV) in patients identified as at high risk for developing PONV. *AANA Journal, 77*(4), 293–299.

Polit, D. F., & Beck, C. T. (2004). *Nursing research: Principles and methods* (7th ed.). Philadelphia, PA: Lippincott Williams & Wilkins.

Prasun, M. A., Kocheril, A. G., Klass, P. H., Dunlap, S. H., & Piano, M. R. (2005). The effects of a sliding scale diuretic titration protocol in patients with heart failure. *Journal of Cardiovascular Nursing, 20*(1), 62–70.

Sackett, D. L., Straus, S. E., Richardson, W. S., Rosenberg, W., & Haynes, R. B. (2000). *Evidence-based medicine: How to practice and teach EBM.* Edinburgh, Scotland: Churchill Livingstone.

OTHER EXPERIMENTAL AND QUASI-EXPERIMENTAL STUDIES

Bakitas, M., Lyons, K. D., Hegel, M. T., Balan, S., Brokaw, F. C., Seville, J., et al. (2009). Effects of a palliative care intervention on clinical outcomes in patients with advanced cancer: The project ENABLE II randomized controlled trial. *JAMA, 302*(7), 741–749.

Brown, S. J., & Schoenly, L. (2004). Test of an educational intervention for osteoporosis prevention with U.S. adolescents. *Orthopaedic Nursing, 23*(4), 245–251.

Bryanton, J., Walsh, D., Barrett, M., & Gaudent, D. (2004). Tub bathing versus traditional sponge bathing for the newborn. *Journal of Obstetric, Gynecological, and Neonatal Nursing, 33*(6), 704–712.

Burke, C. N., Voepel-Lewis, T., Hadden, S., DeGrandis, M., Skotcher, S., D'Agostino, R., et al. (2009). Parental presence on emergence: Effect on postanesthesia agitation and parent satisfaction. *Journal of PeriAnesthesia Nursing, 24*(4), 216–221.

Fink, R. M., Hjort, E., Wenger, B., Cook, P. F., Cunningham, M., Orf, A., et al. (2009). The impact of dry versus moist heat on peripheral IV catheter insertion in a hematology-oncology outpatient population. *Oncology Nursing Forum, 36*(4), E198–E204.

Harrison, M. B., Graham, I. D., Lorimer, K., VandenKerkhof, E., Buchann, M., Wells, P. S., et al. (2008). Nurse clinic versus home delivery of evidence-based community leg ulcer care: A randomized health services trial. *BMC Health Services Research, 8,* 243–254. Retrieved from http://www.biomedcentral.com/1472-6963/8/243

Lautrette, A., Darmon M, Megarbane B, Joly LM, Chevret S, Adrie C, et al. (2007). A communication strategy and brochure for relatives of patients dying in the ICU. *New England Journal of Medicine, 356*(5), 469–478.

CHAPTER EIGHT
Cohort Research

Studying the cause-effect relationship between risk factors and health outcomes presents unique challenges. Random assignment of participants to a risk factor exposure that could result in disease or a poor health outcome ethically is not an option. Thus, cohort studies evolved as a way of studying risk factors associated with heredity, environment, behavior, a particular life experience, or a medical treatment. For instance, a cohort design could be used to study the long-term health effects of elderly persons who were mugged.

Cohort Studies

Design

In a **cohort study**, a sample is drawn from a larger population and classified into two distinct groups: those with the risk factor and those without it. The two groups, called cohorts, are followed over an appropriate length of time to determine how often the outcomes of interest occur in both groups. Cohort studies are like experiments in that they involve comparison of outcomes in contrasting groups of a specified population; however, they are unlike experiments in that the contrasting groups are not created by random assignment. Rather, the groups are formed based on whether or not they have had exposure to a particular risk factor. Typically, the cohorts are identified before the outcomes of interest develop and then followed to determine the rates at which the outcomes occur. A 2 × 2 matrix, which is used to portray the results of cohort a study, is helpful in understanding the logic of cohort design

(Table 8–1). The first division of the sample is into the exposed or not exposed group. Later, when the outcome is measured, everyone in the sample is classified into one of the four groups (a, b, c, or d), which becomes the basis for the analysis of the data.

Cohort studies often use information in health system databases to reconstruct the presence of a risk factor at a point in time or over time and the subsequent development of a particular outcome. A cohort study looked at adverse drug reactions among frail elderly persons after discharge from hospital (Hanlon et al., 2006). Data was collected from patients' healthcare records regarding various risk factors for adverse drug reactions, and patients were followed to determine those who experienced an adverse drug reaction. The main finding was that the number of medications the patient took and the use of the drug warfarin increased the risk of adverse drug events.

Confounding

The major concern in cohort studies is that the two groups could be different in some way other than the presence or absence of the risk factor, and that difference may produce different outcomes for the two groups. For instance, they may have different biophysical characteristics, lifestyles, or experiences. The difference could be something as easy to identify as an age difference or something as buried as different levels of nutrition during youth. If the difference is a determinant of the outcomes being studied and is unequally distributed in the two groups, it is called a confounding variable, or a confounder (Mamdani et al., 2005). Recognizing confounders in advance of doing a

Table 8–1 LOGIC OF A COHORT STUDY

		ADVERSE OUTCOME		
		PRESENT	ABSENT	TOTALS
Exposed to	Yes	a	b	a + b
Risk Factor	No	c	d	c + d
Totals		a + c	b + d	

Exposed Cohort
  a = exposed to risk factor and develop adverse outcome
  b = exposed to risk factor but do not develop adverse outcome
Unexposed Cohort
  c = not exposed to risk factor but develop adverse outcome
  d = not exposed to risk factor and do not develop adverse outcome

study allows researchers to collect data about them and run analyses to check on their influence on the outcome variables. Even when the analysis has ruled out suspected confounders, cohort studies are still vulnerable to unknown confounders. Thus, when reading cohort studies, you must think about whether a confounder other than those considered by the researcher might exist, because it could have had an independent effect on the outcomes, apart from the effect of the risk factor of interest. In the study you will read in this chapter, you will learn about the techniques researchers can take to rule out confounding.

Other Limitations

Cohort studies that follow participants for long periods of time often suffer from high dropout rates. High dropout rates can bias the incidence of the outcome in either or both groups, thus confounding the results. Another limitation of cohort design is that it does not work well if the outcome being studied occurs rarely. A rare outcome would require following a very large number of people to detect a connection between the risk factor and the outcome. Therefore, when the outcome being studied is rare, researchers may use another design, case-control design.

Case-Control Studies

In a sense, a **case-control study** is the opposite of a cohort study. Remember: A cohort study starts by identifying cohorts of persons and then follows them forward to determine if they develop certain outcomes. In contrast, a case-control study starts by identifying persons with and without a particular outcome, for example, a disease, and then looks backward in their history to identify how the two groups were different in regard to suspected causes of the outcome. See Figure 8–1.

Generally, cohort studies are used to study exposures and outcomes that occur rather frequently and outcomes that develop or occur not too long after the risk factor or exposure, whereas case-control studies are used to study outcomes that are rare or take a long time to become evident (e.g., osteoporosis fracture, lung cancer). Case-control studies are even more prone to confounding by unknown factors than are cohort studies. They are highly prone to confounding because the study involves looking back in time and important data may not be available or may be forgotten or distorted by memory.

A case-control study was conducted to determine the association between unplanned extubations in a pediatric intensive care unit and several patient, staffing, and care variables (Marcin, Rutan, Rapetti, Rahnsmayi, & Pretzlaff, 2005). Patients with unplanned extubations were identified, then controls

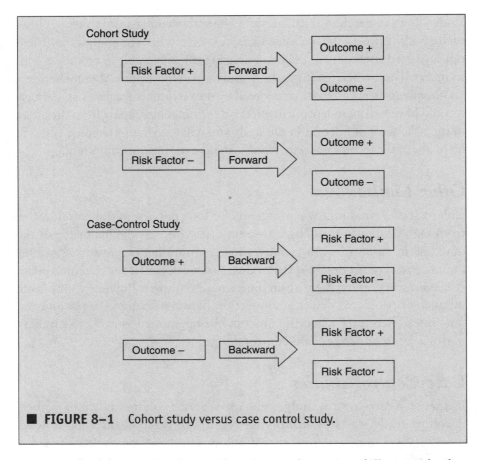

■ FIGURE 8–1   Cohort study versus case control study.

were matched for age, intubation duration, and severity of illness. Fifty-five patients experienced unplanned extubations during the four-year period of the study; they were matched with 165 patients who did not experience the event. Then, looking back at data from the patients' time in ICU, they determined that nurse-to-patient assignment ratios of 1:2 were associated with unplanned extubations, whereas nurses' years of experience in pediatric intensive care nursing, patient restraints, and method of sedation delivery were not associated. Thus, by looking back after the event at four possible risk factors, this case-control study identified one that put patients at risk.

Wrap-Up

Cohort studies provide a way of evaluating risk factors for health conditions or events; they do so by comparing groups with and without exposure to a pre-identified risk factor or factors. Because random assignment is not used to form the comparison groups, cohort studies are prone to confounding, which threatens the validity of study conclusions about the relationship between the risk factor and the outcome of interest. However, cohort studies do provide control over follow-up and diagnosis of the outcome. An alternative design that is used to study risk factors when the outcome of interest is rare is the case-control study, but this design has even greater potential for confounding.

Exemplar

📖 *Reading Tips*

The big phrase in the title of this article, *hemicallotasis technique*, is an orthopaedic surgical procedure performed to straighten knees deformed by arthritis. For our purposes, the exact nature of the surgery is not important except to note that metal pins are inserted into the bone and remain in place until the realigned bones fuse (see Figure 8–2). The pins go into the bone, but the ends remain outside the skin where they are attached to a rigid external frame, which is what provides the immobilization. The pin tract is a potential site for infection.

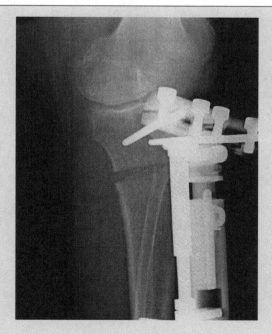

■ **FIGURE 8–2**   Radiograph of high tibial osteotomy.

Source: W-Dahl, A., Toksvig-Larsen, S., & Roos, E. M. (2009). Association between knee alignment and knee pain in patients surgically treated for medial knee osteoarthritis by high tibial osteotomy. A one year follow-up study. *BMC Musculoskeletal Disorders 2009, 10,* 154. doi:10.1186/1471-2474-10-154.

Cigarette Smoking Delays Bone Healing: A Prospective Study of 200 Patients Operated On by the Hemicallotasis Technique

Annette W-Dahl and Soren Toksvig-Larsen

Acta Orthopaedica Scandinavica (2008), 75(3), 347–351.

Department of Orthopedias. University Hospital. Lund. Sweden
Correspondence AWD: anette.w-dahl@ort.lu.se
Submitted 03–04–26. Accepted 03–10–14

Background: Cigarette smoking is known to impede bone healing. The hemicallotasis technique is based on an external fixation and delayed healing prolongs treatment and increases the risk of further complications.

Patients and methods: 200 patients, 34 smokers and 166 nonsmokers, operated on by the hemicallotasis technique in the proximal tibia for deformities of the knee (knee arthrosis in 186 patients) were consecutively studied. We recorded their preoperative smoking habits, postoperative complications and the duration of treatment with external fixation.

Results: Half of the smokers and one fifth of the nonsmokers developed complications. Their mean time in external fixation was 96 (SD 20) days. Smokers required an average of 16 days more in external fixation. Delayed healing and pseudoarthrosis were commoner in smokers than nonsmokers. The risk ratio for smokers to develop complications was 2.5, as compared to nonsmokers.

Tibia osteotomy by the hemicallotasis technique (HCO) is based on external fixation. Delayed healing and nonunion prolong the treatment and increase the risk of further complications.

Studies on rabbits have shown delayed bone healing and decreases in bone mineral density (BMD) and strength in the lengthened tibia caused by cigarette smoking (Ueng et al. 1997, 1999). Smoking was the single most important risk factor for the development of serious postoperative complications after elective arthroplasty of the hip and knee (Moeller et al. 2003).

We studied whether smokers had longer healing times and more complications than nonsmokers who underwent HCO.

Methods

Patients

In a prospective study 200 consecutive patients (119 men), mean age 53 (18–75) years, were operated on by HCO for knee deformities (Tables 1–2).

Table 1   PATIENT CHARACTERISTICS OF THE STUDY GROUP

	NONSMOKERS $n = 166$	SMOKERS $n = 34$
Gender		
Men	102 (61)	17 (50)
Women	64 (39)	17 (50)
Age		
Mean	53	53
SD	10	6
< 50	47 (28)	9 (26)
50–59	77 (46)	22 (65)
60+	42 (25)	3 (9)
Preop HKA-angle in medial cases		
Mean	170°	170°
SD	5°	4°
≤ 189°	17 (11)	2 (3)
> 190°	5 (5)	3 (12)
BMI		
< 25	25 (16)	12 (35)
25–29	77 (48)	13 (38)
30+	58 (36)	9 (27)

Percentages within parentheses
Preop HKA-angle = Preoperative hip-knee-ankle-angle
BMI = Body mass index

Table 2   INDICATION FOR SURGERY IN 200 PATIENTS WHO UNDERWENT HCO

	ALL n = 200	NONSMOKERS/SMOKERS n = 166/34
Knee osteoarthrosis	186	153/32
Medial	163	134/29
Lateral	20	15/5
Pre[a]	2	2/0
Fracture sequelae	8	6/2
Knee deformity	4	4/0
Osteonecrosis	1	1/0
Sequelae of tibia osteotomy	1	1/0

[a]Arthroscopic osteoarthrosis with symptoms but no osteoarthrosis, according to radiographic Ahlback grade I.

The patients' smoking habits (smoker or nonsmoker) were noted preoperatively.

They were called nonsmoker if, at the preoperative examination, they stated that they had never smoked or had stopped smoking more than 6 months previously. Thirty-four (17%) were smokers and 166 (83%) nonsmokers. Seven patients underwent simultaneous bilateral surgery (1 smoker and 6 nonsmokers).

Hemicallotasis Osteotomy

Four conical pins were inserted, 2 hydroxyapatite-coated in the metaphyseal bone and 2 standard pins (Orthofix®, Bussolengo, Italy) in the diaphyseal bone. The Orthofix® T-garche was used. The patients were allowed free mobilization and full weight bearing after the operation.

The distraction started 7–10 days postoperatively. Eight weeks after surgery, the fixation was dynamised to stimulate healing of the bone. The first evaluation of bone healing was done 12 weeks postoperatively. If healing of the osteotomy was deemed satisfactory on both the radiographic and ultrasound examinations, the patient did a weight-bearing test—i.e., walked for a few hours or even some days without the instrument, but with the pins in situ. If no symptoms developed, the pins were removed in the outpatient clinic, but if the patient developed symptoms, the T-garche was applied again for 2–4 weeks.

Outcome

We recorded the duration of external fixation (from surgery until the external pins were removed) and the complications, such as delayed healing (> 16 weeks in external fixation), pseudoarthrosis, septic arthritis, deep venous thrombosis, nerves injury, and interrupted treatment (i.e., loose pins due to a pin site infection).

Statistics

The analysis of variance (ANOVA) test, t-test and Chi-square test were used for the statistical analysis, and the statistical significance was set at $p < 0.05$. A multiple logistic regression analysis (checked for potential confounder) was used to estimate the odds ratio (OR) of complications, delayed healing and pseudoarthrosis.

The study was approved by the Ethics Committee, Lund University, Sweden.

Results

More complications occurred among the smokers than the nonsmokers. Fifty-one patients had one or more complications (delayed healing, pseudoarthrosis, septic arthritis, deep venous thrombosis, nerves injury or interrupted treatment) (34/166 (Table 3) nonsmokers and 17/34 smokers, $p < 0.001$). 12/51 patients had 2 or more complications (7 nonsmokers and 5 smokers, $p = 0.02$). The risk ratio for the smokers who developed complications, as compared to the nonsmokers, was 2.5 (95% CI 1.5–3.9).

Table 3 COMPLICATIONS IN 200 PATIENTS OPERATED ON BY HCO

			RELATIVE RISK	
	NONSMOKERS $n = 166$	SMOKERS $n = 34$	(RR)	(95% CI)[a]
Delayed healing[b]	25	14	2.7	(1.5–4.7)
Pseudoarthrosis	3	5	8.1	(1.8–42)
Septic arthritis	2	1	2.4	(0.1–34)
Deep venous thrombosis	3	2	3.3	(0.4–23)
Nerve injury	1	0	0	(1.0–84)
Interrupted treatment	3	1	1.6	(0.1–17)

[a](95% CI) = 85% confidence interval.
[b]Includes 5 patients who developed pseudoarthrosis after removal of external fixation.

Delayed healing and pseudoarthrosis occurred more often among the smokers. The risk ratio for delayed healing was 2.7 (95% CI 1.5–4.7) in the smokers. Eight patients with delayed healing developed pseudoarthrosis. The risk ratio for smokers to develop pseudoarthrosis was 8.1 (95% CI 1.8–42.0) (Table 3). Six of the patients who developed pseudoarthrosis required additional surgery for healing (5 smokers and 1 nonsmoker) and 2 patients (nonsmokers) healed after low intensity ultrasound stimulation (Exogen®, Tuttlingen, Germany).

In the 3 patients who developed septic arthritis (2 nonsmokers and 1 smoker), the treatment was interrupted and in one patient (non-smoker), the treatment was interrupted due to loose pins. The mean time in external fixation was 96 (SD 20) days in all patients. The mean time in external fixation for nonsmokers was 94 (SD 18) days and 110 (SD 25.2) days for smokers (p < 0.001). The smokers had 16 days (p < 0.001, 95% CI 7.0–25) longer mean time in external fixation than the nonsmokers. In patients with a frame time > 112 days, the smokers had a mean of 17 days more (p = 0.004, 95% CI 5.5–26) in external fixation than the nonsmokers (Table 4). Among the 7 patients who underwent bilateral HCO in one séance, 3 patients had complications—i.e., 2 had delayed healing, 1 smoker and 1 nonsmoker. And 1 (nonsmoker), with osteonecrosis after treatment for leukemia, developed pseudoarthrosis (rapid loss of correction) in one of the osteotomies.

Table 4   FRAME TIME > 112 DAYS IN PATIENTS OPERATED ON BY HCO

	NONSMOKERS	SMOKERS	P-VALUE
Mean (days)	126	143	0.004
SD	13	16	
n	23	11	

The multivariate analysis, used to detect potential confounder, showed that cigarette smoking was the greatest preoperative risk factor for complications OR 5.1 (p = 0.001, 95% CI 2.2–12), delayed healing OR 4.0 (p = 0.004, 95% CI 1.7–9.5), and pseudoarthrosis OR 8.9 (p = 0.02, 95% CI 1.7–47.1) (Table 5).

Table 5   RELATIONSHIP OF RISK FACTORS TO COMPLICATIONS, DELAYED
HEALING AND PSEUDOARTHROSIS IN PATIENTS OPERATED ON BY HCO

	COMPLICATIONS ADJUSTED OR[a]	DELAYED HEALING ADJUSTED OR[a]	PSEUDOARTHROSIS ADJUSTED OR[a]
Gender			
Men[b]	1.0	1.0	1.0
Women	1.4 (0.7–2.9)	1.8 (0.8–4.1)	5.0 (0.8–31)
Age			
< 50[b]	1.0	1.0	1.0
50–59	0.9 (0.4–2.3)	1.0 (0.4–2.6)	0.5 (0.09–3.3)
60+	1.4 (0.5–3.9)	0.9 (0.3–3.0)	1.4 (0.2–12)
BMI			
< 25b	1.0	1.0	1.0
25–29	0.7 (0.3–1.8)	0.7 (0.3–2.1)	0.9 (0.1–6.0)
30+	1.2 (0.5–3.1)	1.1 (0.4–3.1)	0.5 (0.06–3.6)
Preop HKA-angle[c] medial/lateral			
> 171/< 189[b]	1.0	1.0	1.0
< 170/> 190	1.8 (0.9–3.7)	1.7 (0.8–3.8)	3.6 (0.6–21)
Smoking			
Nonsmokers[b]	1.0	1.0	1.0
Smokers	4.1 (1.8–3.7)	3.7 (1.5–8.9)	7.5 (1.4–41)

[a]Odds ratio (OR) adjusted simultaneously for all other risk factors listed and 95% confidence interval in parenthesis.
[b]Reference category.
[c]Hip-knee-ankle-angle preoperatively (varus or valgus).

Discussion

Smokers operated on by HCO for knee deformities needed a longer time in external fixation and had more complications, such as delayed healing and pseudoarthrosis than nonsmokers. Half of the smokers developed complications. The risk for the smokers developing complications was 2.5 times higher than in the nonsmokers.

A recent study by Moeller et al. (2003) on patients operated on for arthroplasty of the hip and knee confirmed our findings—i.e., smoking is the greatest risk factor for developing postoperative complications.

The number of smokers (34 of 200 patients) in our material is similar to the percentage of smokers in the Swedish population, 19% (18% men and 20% women) (Mackay and Eriksen 2002).

The mean time in external fixation in patients operated on by HCO has ranged from 79 to 91 days in various studies (Magyar et al. 1998, Klinger et al. 2001, Gerdhem et al. 2002), as compared to our 96 days. These differences may be due to the time when the first examination for healing was done, the methods used to assess healing, the experience in evaluating the healing on radiographs and perhaps the use of ultrasound. The size of the correction and whether bilateral osteotomies were done in one séance could also account for a longer treatment time. We found no differences between unilateral and bilateral osteotomies or the preoperative HKA-angle, as regards the longer healing time.

Cigarette smoking has been shown to cause slower healing and pseudoarthrosis in tibial fractures, both after closed (Kyro et al. 1993) and surgical treatments (Adams et al. 2001). In closed and grade I open tibial shaft fractures, Schmitz et al. (1999) found statistical differences in clinical and radiographic healing rates in smokers and nonsmokers in patients who underwent intramedullary or external fixation.

Cobb et al. (1994) reported that the relative risk of nonunion after ankle arthrodesis was 4 times higher in smokers. When patients had no known risk factors for nonunion, the risk of nonunion was 16 times higher in smokers.

Examination after a laminectomy and fusion showed more pseudo-arthrosis among smokers than nonsmokers (Brown et al. 1986). After ulna-shortening osteotomy, the smokers had longer healing times and nonunion than the nonsmokers. The mean union rates were 7 months in smokers and 4 months in nonsmokers (Chen et al. 2001). Our study of patients who underwent HCO can be added to the list of treatments showing that smoking is an important risk factor for the development of complications in orthopaedic surgery.

In a preoperative smoking intervention study, cessation of smoking from 6–8 weeks preoperatively and 10 days postoperatively reduced the postoperative complications in patients undergoing hip and knee replacement. The smoking cessation group was compared to one with an at least 50% reduction in smoking. The patients who reduced their smoking did not differ from the smoking group in other respects (Moeller et al. 2002). Patients undergoing arthroplasty of the hip and knee who smoked previously had a better short-term outcome than those who were smoking (Lavernia et al. 1999). Glassman et al. (2000) showed that the cessation of smoking after surgery helped to reverse the effects of cigarette smoking on the outcome of spinal fusion.

These studies indicate that smoking cessations both preoperatively and postoperatively decrease the risk for complications, whereas smoking reduction is not enough to decrease the risk.

The conclusions of the present study were that information about smoking cessations prior to surgery should be an important part of the preoperative information as well as cigarette smoking should be a factor to consider when selecting patients for callus distraction.

References

Adams C I, Keating J F, Court-Brown C M. Cigarette smoking and open tibial fractures. Injury 2001; 32 (1): 61–5.

Brown C W, Orme J T, Richardson H D. The rate of pseudoarthrosis (surgical nonunion) in patients who are smokers and patients who are non-smokers: a comparison study. Spine 1986; 11 (9): 942–3.

Chen F, Osterman A L, Mahony K. Smoking and bony union after ulna-shortening osteotomy. Am J Orthop 2001; 30 (6): 486–9.

Cobb T K, Gabrielsen T A, Campbell D C, Wallrichs S L, Ilstrup D M. Cigarette smoking and nonunion after ankle arthrodesis. Foot Ankle Int 1994; 15 (2): 64–7.

Gerdhem P, Abdon P, Odenbring S. Hemicallotasis for medial gonarthrosis: a short-term follow-up of 21 patients. Arch Orthop Trauma Surg 2002; 12 (3): 134–8.

Glassman S D, Anagnost C S, Parker A, Burke D, Johnson J R, Dimar J R. The effect of cigarette smoking and smoking cessation on spinal fusion. Spine 2000; 25 (20): 2608–14.

Klinger H M, Lorenz F, Harer T. Open wedge tibial osteotomy by hemicallotasis for medial compartment osteoarthritis. Arch Orthop Trauma Surg 2001; 121 (5): 247–7.

Kyro A, Usenius J P, Aarnio M, Kunnamo I, Avikainen V. Are smokers a risk group for delayed healing of tibial shaft fractures? Ann Chir Gynaecol 1993; 82 (4): 254–62.

Lavernia C J, Sierra R J, Gomez-Marin O. Smoking and joint replacement: resource consumption and short-term outcome. Clin Orthop 1999; (367): 172–80.

Mackay J, Eriksen M. The Tobacco Atlas. Myriad Edition Limited. Brighton 2002.

Magyar G, Toksvig-Larsen S, Lindstrand A. Open wedge tibial osteotomy by callus distraction in gonarthrosis. Operative technique and early results in 36 patients. Acta Orthop Scand 1998; 69 (2): 147–51.

Møller A M, Villebro N, Pedersen T, Tonnesen H. Effect of preoperative smoking intervention on postoperative complications: a randomised clinical trial. Lancet 2002; 359 (9301): 114–7.

Møller A M, Pedersen T, Villebro N, Munksgaard A. Effect of smoking on early complications after elective orthopaedic surgery. J Bone Joint Surg Br 2003; 85 (2): 178–81.

Schmitz M A, Finnegan M, Natarajan R, Champine J. Effect of smoking on tibial shaft fracture healing. Clin Orthop 1999; (365): 184–200.

Ueng S W, Lee M Y, Li A F, Lin S S, Tai C L, Shih C H. Effect of intermittent cigarette smoke inhalation on tibial lengthening: experimental study on rabbits. J Trauma 1997; 42 (2): 231–8.

Ueng S W, Lin S S, Wang C R, Liu S J, Tai C L, Shih C H. Bone healing of tibial lengthening is delayed by cigarette smoking: study of bone mineral density and torsional strength on rabbits. J Trauma 1999; 46 (1): 110–5.

Profile & Commentary

WHY *Study Purpose*

This study was conducted to determine if cigarette smokers and nonsmokers had the same rates of healing and complications after having an orthopaedic surgical procedure called tibial hemicallotasis osteotomy.

In brief, then:

- Population: Persons having this orthopaedic surgical procedure
- Risk cohorts: Smokers and nonsmokers—note the definition of smoker
- Outcome variables: Complications, delayed bone healing, infection, loose pins

HOW *Design*

The design of this study is a consecutive series, prospective cohort design. *Consecutive series* indicates that the sample was created by asking a series of patients who were having the surgical procedure to participate in the study. *Prospective* indicates that the participants were entered into the study and followed to determine how many developed complications after the surgery. In fact, this study design is the only way to compare complication rates in smokers and nonsmokers after surgery because random assignment to a smoking or not smoking group is not logistically possible.

Risk Factor of Interest

Prior research indicates that a history of recent smoking and current smoking slow, and in some cases prevent, bone healing after orthopaedic surgeries. This is the first study examining the effects of smoking with this particular procedure. Note that the definition of who was considered a non-smoker depended on the patient's report. Many cohort studies rely on patient reports regarding exposure to the risk factor, although some cohort studies use a very rigorously applied set of criteria to classify patients into one risk group or the other. I assume from the definition of nonsmoker that persons who were categorized as smokers preoperatively continued to smoke postoperatively—although this was not explicitly stated.

Sample

The target population was persons having a particular knee reconstruction procedure. The researchers obtained a sample of this population by studying 200 consecutive patients in one Swedish hospital. Enrolling consecutive patients is a reasonably unbiased way of obtaining a sample because it does not allow anyone on the research team to pick and choose who is in the study. In this study, consecutive enrollment of patients does not present any obvious concerns about the sample being different from persons who have the surgery at other times. The smokers cohort comprised 17% of the sample and the nonsmokers cohort made up the rest (83%).

Outcomes

Note how the outcomes were measured and the timing of the measurements. The outcome of time in external fixation was measured using an interval scale (days). Other outcomes (various complications) were measured as dichotomous outcomes, that is: The complication either occurred or didn't occur. The overall complication rate (one or more complications) was measured as well as the rate of each of six complications.

WHAT Results

In a cohort study, the first table often profiles the two cohorts as a first step in identifying potential confounders. Accordingly, Table 1 provides a profile of the smoker and nonsmoker groups with specifics about variables the researchers think could have an influence on the occurrence of complications. We note that there are differences between the composition of the two groups, particularly in terms of gender and proportion of persons over age 60. This raises a concern that perhaps these differences influenced the occurrence of complications and contributed to the differences found. At this point, the differences just send up a red flag and remind us to note whether the researchers deal with them during data analysis.

Dichotomous Outcomes   In the narrative, the researchers tell us that 20% of nonsmokers (34/166) and 50% of smokers (17/34) had one or more complications; thus, the absolute difference in the complication rates of the two groups is 30% (50% minus 20%). Further, the *p*-value associated with this difference indicates that this is a real difference, not a chance difference (*p* < .001). To provide additional clinical perspective on the risk of one or more complications, the risk for smokers to develop complications was compared to the risk for nonsmokers. This was reported as relative risk (RR), which is the ratio between risk in the smoker group and risk in the nonsmoker group.[1] Because the risk of the smoker group was 50% and the risk of the nonsmoker group was 20%, the ratio was 50:20 = 2.5.

To understand the meaning of this RR, you need to know that an RR greater than 1.0 indicates the smoker group had a higher risk of the complication than did the nonsmoker group, whereas an RR of less than 1.0 would mean that the smoker group had a lower risk of complication than did the nonsmoker group. If the two groups had equal risk, the RR would be 1.0.

Thus, the RR = 2.5 for smokers having at least one complication means that the risk for smokers developing complications was 2.5 times higher than was the risk for nonsmokers.

Relative risk (RR) was also used in Table 3 to portray the risk of smokers in relation to nonsmokers for six poor outcomes. From this table, you can tell that being a smoker puts persons at much higher *relative risk* (8.1) of developing pseudoarthrosis and a lower level of *relative risk* of delayed healing (2.7). This means that the risk of smokers developing pseudoarthrosis was 8 times that of nonsmokers, and their risk of developing delayed healing was 2.7 times that of nonsmokers. When interpreting RR, the operative word is *relative*—glossing over it can easily lead to misinterpretations of RR.

---

[1]

$$\text{Risk} = \frac{\text{Number in the group who have the complication}}{\text{Total number in group}}$$

$$\text{Relative Risk} = \frac{\text{Risk of smoker group}}{\text{Risk of nonsmoker group}}$$

Table 8–2	COMPLICATION IN 200 PATIENTS OPERATED BY HCO			
OUTCOME	RISK NONSMOKERS $n = 166$	RISK SMOKERS $n = 34$	ABSOLUTE DIFFERENCE IN RISK	RELATIVE RISK
Delayed healing	25 (15%)	14 (41%)	26%	2.7
Pseudoarthrosis	3 (1.8%)	5 (14.6%)	12.8%	8.1

Source: Adapted from W-Dahl, A., & Toksvig-Larsen, S. (2004). Cigarette smoking delays bone healing: A prospective study of 200 patients operated on by the hemicallotasis technique. Acta Orthopaedica Scandinvavica, 75(3), 347–351.

RR allows a comparison of smokers' relative risks for several outcomes. Comparing smokers' RRs for delayed healing (2.7 and pseudoarthrosis (8.1) tells us that being a smoker increases the risk of pseudoarthrosis more than it increases the risk of delayed healing (note the relative word *more*). When looking at smokers' RRs for delayed healing and pseudoarthrosis, *do not* make the mistake of interpreting it to mean that smokers are at a higher risk of pseudoarthrosis than they are of delayed healing. Because this can be confusing, I like to see the absolute rates and the RRs together, so I did my own fiddling with Table 3 (see Table 8–2). This display reminds me that the absolute risk rate of a complication in a group and its relative rate when compared to another group are quite different takes on the data.

That explanation may have been difficult to grasp and RRs can be misleading if you don't work with them frequently. My thinking regarding RR is this: If you do not regularly read reports with RR statistics, don't worry about understanding all the implications of RR beyond knowing that it is a way of comparing the risk of two groups for an outcome. Rather, focus on the absolute difference in the risk rates of the two groups for each outcome. They make sense in a very straightforward way and are less likely to lead you to wrong conclusions than RRs are. If your clinical field requires that you read reports that use RR, then get a good source book and get a handle on just what RR means. As a starting point, I would recommend a short but clear article by Sheldon (2000).

Interval Level Outcomes   Switching to the analysis of days in external fixation, which is an interval level outcome, the mean days in external fixation for smokers and nonsmokers were compared. In the Results section, we learn that the difference between smokers' and nonsmokers' time in external fixation was 16 days (110 minus 94). From a clinical perspective, this is a clinically significant difference because it represents two fewer weeks of being in the fixation device. The *t*-test comparing the two means was statistically significant at the *p* < .001 level. This means that there is less than 1 chance in 1,000 that a difference as large as the one found could have occurred just by chance—a difference that is likely to exist in the larger population as well as in this sample.

Note in the text that the 95% **confidence interval (CI)** for the *difference* in days in external fixation is 7.0–25.0, which means that if this study were repeated 100 times with similar samples, the mean difference for 95 of the 100 studies could be between 7 and 25. This added information changes our take on the clinical meaning of the result a bit because it tells us that in the target population smokers could spend as much as 25 days or as few as 7 days more in external fixation than nonsmokers do. Unfortunately, this CI is rather wide (because the sample size of the study was not large); a wide CI provides a less precise estimate of what might actually occur in the population than does a narrow one.

If you do not understand confidence intervals, you should go back to your statistical text because you are likely to encounter them when reading research reports and SRs. They are of practical, clinical value because they provide estimates of the likely results that will be realized when applying the study's intervention in everyday practice.

Looking for Potential Confounders   The researchers were aware that smoking was not the only risk factor for complications and that the smoking and nonsmoking groups could be different in ways other than just their smoking status. And we remember that Table 1 revealed some of those differences, for example, greater percentage of women in the smoker group and greater percentage of people over age 60 years in the nonsmoker group. To more definitively address the possibility that differences between smokers and nonsmokers on these other risk factors could have influenced the occurrence of complications, the researchers ran a multiple logistic regression analysis.

The results, shown in Table 5, were reported using a statistic called odds ratio. First, let's consider the concept of odds and how it compares to risk. Odds of a complication are similar to risk of a complication but slightly different. A risk is the likelihood (i.e., probability) of something occurring in relation to the number of times it could have occurred. You roll a dice and are hoping to roll a five. There is one in six chances that you will get a five; thus, the risk of a five is 1 in 6, which is 0.17 when converted as a decimal. In contrast, odds are the chances of something occurring in relation to the chances of it not occurring; thus, the odds of rolling a five are 1 to 5 or .20.

The numerator is the same in both calculations, but the denominator is different (compare the formula below[2] to the one given earlier for risk).

Like relative risk, an odds ratio is a ratio, specifically the odds of a particular outcome occurring in a comparison group (the numerator) relative to the odds of it occurring in the reference group (the denominator). It is interpreted like relative risk (RR). An odds ratio of 1 means the two groups have the same odds of experiencing the particular outcome. For a further explanation of odds ratios, I again refer you to Sheldon (2000) and to the link provided in the Chapter 8 folder at the companion website for this book, which can be accessed at ⌐ **go.jblearning.com/brown**. Also note that odds ratios are appearing with increased frequency in the nursing literature.

An odds ratio (OR) is used instead of RR in some analyses for technical reasons. As a clinical reader, you are not expected to know when one or the other should be used. The researcher and the peer review team are responsible for getting this right. One other point is that an adjusted OR is an OR that takes into account the other variables in the analysis; the adjustment essentially holds the other variables constant while calculating the OR of each variable.

Getting back to the study results, in Table 5 we notice that the smokers were the only subgroup having an odds ratio (adjusted OR) significantly larger than 1.0; their confidence intervals were the only ones that did not include 1.0. Therefore, being a smoker is the only risk factor that determined whether each of the complications occurred. This analysis in essence ruled out the other risk factors as confounders, leaving smoking as the best explanation for why complications occurred at different rates in the smoker and nonsmoker groups.

I would add here that potential confounding influences could have been controlled by inclusion criteria that allowed into the study only persons who don't have a particular characteristic. So, in this study the researchers could have excluded people over age 60 if they thought that the smoking group might be older and that age would have a great influence on complications after surgery. This would have had the effect of reducing the number of people eligible for the study and would have produced findings that were

---

[2]
$$Odds = \frac{Number\ in\ group\ with\ complication}{Number\ in\ group\ without\ complication}$$

$$Odds\ Ratio = \frac{Odds\ of\ complication\ in\ smokers}{Odds\ of\ complication\ in\ nonsmokers}$$

less generalizable. Moreover, the results bear out that it was not necessary to exclude this group because the risk factor of age over 60 did not predict any of the three complications (all three 95% CIs include 1.0).

Discussion

Importantly, the researchers placed their findings in the context of other work that has been done on the subject and concluded that the findings of this study add to the list of studies showing that smoking is a risk factor for postoperative complications after orthopaedic surgery.

REFERENCES

Hanlon, J. T., Pieper, C. F., Hajjar, E. R., Sloane, R. J., Linblad, C. I., Ruby, C. M., & Schmader, K. E. (2006). Incidence and predictors of all preventable adverse drug reactions in frail elderly persons after hospital stay. *Journals of Gerontology. Series A, Biological Sciences and Medical Sciences, 61*(5), 511–515.

Mamdani, M., Skyora, K., Li, P., Normand, S. L., Streiner, D. L., Austin, P. C., Rochon, P. A., & Anderson, G. M. (2005). Reader's guide to critical appraisal of cohort studies: 2. Assessing potential for confounding. *British Medical Journal, 330,* 960–962.

Marcin, J. P., Rutan, E., Rapetti, P. M., Rahnsmayi, R., & Pretzlaff, R. K. (2005). Nurse staffing and unplanned extubation in the pediatric intensive care unit. *Pediatric Critical Care Medicine, 6*(3), 254–257.

Sheldon, T. (2000). Statistics for evidence-based nursing. *Evidence-Based Nursing, 3,* 4–6.

W-Dahl, A., & Toksvig-Larsen, S. (2004). Cigarette smoking delays bone healing: A prospective study of 200 patients operated on by the hemicallotasis technique. *Acta Orthopaedica Scandinavica, 75*(3), 347–351.

IN-DEPTH READING ABOUT COHORT STUDIES

Mamdani, M., Skyora, K., Li, P., Normand, S. L., Streiner, D. L., Austin, P. C., Rochon, P. A., & Anderson, G. M. (2005). Reader's guide to critical appraisal of cohort studies: 2. Assessing potential for confounding. *British Medical Journal, 330,* 960–962.

Montero-Odasso, M., Schapira, M., Soriano, E. R., Varela, M., Kaplan, R., Camera, L. A., & Mayorga, L. M. (2005). Gait velocity as a single predictor of adverse events in healthy seniors aged 75 years and older. *Journals of Gerontology. Series A, Biological Sciences and Medical Sciences, 60*(10), 1304–1309.

Rochone, P. A., Gurwitz, J. H., Skyora, K., Mamdani, M., Streiner, D. L., Garfinketl, S., et al. (2005). Reader's guide to critical appraisal of cohort studies: 1. Role and design. *British Medical Journal, 330,* 895–897.

CHAPTER NINE

Systematic Reviews

Once several, or many, studies have been conducted on an issue, clinicians or researchers will feel the need to pull together the findings of the various studies into one document so as to see the bigger picture. This pulling together has to be done systematically and carefully so as to not introduce bias into the conclusions. For that reason, the methods for conducting systematic reviews have been explicitly set forth by the healthcare disciplines. When done well, a systematic review helps clinicians and researchers identify what is known with certainty, what is tentatively known, and what the gaps in knowledge are regarding an issue.

Types of Systematic Reviews

The overarching goal of systematic reviews is to reach conclusions regarding specified issues by compiling and analyzing findings from several (or many) studies. There are three ways of accomplishing this: **integrative research reviews, meta-analysis,** and **metasynthesis** (Whittemore, 2005). Integrative research reviews are narrative summaries of past research in which the reviewer extracts findings from original studies, creates findings tables, and uses analytical reasoning to produce conclusions about the findings of a body of research. The meta-analysis method of summarizing research findings uses statistical techniques to combine the results of studies from several or many intervention studies. This statistical combining can often reveal intervention effectiveness that was not detectable in smaller, original studies. A metasynthesis combines results or findings from several or many qualitative studies.

Meta-analyses and metasyntheses are appearing with increased frequency in the nursing literature. However, for now, your focus should be on integrative research reviews (IRRs), which are the central interest of this chapter. A meta-analysis and a metasynthesis article are listed at the end of the chapter.

Importantly, healthcare organizations around the world produce and index systematic reviews. Thus, often one or more systematic reviews are available to agency project groups revising clinical protocols. When you have chosen your clinical field of practice, you will learn which sites have systematic reviews relevant to your area of practice.

> ### Systematic Reviews
>
> - Integrative research reviews
> - Meta-analysis
> - Metasynthesis

Before heading into a description of IRRs, I would point out that all three types of systematic reviews are different from "literature reviews" in several ways (see also Table 9–1):

- All systematic reviews have prescribed criteria regarding how the steps of the review process should be done. No process is prescribed for literature reviews; rather they are done according to the reviewer's predilections. Moreover, systematic review reports include explicit and detailed descriptions of how each step was done; no such expectation exists for literature reviews.
- Systematic reviews incorporate only research reports and sometimes data from large databases. Literature reviews can include a wide variety of types of articles including experiential accounts, opinion, and essay articles.
- Systematic reviews are based on a wide and diligent search for studies, whereas literature reviews can be, and often are, selective in what they report.

Integrative Research Reviews

Integrative research reviews (IRRs) are also called state-of-the-science summaries, narrative reviews, and qualitative systematic reviews (to differentiate them from quantitative research reviews, that is, meta-analyses).

Table 9–1	DIFFERENCES BETWEEN SYSTEMATIC REVIEWS AND LITERATURE REVIEWS	
FEATURE	SYSTEMATIC REVIEW (SR)	LITERATURE REVIEW
Purpose	Thorough examination of an issue (narrow or broad)	Highlights of an issue; varying degrees of thoroughness
Production process	Standards exist and the process used is described in report	No standards; process not described
Search	As exhaustive as possible	Often limited
Inclusion	Original study reports, previous SRs, information from large databases	Original study reports, theoretical literature, essays, opinion articles
Selection	Often uses a quality appraisal filter	Quality filter not used
Report	Inclusive of all qualifying studies	Often selective based on purpose

Scope

Panels or individuals with expertise in the issue of interest conduct integrative research reviews. The word *conduct* is used because doing an IRR is a demanding and rigorous undertaking. Like research, it requires that steps be taken to control error and bias in: (a) the selection of original studies included in the review, (b) the extraction of data from the original studies, (c) the analysis of findings, and (d) the conclusions. A review panel has greater potential to conduct an IRR that is free of error and bias than does an individual—the panel members act as checks-and-balances to each other's work and uncover unconscious biases.

The review panel starts by identifying a topic, issue, or problem it believes is in need of summarization. Sometimes, the topic is broad, other times the issue is quite narrow. A broad topic addresses several aspects of an issue, whereas a narrow topic focuses on one particular aspect; this is the IRR's **scope**. A review of studies about "preventing falls in the elderly" would be broader than is a review about "preventing falls in the home-dwelling elderly." A review titled "Environmental alterations to prevent falls in home-dwelling elders" would be even narrower.

Broad and narrow scope is not a good–bad issue; rather, broad topics require retrieving and appraising a greater number of studies than do narrow topics. A review about preventing falls in community-dwelling elders would have to include studies regarding the functional status of patients (e.g., balance and gait), the role of medications, orthostatic hypotension, environmental issues, and more. In contrast, an IRR about environmental alterations to prevent falls in the home could focus on a smaller subset of studies having to do with floor surfaces, grab bars, lighting, etc. Similarly, a review of smoking cessation interventions would be quite broad, but by specifying a population, such as adolescents, the review becomes considerably narrower. The broader the issue or topic, the more resources required to do the review, the more difficult the summary is to produce, and the longer the report.

Early on, reviewers consider the kinds of studies they will include in the review and how far back they will go in the search for studies. Sometimes changing technology or patterns of care mean that it does not make sense to go back beyond a certain date.

The reviewers also decide whether studies using the full range of designs will be included or just those with certain design characteristics. For instance, a physician group interested in reviewing interventions for urinary incontinence in nursing home residents included only randomized trials (Fink, Taylor, Tacklind, Rutks, & Wilt, 2008). In contrast, a nurse reviewer interested in women's experiences of cardiac pain included only qualitative studies because she was interested in understanding the women's perspective (O'Keefe-McCarthy, 2008). The difference in the types of studies included in the two reviews was determined by the clinical issue. RCTs are the best way to evaluate the cause and effect relationships involved in evaluating intervention effectiveness, whereas qualitative studies are the best way to gain insight about people's lived experiences.

Early on, review panels decide how they will handle studies that are of dubious methodological quality. Some panels will include them but note their poor or modest quality, whereas other panels will eliminate them altogether. Still others will analyze the results of low-quality and high-quality studies together and then separately to determine if study quality affects the conclusions.

Search for Studies

When the topic and scope have been clearly delineated, the search for studies begins. Many review panels include a health science librarian who has expertise in identifying and retrieving articles. The most common search-starting place is the computerized databases of the published clinical literature.

Reviewers typically search several healthcare databases using a variety of search terms, combinations of search terms, and search options.

Usually, the panel's goal is to include all the eligible studies on the issue; however, database indexing and retrieval may fail to identify some eligible studies, which can be a source of bias. Moreover, databases include only published studies, and some studies may have been done but were never published. This too can be a source of bias because published studies tend to be larger and have more dramatic results than unpublished studies do (Soeken & Sripusanapan, 2003). Thus, retrieval of eligible studies from databases is only a starting point. The panel should go on to peruse reference lists, go to research registries, contact colleagues, and even run searches using Web search engines.

Sifting and Sorting

At this point in conducting a review, hundreds of articles may be under consideration. Careful review of the abstracts can reduce the number by eliminating those that are not research articles or do not actually address the topic. Then, all relevant research articles are retrieved. Using a prespecified set of inclusion criteria, two persons (ideally) decide which studies qualify for full review. Often, the number of studies included in the full review is fewer than 50, or even 20, depending on the topic and how much research has been done on it.

The panel will then sort the articles into stacks by subtopics, such as those using similar forms of the intervention, those with similar populations, or those evaluating a particular clinical outcome. For instance, in a study of parenting in the neonatal intensive care unit (Cleveland, 2008), studies were grouped by whether they examined the learning needs of parents or support of parents. A separate evidence table was created for each subtopic.

Analysis of Findings

Panel members read each report and extract basic information about design, sample, variables, and results. They then enter the information into tables and create lists to help them identify differences, commonalities, and patterns across the studies. Different research questions, ways of measuring a variable, or timing of the outcome measurement are noted. Similarities and differences in results and findings would be identified and reasons for the differences explored.

The goal of analysis is to reach conclusions that represent the findings of the individual studies as a body of findings, which is different from looking at each one in isolation from the others. This combining of findings from many studies in the form of conclusions is often referred to as *synthesis* because new knowledge claims are produced—claims that go beyond what any single study produced. The term synthesis makes the process of bringing research findings together sound quite exacting—which it is not. In all three forms of systematic reviews, interpretation enters the process; assumptions, decisions, and missteps can affect the conclusions—and even produce misleading ones. However, these sources of bias can be minimized by following recognized ways of conducting reviews.

IRR Reports

IRR reports open by stating the issue they examine and why the reviewers think it is important. You should note if the review focused on a certain population or setting, and whether it is focused on one or several outcomes. For instance, a review about the effectiveness of relaxation techniques could focus just on the outcome of pain, or it could also include studies that examined relaxation techniques for anxiety, onset of panic attacks, or smoking cessation.

Next, the process that was used to search for study reports is described in detail, including databases searched, key terms used, and any inclusion or exclusion criteria used. The process used to extract information from the reports and the methods used to evaluate the quality of the studies are also described.

Typically, tables display much abbreviated profiles of the studies and the findings. Table 9–2 is part of an evidence table from a review of interventions to prevent disability in frail community-dwelling elderly (Daniels, van Rossum, de Witte, Kempen, & van den Heuvel, 2008). Note how this table provides a quick overview of the methods and the results of the studies.

In the text, findings that are consistent, conflicting, and equivocal, as well as gaps in the research base, are reported, and bottom-line conclusions are set forth. Finally, the panel or authors indicate whether and how their conclusions square with any prior summarization work that has been done on the topic, summarize the limitations of the body of research, and offer opinions regarding the ramifications of the conclusions.

Table 9-2 EXAMPLE OF A FINDINGS TABLE FROM AN IRR

Study	N Randomized/ Followed-up*	Participants Inclusion criteria and mean age	Interventions	Primarily aimed at[‡]	Follow-up[‡]	Outcome measures[§]	Results[+]
Binder, 2002, USA	IG: 69/66 CG: 50/49	Two out of three criteria: Score between 18–32 on Modified PPT, peak oxygen uptake between 10–18 mL/kg/min, self-reported difficulty in max. 2 ADLs or 1 IADL (Mean age: 83)	IG: 9-month program provided by physiology exercise technicians consisting of three phases of each 36 sessions. Phase 1: Group format: 22 exercises on flexibility, balance, coordination, speed of reaction and strength. Phase 2: Progressive resistance training combined with shortened version of phase 1 exercises. Phase 3: Endurance training combined with shortened version of phase 1 and phase 2 exercises. CG: 9-month home exercise program including 9 of the 22 exercises from phase 1. Participants were asked to perform exercises 2–3 times a week and attended a monthly class.	Reduce or delay frailty	3, 6, and 9 months	Self-reported use of assistance or assistive technology (OARS ADL and IADL scale) Self-reported difficulty with ADL and IADL (Physical Function subscale of FSQ) Modified PPT items Knee extension/ flexion strength VO_2-peak Balance Body weight	No differences between groups (data not presented). Difference (SS) in favor of IG. Differences (SS) in favor of IG for modified PPT score, knee strength, VO_2-peak and balance. No SS difference for body weight (data not shown).

(continues)

Table 9-2 EXAMPLE OF A FINDINGS TABLE FROM AN IRR *(continued)*

Study	N Randomized/ Followed-up*	Participants Inclusion criteria and mean age	Interventions	Primarily aimed at†	Follow-up‡	Outcome measures§	Results⁺
Boshuizen, 2005, Netherlands	IG: High guidance (HG) 24/16 IG: Medium guidance (MG) 26/16 CG: 22/17	Experiencing difficulty in rising from chair and maximum knee extensor torque < 87.5 N-m (Mean age: ~79)	IG: *High-guidance:* 10-wk exercise program, each week two group sessions (60 min) by PT and one unsupervised home session. Focus on exercises with a variation in concentric, isometric, and eccentric knee-extensor activity. IG: *Medium-guidance:* Same program, though each week one supervised session and two unsupervised home sessions. CG: No training or other encouragement	Increasing strength knee extensors	10–12 weeks	Self-reported performance in activities of daily living (GARS) Knee extensor strength Walking function Balance Box stepping Timed Up and Go	No differences between groups. Difference (SS) in knee strength and walking function for HG group compared to CG. Differences (NS) between HG and MG for walking function in favor of HG.

Table 9–2 EXAMPLE OF A FINDINGS TABLE FROM AN IRR (continued)

Study	N Randomized/ Followed-up*	Participants Inclusion criteria and mean age	Interventions	Primarily aimed at[†]	Follow-up[‡]	Outcome measures[§]	Results[◆]
Chandler, 1998, USA	IG: 50/44 CG: 50/43	Inability to descend stairs step over step without holding the railing (Mean age: ~78)	IG: 10-wk exercise program, each week three individual in-home sessions by PT. Focus: Progressive resistive lower extremity exercises with Thera-Band. CG: No training or any encouragement.	Increasing lower extremity strength	10 weeks	Self-reported limitations in physical activities (MOS-36 physical functioning subscale) Lower extremity strength Physical performance	No significant differences between groups (data not presented). Greater lower extremity (SS) strength gain in favor of IG (data on physical performance not presented).

Source: Adapted from Daniels, R., van Rossum, E., de Witte, L., Kempen, G. I., & van den Heuvel, W. (2008). Interventions to prevent disability in frail community-dwelling elderly: A systematic review. *BMC Health Services Research, 8,* 278. Retrieved from http://www.biomedcentral.com/content/pdf/1472-6963-8-278.pdf

*Randomized relates to the number of participants randomized to intervention guidance (IG) and control group (CG). Followed-up relates to the numbers of participants taken into data analysis.

[†] Outcome that the authors primarily aimed to improve by conducting the intervention.

[‡] Follow-up measurement in weeks or months after randomization.

[§] Measured disability concept and instrument, followed by outcome measures for frailty components.

[◆] SS = Statistically significant difference if $p < .05$; NS = Not statistically significant.

Use of IRRs

IRRs are being published in clinical journals with increasing frequency, which is very helpful to clinician teams designing nursing protocols. Locating a well-conducted, recent IRR saves a clinical project team all the work of identifying, retrieving, analyzing, and summarizing the research findings pertaining to the protocol they are designing.

At the same time, users of IRRs need to keep in mind that the conclusions are interpretations of findings, and as such they are prone to unidentified assumptions, oversight, and unconscious bias. Two review groups examining the same body of research findings could arrive at different conclusions. Starting with the **appraisal** of the quality of the individual studies and on through the conclusions, there are numerous points at which the opinion of two review groups could differ. One group may discount the findings of a study that another group thinks is important. One group may focus on one outcome, while another group thinks another outcome is more important.

Exemplar

⌒ *Reading Tips*

I would like to provide some background and add an addendum to this reprint. Because the synthesis of this review is so strong, this IRR interested me. However, the lack of information about the methods used to produce it was of concern. So, I wrote to the lead author, and he kindly responded with the information about methodology, which is provided in Box 9–1 (Dr. Fadi Khraim, personal communication, March 7, 2010). This additional information assured me that this IRR was soundly conducted.

You may have noticed that this is the second time I have mentioned contacting an author and getting an answer. You may also have noted that most articles contain an e-mail address for the corresponding author. Most authors are pleased to have interest in their article and to provide the requested information—to students as well as book authors!

Box 9–1   ADDITIONAL INFORMATION ABOUT THE KHRAIM AND CAREY IRR

Selection and Inclusion

To identify the relevant literature, the following keywords were searched in combination with acute myocardial infarction or heart attack: attitude to illness/health, health beliefs, help or health seeking behavior, health behavior, psychosocial factors, treatment delay, socioeconomic factors, time factors, prehospital delay, and symptoms. This search of the databases yielded more than 50 articles. Of these, only articles reporting original research were included (40 papers); commentaries, review papers, letters to editors, etc. were excluded. The 40 original research articles were further scrutinized, and only the articles reporting research on factors or predictors of prehospital delay were included. The result was 26 articles.

Analysis

The identified studies were explored for similarities and dissimilarities concerning the type of prehospital delay predictors that were investigated, which eventually resulted in the six major categories identified under the subheading titled 3.3. Factors Associated with Pre-hospital Delay.

Evidence Table

Due to lack of space, an evidence table was not included in the article. The authors felt that including such a table would essentially require trimming the analysis to maintain the journal's prespecified paper length. Therefore, this was deemed unwarranted because the focus was providing a thorough analysis of the subject matter.

(Dr. Fadi Khraim, personal communication, March 7, 2010)

Predictors of Pre-hospital Delay Among Patients with Acute Myocardial Infarction

Fadi M. Khraim and Mary G. Carey

Patient Education and Counseling (2008), 75(2), 155–161.

Key Words

Acute myocardial infarction, decision delay, healthcare seeking behavior, time factors

Abstract

Objective: To evaluate current literature on predictors of pre-hospital delay among patients with acute myocardial infarction (AMI).

Methods: Medline, CINHAL, and Psych Info databases were searched using keywords: attitude to illness/health, health beliefs, help/health seeking behavior, health behavior, psychosocial factors, treatment delay, socioeconomic factors, time factors, pre-hospital delay, and symptoms. These keywords were combined with AMI to identify literature published during 1995–2008.

Results: Twenty-six data-based research articles were identified. Delay varied across literature and median pre-hospital delay was often reported due to distribution skewness resulting from extremely prolonged values (1.5–15.2 h). Six categories of predictors influenced pre-hospital delay; socio-demographic, symptom onset context, cognitive, affective/psychological, behavioral, and clinical factors. Pre-hospital delay was shortest when the decision to seek healthcare was facilitated by family members or coworkers and when symptoms suggestive of heart attack were continuous and severe.

Conclusion and practice implications: Developing interventions programs to reduce pre-hospital delay for high-risk patients is warranted. Because decision delay is the only modifiable part by intervention, it is recommended that future investigations and interventions attend to decision time as the primary variable of interest instead of combining it with transportation time. Moreover, content of patient education need to emphasize on symptom awareness and recognition, and prompt and proper patient actions for optimum results. Also, in order to eliminate sampling bias resulting from investigating surviving AMI patients, it is recommended that future studies incorporate data from both surviving and surrogates of non-surviving AMI patients.

1. Introduction

Coronary heart disease (CHD) is the number one killer for both men and women in the United States accounting for 1 of every 5 deaths [1]. Based on the American Heart Association calculations, it is estimated that every 26 s an American will suffer a coronary event, and about every minute someone will die from one. About 38% of the people who experience a coronary event in a given year will die from the event [2]. In 2004, mortality from CHD as an underlying or contributing cause of death was 607,000, out of which one-third were attributed to acute myocardial infarction (AMI) [1].

1.1. Background and significance

Longer delay from the onset of AMI symptoms to the delivery of emergency medical care negatively affects patients' prognosis [3–5]. It is estimated that of all patients who die within 28 days after onset of AMI symptoms, about two-thirds die before accessing healthcare facility [6]. A delay of as little as 30 min in the administration of reperfusion therapy for ST segment elevation myocardial infarction raises mortality risks [5,7] and reduces life expectancy by an average of 1 year [8]. The American College of Cardiology and American Heart Association recommend administration of reperfusion therapy to all patients who show symptoms suggestive of AMI, changes in the electrocardiography characterized by ST segment elevation or left bundle branch block, and have no contraindications irrespective to their race, gender, and age [9].

The body of research that illustrates the importance of early reperfusion therapy for AMI is mounting. Investigations of the importance of various reperfusion therapies revealed that timely interventions were warranted in order to reduce mortality and morbidity [10–13]. Although treatment trends may favor one reperfusion modality over another (coronary angioplasty vs. thrombolytic reperfusion), reduced time-to-intervention remains one of the most important factors that determines realization of reperfusion benefit regardless of what reperfusion modality used [12–14].

1.2. Pre-hospital and in-hospital delay

Delay before the initiation of reperfusion therapy for AMI can be divided into two distinct time periods: pre-hospital delay and in-hospital delay. Pre-hospital delay is the time from onset of symptoms to arrival to hospital. In-hospital delay, also known as door-to-treatment, is defined as time from arriving to the hospital to initiation of reperfusion therapy. Pre-hospital delay can be divided into two time periods: decision delay time and transportation delay time. Decision delay is time from onset of symptoms to making the initial decision to seek professional healthcare, and transportation delay is the time from making the initial decision to seek professional healthcare to arrival to hospital. Data from the National Registry of Myocardial Infarction indicates that median in-hospital delay time for thrombolytic therapy was significantly reduced by nearly half, from 61.8 to 37.8 min, during the last few years [15]. This reduction occurred due to following stringent policies of intervention initiation. Moreover, many hospitals are still working to meet the goal of 30 min set in 1991 [15]. Understanding predictors of pre-hospital delay is important and will provide the essential assets for interventions to modify individuals' behaviors targeting reduced delay. This review evaluates current literature on predictors of pre-hospital delay among patients with acute myocardial infarction.

2. Methods

In order to evaluate literature on pre-hospital delay, Medline, CINHAL and Psych Info databases were searched. Keywords used in this search were attitude to illness/health, health beliefs, help/health seeking behavior, health behavior, psychosocial factors, treatment delay, socioeconomic factors, time factors, pre-hospital delay, and symptoms. Those keywords were combined with acute myocardial infarction or heart attack that is found in literature published in the period of 1995–2008.

3. Results

Twenty-six articles were identified as research papers, most of which had utilized a cross-sectional correlational quantitative design, and few used qualitative or mixed designs. Pre-hospital delay varied across literature reviewed. Median delay was often reported due to distribution skewness resulting from extremely prolonged delay values. While the majority of authors who described the distribution of delay times reported skewness toward longer delay values [16–24], McKinley et al. [25], who studied treatment seeking behavior among a cohort of Australians and North Americans, reported skewness toward short values.

Pre-hospital delay medians ranged from 1.5 h in North American and Australian cohort [25] to 15.2 h in Hong Kong Chinese patients [26]. When pre-hospital delay is added to in-hospital delay, the sum is typically substantial delay before definitive treatment is started. Extensive delay results in higher morbidity, mortality and higher cost of healthcare [4,27].

3.1. Theoretical frameworks utilized

Half of the articles reviewed did not report using a conceptual framework to define the variables of interest in their studies [16,19,20,22,26,28–35]. Of the ones that reported using a conceptual framework, eight [18,21,23,25,36–39] have used Leventhal's model [40]. Leventhal's model was used in conjunction with another conceptual framework in three of the studies: Grounded Theory [36], Thematic Framework [37], and Dispositional Optimism [23]. Other theories that were reported: Bandura's Social Cognitive Theory [24], Symbolic Interactionism (Grounded Theory) [41], Individualism–Collectivism Theory [17], feminist approach [42], and epidemiological research paradigm [43]

3.2. Instruments

Investigators have used various instruments for measurement (Table 1).

Table 1   LIST OF INSTRUMENTS USED

1. The Response to Symptoms Questionnaire [16,17, 19–21, 25, 31,34]
2. The Symptom Representation Questionnaire [23]
3. Illness Perception Questionnaire [18]
4. Myocardial Infarction Symptom Survey [24]
5. Interpersonal Relationship Inventory [24]
6. Mastery Scale of Personal Control [24]
7. Heart Disease Threat Scale [24]
8. Eysenck Personality Questionnaire [24]
9. Independent and Interdependent Construal of Self [17]
10. Representation of Heart Attack Symptoms Questionnaire [39]
11. McSweeney Acute and Prodromal Myocardial Infarction Symptom Survey [32]
12. Perceived Racism Scale [16]
13. Life Orientation Test [23]
14. Morgan Incongruency of Heart Attack Symptoms Index [35]

3.3. Factors associated with pre-hospital delay

Researchers have identified different variables that influence pre-hospital delay. These variables can be grouped under six major categories. The grouped categories are; (1) socio-demographic: gender, age, socio-economic status, race, marital status, and health insurance; (2) contextual: onset while at home/being alone; (3) cognitive: match/mismatch of symptoms expected and symptoms experienced, perceived control over symptoms, knowledge of AMI, and perceived threat (susceptibility and seriousness); (4) affective/psychological: fear of consequences and denial, fear of troubling others, and embarrassment of seeking care; (5) behavioral: waiting for symptoms to go away/trying to relax, telling someone about symptoms, calling the emergency medical services, calling or visiting the primary care provider; and (6) clinical factors: past medical history/coexisting morbidities, and nature of symptoms.

3.3.1. Socio-demographic factors

Investigators who studied gender differences reported conflicting results of whether women delay significantly longer than men upon experiencing AMI symptoms. Several investigators reported that female gender was a significant variable in predicting delay [28,30,42,43]. In contrast, many others found no significant gender differences [16,18,20,21,25,31].

Increased age was associated with longer pre-hospital delay in many of the studies [20,25,30,31,42,43]. Sheifer et al. [43] reported a positive linear relationship between age and pre-hospital delay. However, other researchers did not find statistical significance result for age's influence on delay [16,18,23,28].

Three studies reported little or no relation between pre-hospital delay and socio-economic status (SES) [18,20,23]. Nonetheless, Okhravi [22], who looked at reasons for pre-hospital delay in AMI patients in Tehran, capital of Iran, found that patients who delayed more than 6 h after the onset of symptoms were characterized by low income and low-education levels. Similarly, Sheifer et al. [43] reported that low SES, measured by zip-code residency, was a significant determinant of longer pre-hospital delay; however, due to the large sample size ($n = 102,339$) in the study, reporting type I error or false positive results becomes inevitable.

Quinn [23] found no racial differences that could explain longer delay prior to arriving to emergency room. However, Caucasians comprised 92% of the total sample ($n = 100$), therefore, the author may have had reported false negative results. In contrast, Sheifer et al. [43] reported that White race, compared to Black or other races, was associated with significantly shorter delay. The authors also reported that race had an interaction effect with both SES and gender; White males who were not poor had shortest delay after onset of symptoms. Additionally, Banks and Dracup [16] reported that African-Americans had prolonged pre-hospital delay (mean delay = 13.5 ± 19.5 h, median = 4.25) but maintained that perceived racism was not associated with a different delay pattern among this minority population in the United States.

Results about marital status were as conflicting as other socio-demographic variables. While McKinley et al. [25], and Banks and Dracup [16] found that married people delayed significantly shorter than single people, other investigators found no difference [21,31].

Investigators reported that patients having health insurance were not different from those without insurance with regard to early presentation to hospital [20,35]. O'Donnell et al. [42], however, reported that having private insurance was associated with shorter delay. Banks and Dracup [16] found that African-Americans who did not have medical insurance had shorter delay relative to those who were medically insured; however, these results can be misleading due to the small proportion of insured ($n = 9$) to the uninsured ($n = 52$). On the other hand, McSweeney et al. [32] reported that African-American women who are eligible for public insurance such as Medicare or Medicaid (a proxy variable measured based on income and age) were 2.3 times as likely to get treatment for AMI within 2 h of symptom onset.

3.3.2. Contextual factors

Lebanese women who experienced symptoms during weekdays delayed longer than those who experienced onset during week-ends [34]. Furthermore, researchers reported that having symptom onset at home was associated with longer pre-hospital delay [16,25,31]. Conversely, African-Americans experiencing symptoms alone delayed longer than when with company [16].

3.3.3. Cognitive factors

Horne et al. [18] reported that 58% of patients with AMI reported a difference between symptoms experienced and symptoms expected. Zerwic [39] surveyed the public and reported that people have different and diversified perceptions of AMI symptoms. Patients may explain their symptom representation as a heartburn or indigestion [31] and would not attribute their symptoms as an AMI unless symptoms classically present in a "Hollywood style heart attack" in typical crushing chest pain [30,36]. This mismatch in symptom representation was found to be associated with significant delay deciding to seek treatment [18–21,25,31,35–37]. On the other hand, patients who compared their symptoms presentation with others' experience of AMI, were more likely to seek care early [37,41]. This comparison helped AMI victims cognitively draw a picture or label for the illness [26]. Banks and Dracup [16] reported that matching of symptom experience with expectation among African-Americans ($n = 61$) did not result in reduced delay. Nonetheless, in a multi-center study in eight states, McSweeney et al. [32] reported that African-American women ($n = 509$) and White women ($n = 500$) who attributed their symptoms to AMI were 3 and 4 times (respectively) as likely to get treatment within 2 h following symptoms onset.

Patients perceived ability to cope with [26] or control symptoms [19,35] was associated with increased delay. Rosenfeld [24] reported a similar pattern in delay of women who perceived control over their symptoms. Additionally, Dempsey et al. [36] reported longer delay when women used symptom alleviation strategies that worked in the past to control for current similar symptoms. Furthermore, patients who used different drugs such as Tylenol or antacids in an attempt to control their symptoms delayed longer due to their perception of illness control using self-treatment [20,31].

Dracup and Moser [31] reported no significant association between knowledge of AMI symptoms and early presentation to hospital. However, 9 years later, the authors reported that men with knowledge of thrombolytic therapy and its effectiveness delayed less than those who did not have knowledge. In contrast, women knowledge regarding thrombolytics did not result in reduced delay [20].

Unsurprisingly, lack of perceived seriousness of symptoms [17,19–22, 25,28,29,31,34,35,41] and lack of perceived susceptibility to heart disease [24,36,37] was associated with longer delay. In contrast, understanding of symptoms significance was associated with readiness to seek care [41].

3.3.4. Psychological and affective factors

Acute myocardial infarction is an illness that is associated with possible unpleasant life modifications and limitations to lifestyle [44,45]. Therefore, delayers often feared seeking care for their symptoms [20,31,36]. This can be explained in a context of denial as a self-defense mechanism toward illness because people tend to reject ideas that are associated with possible unpleasant experiences or feelings [46].

Longer pre-hospital delay was perpetuated by the fear of troubling other family members or significant others [17,25,31]. Women, particularly, did not want to worry others about their illness or symptoms due to lack of perceived threat or feeling of their illness as trifling [20,21,26,36].

Patients who were embarrassed to seek care often delayed doing so for their symptoms [17,19,25]. Embarrassment seemed to be related to the perception of lack of seriousness and susceptibility to AMI. Patients avoided going to the emergency room to avoid embarrassment if symptoms were benign or not life-threatening. Feeling embarrassed to call the ambulance was associated with increased pre-hospital delay [29].

3.3.5. Behavioral factors

The decision-making process of seeking healthcare appears to be influenced by the initial actions of patients. The interplay between psychological and cognitive variables shaped the behaviors of patients toward promptly seeking care or delaying. Patients who waited for symptoms to go away or tried to relax, based on past experiences or denial of illness, were more likely to delay longer than people whose initial behavior was toward seeking professional healthcare [19,21,22,25,28,31,34,36].

Researchers found that the sooner a family member or a coworker was informed about symptoms, the faster the decision was made to seek professional help. Calling the emergency medical services (EMS) was often associated with advice from a spouse or a friend [28,36]. Dempsey et al. [36] theorized that when methods of gaining control over symptoms such as waiting for symptoms to go away or relaxing fail, women seek to relinquish control by consulting a family member or friend to help them make the decision to seek care.

While a small proportion of AMI patients called for an ambulance as a first response, investigators found that calling the EMS immediately was associated with significantly shorter delay [16,18,19,28–30]. O'Donnell et al. [42] reported that those who drove themselves to the hospital also arrived significantly early. However, calling [28,29,33,42], or visiting [21,22,43] the primary care provider (PCP) was associated with significant delay. Alonzo [33] reported that the median pre-hospital delay for those who called their PCP was 4 times longer than non-callers.

3.3.6. Clinical factors

Investigators reported that patients with history of AMI [30,43] or a history of cardiac interventions such as percutaneous transluminal coronary angioplasty/stent or coronary artery bypass graft [43] experienced reduced pre-hospital delay. Moser et al. [20] reported significant shorter delay in men rather than women with previous AMI. On the other hand, four other studies found that previous AMI was not related to pre-hospital delay [16,23,28,31]. Similarly, researchers who looked at other comorbidities such as history of angina [16,25,43], diabetes mellitus [16,20,22,25,30,31,43], and hypertension [20,25,31] reported conflicting results of whether patients with these comorbidities experience reduced delay or not.

The nature of symptoms presentation affected the healthcare seeking behavior. Increased symptom intensity [16–18,34], having symptoms of continuous nature [19–21,25], increased anxiety due to continuing symptom presentation [20,31,35,36], and having fast onset symptoms (symptoms that develop rapidly) [18] were associated with shorter pre-hospital delay. Johansson et al. [28] reported that increased intensity of symptoms such as increased levels of chest pain was associated with calling for an ambulance. In contrast, Noureddine et al. [21] found no correlation between Lebanese patients' pain levels and early or late presentation to hospital.

4. Discussion and conclusion

4.1. Discussion

In general, this review of current literature on predictors of pre-hospital delay among patients with AMI reveals that researchers utilized different research approaches in variety of cultures or ethnic backgrounds. Therefore, researchers in one study often reported results that are contradictory in nature to results in another study. Nonetheless, research described succeeded in identifying factors that predict pre-hospital delay among various populations. These predictors will help healthcare professionals and policy makers put tangible remedies to target respective populations in order to reduce delay.

Research reviewed suffers from various methodological shortcomings. One of the most important methodological shortcomings is lack for power needed to detect significance in studies that looked at subgroup difference. In such studies [18,21,25], comparisons were made based on underpowered group sizes leading to a possibility of reporting false negative results. For example, Noureddine et al. [21] reported longer mean delay for women than men (18.47 ± 33.48 h vs. 14.5 ± 26.41 h, respectively) that is of clinical significance, yet did not have enough power in the female comparison group in order to elicit statistical significance (females = 56 vs. males = 148).

Additionally, literature has shown selection bias in the sampled populations. Due to the nature of the problem, investigators were only able to sample from individuals who survived and could be interviewed following AMI. No attempts were made to investigate predictors of delay for those who did not survive AMI utilizing their surrogates. Therefore, generalization of these results on all AMI patients would be misleading as current literature only pertained to survivors. Although one may argue that some patients who die due to a coronary event do not share their symptom experience with others or die alone, many others share this important piece of information with a family member or a significant other. Therefore, it is essential for future investigations to plan on interviewing surrogates of those who did not survive AMI or those who cannot be interviewed whenever possible in order to elicit generalizable data to all AMI patients.

Moreover, research that investigated healthcare seeking behavior among AMI patients only looked at pre-hospital delay as the dependent variable of interest. Only Morgan [35] attended to decision delay that is principally determined by the decision-making process and influences pre-hospital delay as a whole. The assumption here is that patients with AMI have little or no control over the transportation time once they decide to make the initial attempt to seek professional help. Therefore, it is important to focus future investigations on decision delay time which is reflected by healthcare seeking decision process.

Most studies reported pre-hospital delay that is skewed toward longer values indicating prolonged delay time in populations studied. Only one paper reported skewness toward shorter delay values and shorter median of pre-hospital delay [25]. This different trend of skewness of delay distribution may have occurred due to sampling bias resulting from either different inclusion criteria utilized among the two sample populations (North Americans and Australians), or lack of sample heterogeneity.

Different factors that influence pre-hospital delay were identified. Studies that investigated socio-demographic variables reported conflicting results due to studying different sample populations. Women often have different symptom cluster than men reporting chest pain less frequently [47–50]. Experiencing other symptoms than chest pain confuses women in identifying the symptoms as those of AMI and therefore, leads to longer delay seeking healthcare. Similarly, older persons and racial minorities are more likely to delay longer due to experiencing of different AMI symptom clusters [49,50]. In addition to that, racial minorities may also have certain ethno-cultural health beliefs and perceptions related to healthcare seeking behavior which may lead to longer delay [51].

Healthcare seeking behavior is often shared decision with friends or family members. Sharing the experience of symptoms with significant others or coworkers helped victims appraise their symptoms as serious leading to faster decision to seek professional help [28,36]. Significant others and coworkers appear to have a catalyst role in the healthcare seeking decision-making process that helps victims overcome their fear or denial of illness. Therefore, successful intervention strategies should employ spouses or significant others in the education process aiming to reduce delay [52].

Victims, who drew correct cognitive pictures of symptoms, were less likely to delay [18–21,25,31,36,37]. Knowledge of AMI symptoms and treatment combined with correct attribution of symptoms indicted shorter delay [34]. Understanding of the threat of illness is a logical prerequisite for victims to make informed decision of seeking professional healthcare. These individual perceptions of illness threat and benefits of treatment are explained in value expectancy models such as the Health Belief Model (HBM) [53]. This model proposes that an individual needs adequate level of perceived illness threat and perceived benefit of treatment in order to seek help. It is thought that an individual subconsciously analyzes the risk-benefit that entails a certain health behavior [54].

Psychological factors such as fear of consequences, denial of AMI, and fear of troubling others were found to cause considerable pre-hospital delay. Women who did not perceive their illness as serious and felt they were invulnerable to AMI, usually did not want to worry others about their illness or symptoms, therefore, delayed longer [20]. Long delayers were also those who avoided embarrassment especially if symptoms are deemed to be benign or not life-threatening [17,19,25]. Embarrassment also affected the decision to call for an ambulance leading to longer delay [29].

Both psychological and cognitive factors have shaped the behavioral responses to AMI symptoms. As expected, actions directed toward promptly seeking professional help (e.g., calling EMS) yielded the shortest delay [19,21,22,25,29,31,34,36]. On the other hand, actions that originated from intermediate level of illness appraisal (calling or visiting the PCP) were associated with substantially long pre-hospital delay. This trend of delay may have resulted from long waiting time before victim gets attention when visiting the PCP's office or the time taken before the healthcare provider could actually return a call from a patient. Additionally, the PCP may not appraise the symptoms as serious based on patient's telephonic description leading to much longer delay and possible misdiagnosis.

Due to studying different sample populations and/or lack of statistical power to detect difference, literature reported conflicting results of whether having history of previous comorbidities predicted long, short, or had no effect on pre-hospital delay. In sample populations where history of AMI predicted short delay, experience of previous AMI appears to provide knowledge and critical appraisal of own symptoms, and therefore prompted patients to seek help faster.

On the other hand, patients with history of anginal pain experienced long pre-hospital delay. In such sample populations, it appears that patients acquired the belief that their symptoms will not last long especially if certain measures were taken (e.g., taking nitroglycerin, resting). Therefore, patients' acquired sense of control over symptoms contributed to long delay. Conversely, longer pre-hospital delay for those with diabetes is possibly explained by the fact that diabetics may suffer from neuropathies affecting their pain receptors which result in an ill-defined or silent symptom profile [55].

The nature of symptoms presentation was found to influence pre-hospital delay. While having continuous or high level of symptoms intensity predicted short pre-hospital delay [16–18,28], having intermittent or low-intensity symptoms predicted longer delay [19–21,25]. Continuous and intense level of AMI symptoms appears to produce high level of anxiety leading to early hospital presentation [20,31,35,36]. Increased intensity of anxiety heightens individual perceptions of illness threat and therefore leads to faster healthcare seeking [53]. Because of varying degrees of symptom presentation and intensity experienced by patients, it is a crucial implication for any program aiming at intervening to reduce delay to include education about various symptoms of AMI.

4.2. Conclusion
4.2.1. Implications to research
Future investigations aiming to study predictors of pre-hospital delay or designing interventions to reduce delay should take in consideration the following recommendations:

1. Researchers need to adequately power their analysis of sample subgroups, especially genders or ethnic minorities.

2. It is estimated that of all AMI patients who die within 28 days after onset of AMI symptoms, about two-thirds die before accessing a healthcare facility [6], therefore, interviewing only AMI survivors results in intrinsic bias. Although extremely challenging, it is recommended that future studies incorporate data from both surviving and surrogates of non-surviving AMI patients in order to further our understanding of delay predictors.

3. Although literature consistently defined pre-hospital delay as time from onset of symptom to admission to hospital, it is important to reiterate that focus of patient education and counseling is to reduce delay by prompting the decision to seek professional healthcare. The nature of the decision made by the patient determines mode of transportation and its delay time; if a prompt decision was made to call EMS, then transportation delay is short. Furthermore, decision delay is the only part that can be modified by intervention; therefore, it is recommended that future investigations and interventions attend to decision time as the primary variable of interest instead of combining it with transportation time.

4.3. Implications to practice
Long pre-hospital delay is associated with increased mortality and morbidity [4,27,49], therefore, increased delay plays a significant role in survival and planning treatment options for patients. Various factors have been identified in literature to affect the decision-making process of healthcare seeking behavior among AMI patients. Based on the understanding of predictors of pre-hospital delay, it is important to implement interventions that focus on the importance of early symptom recognition and prompt care seeking. In doing so, it should be recognized that mass community education programs designed to educate the public about the importance

of responding quickly to acute coronary events did not produce encouraging results [56,57]. Kainth et al. explained that lack of success of public campaigns is due to utilizing poor methodological approaches. The authors maintained that it is useful to assess the decision-making process to call for help that patients and their family use before advocating interventions [57]. Alonzo and Reynolds reported that educating the public is a complex process due to various socio-psychological difficulties [58]. The authors explain that preparing the public for an event that could be disabling or potentially embarrassing if the event is a false alarm is usually a difficult task to achieve. Additionally, because people tend to normalize unpleasant information, it is not easy to keep the desired awareness level for a long period time [58]. Therefore, individual-based "face-to-face" intervention strategy for those at high risk of AMI or those who have had an AMI is more likely to produce positive results [52,56]. These two groups of "vulnerable patients" are more likely to get the benefit of this program and become more sensitized and aware of the nature of their illness and its serious outcomes. And because the aim of such program is to reduce delay and promote accurate management of AMI symptoms, content of the program should focus on awareness and recognition of AMI symptoms and importance of seeking help quickly by calling for an ambulance. The incorporation of the literature defined cognitive-psychological processes of healthcare seeking behavior among AMI patients in the content of the program is essential for success.

With immense evidence supporting benefits of early intervention on patients experiencing symptoms of AMI, health insurance organizations could take part in facilitating intervention programs. And because implementation of such programs can be done as a usual healthcare education for high-risk individuals, education can be incorporated in context of health promotion and risk reduction activities sponsored or covered by health insurance organizations. Therefore, utilization of available health maintenance and risk reduction coverage will significantly improve cost-effectiveness of intervention implementation.

Conflict of interest

No actual or potential conflict of interest of any kind had inappropriately influenced the preparation of this manuscript.

Acknowledgement

Funding: No funding source(s) had any involvement in preparing this manuscript.

References

[1] National Center for Health Statistics. Centers for Disease Control and Prevention. Compressed mortality file: underlying cause of death, 1979 to 2004. Atlanta, GA: Centers for Disease Control and Prevention.

[2] Rosamond W, Flegal K, Furie K, Go A, Greenlund K, Haase N, Hailpern S, Ho M, Howard V, Kissela B, Kittner S, Lloyd-Jones D, McDermott M, Meigs J, Moy C, Nichol G, O'Donnell C, Roger V, Sorlie P, Steinberger J, Thom T, Wilson M, Hong Y. Heart disease and stroke statistics—2008 update: a report from the American Heart Association Statistics Committee and Stroke Statistics Subcommittee. Circulation 2008;117:e25–146.

[3] Goldberg RJ, Steg PG, Sadiq I, Granger CB, Jackson EA, Budaj A, Brieger D, Avezum A, Goodman S. Extent of, and factors associated with, delay to hospital presentation in patients with acute coronary disease (the GRACE Registry). Am J Cardiol 2002;89:791–6.

[4] Grace SL, Abbey SE, Bisaillon S, Shnek ZM, Irvine J, Stewart DE. Presentation, delay, and contraindication to thrombolytic treatment in females and males with myocardial infarction. Women Health Issues 2003;13:214–21.

[5] De Luca G, Suryapranata H, Ottervanger JP, Antman EM. Time delay to treatment and mortality in primary angioplasty for acute myocardial infarction: every minute of delay counts. Circulation 2004;109:1223–5.

[6] Chambless L, Keil U, Dobson A, Mahonen M, Kuulasmaa K, Rajakangas A-M, Lowel H, Tunstall-Pedoe H. Population versus clinical view of case fatality from acute coronary heart disease: results from the WHO MONICA Project 1985–1990. Circulation 1997;96:3849–59.

[7] French WJ. Trends in acute myocardial infarction management: use of the National Registry of Myocardial Infarction in quality improvement. Am J Cardiol 2000;85:5–9.

[8] Rawles JM. Quantification of the benefit of earlier thrombolytic therapy: five-year results of the Grampian Region Early Anistreplase Trial (GREAT). J Am Coll Cardiol 1997;30:1181–6.

[9] Antman EM, Anbe DT, Armstrong PW, Bates ER, Green LA, Hand M, Hochman JS, Krumholz HM, Kushner FG, Lamas GA, Mullany CJ, Ornato JP, Pearle DL, Sloan MA, Smith Jr SC, Alpert JS, Anderson JL, Faxon DP, Fuster VG, Raymond JG, Gabriel H, Jonathan L, Hiratzka LF, Hunt SAJ, Alice K. ACC/AHA Guidelines for the Management of Patients with ST-Elevation Myocardial Infarction—executive summary: a report of the American College of Cardiology/American Heart Association Task Force on Practice Guidelines (Writing Committee to revise the 1999 Guidelines for the Management of Patients With Acute Myocardial Infarction). Circulation 2004;110:588–636.

[10] Boersma E, Maas AC, Deckers JW, Simoons ML. Early thrombolytic treatment in acute myocardial infarction: reappraisal of the golden hour. Lancet 1996;348:771–5.

[11] Faxon DP. Early reperfusion strategies after acute ST-segment elevation myocardial infarction: the importance of timing. Nat Clin Pract Cardiovasc Med 2005;2:22–8.

[12] Nallamothu BK, Bates ER. Percutaneous coronary intervention versus fibrinolytic therapy in acute myocardial infarction: is timing (almost) everything? Am J Cardiol 2003;92:824–6.

[13] Boersma E. The Primary Coronary Angioplasty vs. Thrombolysis-2 Trialists' Collaborative G. Does time matter? A pooled analysis of randomized clinical trials comparing primary percutaneous coronary intervention and in-hospital fibrinolysis in acute myocardial infarction patients. Eur Heart J 2006;27:779–88.

[14] Brener SJ, Moliterno DJ, Aylward PE, van't Hof AWJ, Ruzyllo W, O'Neill WW, Hamm CW, Westerhout CM, Granger CB, Armstrong PW. Reperfusion after primary angioplasty for ST-elevation myocardial infarction: predictors of success and relationship to clinical outcomes in the APEX-AMI Angiographic Study. Eur Heart J 2008;29:1127–35.

[15] Thom T, Haase N, Rosamond W, Howard VJ, Rumsfeld J, Manolio T, Zheng Z-J, Flegal K, O'Donnell C, Kittner S, Lloyd-Jones D, Goff Jr D, Hong Y, Adams R, Friday G, Furie K, Gorelick P, Kissela B, Marler J, Meigs J, Roger V, Sidney S, Sorlie P, Steinberger J, Wasserthiel-Smoller S, Wilson M, Wolf P. Heart disease and stroke statistics—2006 update: a report from the American Heart Association Statistics Committee and Stroke Statistics Subcommittee. Circulation 2006;113:85–151.

[16] Banks AD, Dracup K. Factors associated with prolonged prehospital delay of African Americans with acute myocardial infarction. Am J Crit Care 2006;15:149–57.

[17] Fukuoka Y, Dracup K, Rankin SH, Froelicher ES, Kobayashi F, Hirayama H, Ohno M, Matsumoto D. Prehospital delay and independent/interdependent construal of self among Japanese patients with acute myocardial infarction. Soc Sci Med 2005;60:2025–34.

[18] Horne R, James D, Petrie K, Weinman J, Vincent R. Patients' interpretation of symptoms as a cause of delay in reaching hospital during acute myocardial infarction. Heart 2000;83:388–93.

[19] McKinley S, Dracup K, Moser DK, Ball C, Yamasaki K, Kim CJ, Barnett M. International comparison of factors associated with delay in presentation for AMI treatment. Eur J Cardiovasc Nurs 2004;3:225–30.

[20] Moser DK, McKinley S, Dracup K, Chung ML. Gender differences in reasons patients delay in seeking treatment for acute myocardial infarction symptoms. Patient Educ Couns 2005;56:45–54.

[21] Noureddine S, Adra M, Arevian M, Dumit NY, Puzantian H, Shehab D, Abchee A. Delay in seeking health care for acute coronary syndromes in a Lebanese sample. J Transcult Nurs 2006;17:341-8.

[22] Okhravi M. Causes for pre-hospital and in-hospital delays in acute myocardial infarction at Tehran teaching hospitals. Aust Emerg Nurs J 2002;5:21-6.

[23] Quinn JR. Delay in seeking care for symptoms of acute myocardial infarction: applying a theoretical model. Res Nurs Health 2005;28:283-94.

[24] Rosenfeld AG. Treatment-seeking delay among women with acute myocardial infarction: decision trajectories and their predictors. Nurs Res 2004;53:225-36.

[25] McKinley S, Moser DK, Dracup K. Treatment-seeking behavior for acute myocardial infarction symptoms in North America and Australia. Heart Lung 2000;29:237-47.

[26] Kaur R, Lopez V, Thompson DR. Factors influencing Hong Kong Chinese patients' decision-making in seeking early treatment for acute myocardial infarction. Res Nurs Health 2006;29:636-46.

[27] GISSI-Avoidable Delay Study Group. Epidemiology of avoidable delay in the care of patients with acute myocardial infarction in Italy. Arch Intern Med 1995;155:1481-8.

[28] Johansson I, Stromberg A, Swahn E. Factors related to delay times in patients with suspected acute myocardial infarction. Heart Lung 2004;33:291-300.

[29] Johansson I, Stromberg A, Swahn E. Ambulance use in patients with acute myocardial infarction. J Cardiovasc Nurs 2004;19:5-12.

[30] Meischke H, Larsen MP, Eisenberg MS. Gender differences in reported symptoms for acute myocardial infarction: impact on prehospital delay time interval. Am J Emerg Med 1998;16:363-6.

[31] Dracup K, Moser DK. Beyond sociodemographics: factors influencing the decision to seek treatment for symptoms of acute myocardial infarction. Heart Lung 1997;26:253-62.

[32] McSweeney JC, Lefler LL, Fischer EP, Naylor AJ, Evans LK. Women's prehospital delay associated with myocardial infarction: does race really matter? J Cardiovasc Nurs 2007;22:279-85. quiz 86.

[33] Alonzo AA. The effect of health care provider consultation on acute coronary syndrome care-seeking delay. Heart Lung 2007;36:307-18.

[34] Noureddine S, Arevian M, Adra M, Puzantian H. Response to signs and symptoms of acute coronary syndrome: differences between Lebanese men and women. Am J Crit Care 2008;17:26-35.

[35] Morgan DM. Effect of incongruence of acute myocardial infarction symptoms on the decision to seek treatment in a rural population. J Cardiovasc Nurs 2005;20:365–71.

[36] Dempsey SJ, Dracup K, Moser DK. Women's decision to seek care for symptoms of acute myocardial infarction. Heart Lung 1995;24:444–56.

[37] Macinnes JD. The illness perceptions of women following symptoms of acute myocardial infarction: a self-regulatory approach. Eur J Cardiovasc Nurs 2006;5:280–8.

[38] Ryan CJ, Zerwic JJ. Knowledge of symptom clusters among adults at risk for acute myocardial infarction. Nurs Res 2004;53:363–9.

[39] Zerwic JJ. Symptoms of acute myocardial infarction: expectations of a community sample. Heart Lung 1998;27:75–81.

[40] Hale ED, Treharne GJ, Kitas GD. The Common-Sense Model of self-regulation of health and illness: how can we use it to understand and respond to our patients' needs? Rheumatology 2007;46:904–6.

[41] Brink E, Karlson BW, Hallberg L. To be stricken with acute myocardial infarction: a Grounded Theory Study of Symptom Perception and Care-Seeking Behaviour. J Health Psychol 2002;7:533–43.

[42] O'Donnell S, Condell S, Begley C, Fitzgerald T. Prehospital care pathway delays: gender and myocardial infarction. J Adv Nurs 2006;53:268–76.

[43] Sheifer SE, Rathore SS, Gersh BJ, Weinfurt KP, Oetgen WJ, Breall JA, Schulman KA. Time to presentation with acute myocardial infarction in the elderly: associations with race, sex, and socioeconomic characteristics. Circulation 2000;102:1651–6.

[44] Westin L, Carlsson R, Israelsson B, Willenheimer R, Cline C, McNeil TF. Quality of life in patients with ischaemic heart disease: a prospective controlled study. J Intern Med 1997;242:239–47.

[45] McBurne CR, Eagle KA, Kline-Rogers EM, Cooper JV, Mani OCM, Smith DE, Erickson SR. Health-related quality of life in patients 7 months after a myocardial infarction: factors affecting the Short Form-12. Pharmacotherapy 2002;22:1616–22.

[46] Stenstrom U, Nilsson AK, Stridh C, Nijm J, Nyrinder I, Jonsson A, Karlsson JE, Jonasson L. Denial in patients with a first-time myocardial infarction: relations to pre-hospital delay and attendance to a cardiac rehabilitation programme. Eur J Cardiovasc Prev Rehabil 2005;12:568–71.

[47] Patel H, Rosengren A, Ekman I. Symptoms in acute coronary syndromes: does sex make a difference? Am Heart J 2004;148:27–33.

[48] Pilote L, Dasgupta K, Guru V, Humphries KH, McGrath J, Norris C, Rabi D, Tremblay J, Alamian A, Barnett T, Cox J, Ghali WA, Grace S, Hamet P, Ho T, Kirkland S, Lambert M, Libersan D, O'Loughlin J, Paradis G, Petrovich M, Tagalakis V. A comprehensive view of sex-specific issues related to cardiovascular disease. CMAJ 2007;176:S1–44.

[49] Goldberg R, Goff D, Cooper L, Luepker R, Zapka J, Bittner V, Osganian S, Lessard D, Cornell C, Meshack A, Mann C, Gilliland J, Feldman H. Age and sex differences in presentation of symptoms among patients with acute coronary disease: the REACT Trial. Rapid Early Action for Coronary Treatment. Coron Artery Dis 2000;11:399–407.

[50] Ryan CJ, DeVon HA, Horne R, King KB, Milner M, Moser DK, Quinn JR, Rosenfeld AG, Hwang SY, Zerwic JJ. Symptom clusters in acute myocardial infarction: a secondary data analysis. Nurs Res 2007;56:72–81.

[51] Klingler D, Green-Weir R, Nerenz D, Havstad S, Rosman HS, Cetner L, Shah S, Wimbush F, Borzak S. Perceptions of chest pain differ by race. Am Heart J 2002;144:51–9.

[52] Dracup K, McKinley S, Riegel B, Mieschke H, Doering LV, Moser DK. A nursing intervention to reduce prehospital delay in acute coronary syndrome: a randomized clinical trial. J Cardiovasc Nurs 2006;21:186–93.

[53] Rosenstock IM. The Health Belief Model: explaining health behavior through expectancies. In: Glanz K, Lewis FM, Rimer BK, editors. Health behavior and health education: theory, research and practice. San Francisco: Jossey-Bass; 1990. pp. 39–62.

[54] Bowers KA. Explaining health behavior: the health belief model. Nurs Adm Q 1980;4:41–6.

[55] DeVon HA, Penckofer S, Larimer K. Midwest nursing research society sage best paper award: the Association of Diabetes and Older Age With the Absence of Chest Pain During Acute Coronary Syndromes. West J Nurs Res 2008;30:130–44.

[56] Caldwell MA, Miaskowski C. Mass media interventions to reduce help-seeking delay in people with symptoms of acute myocardial infarction: time for a new approach? Patient Educ Couns 2002;46:1–9.

[57] Kainth A, Hewitt A, Sowden A, Duffy S, Pattenden J, Lewin R, Watt I, Thompson D. Systematic review of interventions to reduce delay in patients with suspected heart attack. Emerg Med J 2004;21:506–8.

[58] Alonzo AA, Reynolds NR. Responding to symptoms and signs of acute myocardial infarction—how do you educate the public? A social-psychologic approach to intervention. Heart Lung 1997;26:263–72.

Profile & Commentary

WHY *Purpose*

This integrative research review was not explicitly identified as such, but clearly only research articles were included. The purpose is stated as an examination of the research on predictors of prehospital delay among patients with acute myocardial infarction. A solid case is made for the claim that understanding this issue and ultimately addressing it is important to reducing deaths related to acute myocardial infarction (AMI).

Interestingly, the division of the time from the onset of symptoms to reperfusion therapy is divided into prehospital delay and hospital delay. Prehospital delay is then divided into two time periods: decision delay and transportation delay. One gets the sense that the authors are really interested in decision delay, but this has not been studied by itself; instead it has been examined within the larger context of prehospital delay. In the Discussion section, they inform us that only one study focused exclusively on decision delay.

HOW *Methodology*

In the addendum provided by the lead author (Box 9–1), the database search was described and the years in which articles were published were stated. There, we also learn the search terms used and the retrieval yield. In essence, the original 50 possible articles were distilled to 26 research articles that were on-topic.

Scrutiny of these study reports resulted in the identification of the six categories of prehospital delay factors that were used to organize the findings. Importantly, a strong synthesis of the findings within the six predictor areas was produced. Note that the authors do not just go over the study results one by one. Instead, they identify studies with similar findings, those with contradictory findings, and offer reasons why the contradictory findings may have occurred. They also link findings from several studies to create a composite portrayal of an issue—this is synthesis.

WHAT *Results*

Results are reported according to six factors that have been found to be associated with prehospital delay. Quite a few studies have been done for some predictor factors, e.g., cognitive factors and clinical factors. In contrast, little research has been done on contextual factors. Also, the results for some factors are quite mixed, such as for sociodemographic factors. *Mixed* means some studies found an association between the factor and delay but other studies did not find an association. For other factors, the results are more consistent, for example, cognitive factors where a mismatch between people's expectations of what AMI symptoms are like and what they actually experience was found in several studies to be associated with prehospital delay.

Interestingly, patients' history of cardiac disease was not consistently related to shorter prehospital delay. Notice how the authors present findings in this regard—"Investigators [2] reported"; "Moser reported"; "on the other hand, four other studies found"—again, this is synthesis. The inconsistency in the findings under several of the six categories is undoubtedly due to the diversity of populations studied. I determined this diversity by looking at the titles of the articles referenced.

Discussion

The authors create composite portrayals of how the six categories of predictors influence prehospital delay. They also note that quite a few studies suffered from lack of statistical power to detect significant differences between groups. This could have caused factors that really are associated with delay not being identified as such because of an inadequate sample size. Just as importantly, only living persons were interviewed. This may seem obvious but can easily be forgotten when immersing oneself in the results.

In summarizing the results for each of the six predictor categories, the authors turn their attention to thinking about how interventions could be designed to influence the factors that increase the prehospital delay. It is a challenge. There is a need for knowledge about the symptoms of AMI among the general population, but perhaps more importantly for awareness and preplanned action among high-risk individuals. The authors suggest that this could be done within the context of the education about health promotion and risk reduction that is often provided to those who are at high risk of having an AMI.

REFERENCES

Cleveland, L. M. (2008). Parenting in the neonatal intensive care unit. *Journal of Obstetric, Gynecologic, and Neonatal Nursing, 37,* 666–691.

Daniels, R., van Rossum, E., de Witte, L., Kempen, G. I., & van den Heuvel, W. (2008). Interventions to prevent disability in frail community-dwelling elderly: A systematic review. *BMC Health Services Research, 8,* 278. Retrieved from http://www.biomedcentral.com/content/pdf/1472-6963-8-278.pdf

Fink, H. A., Taylor, B. C., Tacklind, J. W., Rutks, I. R., & Wilt, T. J. (2008). Treatment intervention in nursing home residents with urinary incontinence: A systematic review of randomized trials. *Mayo Clinic Proceedings, 83*(12), 1332–1343.

Khraim, F. M., & Carey, M. G. (2008). Predictors of pre-hospital delay among patients with acute myocardial infarction. *Patient Education and Counseling, 75*(2), 155–161.

O'Keefe-McCarthy, S. (2008). Women's experiences of cardiac pain: A review of the literature. *Canadian Journal of Cardiovascular Nursing, 18*(3), 18–25.

Soeken, K. L., & Sripusanapan, A. (2003). Assessing publication bias in meta-analysis. *Nursing Research, 52,* 57–60.

Whittemore, R. (2005). Combining evidence in nursing research: Methods and implications. *Nursing Research, 54*(1), 56–62.

OTHER SYSTEMATIC REVIEWS

Bausewein, C., Booth, S., Gysels, M., & Higginson, I. J. (2008). Non-pharmacological interventions for breathlessness in advanced stages of malignant and non-malignant diseases. *Cochrane Database of Systematic Reviews, 2.* doi: 10,1002/14651858.CD005623.pub2

Eastridge, D. K. (2009). An integrative review of interventions to reduce peripheral arterial disease risk factor in African Americans. *Journal of Vascular Nursing, 27*(2), 31–45.

Hart, P. L. (2005). Women's perceptions of coronary heart disease: An integrative review. *Journal of Cardiovascular Nursing, 20*(3), 170–176. [Posted with a Profile & Commentary at the companion website for this book, ***go.jblearning.com/brown.***]

Kropski, J. A., Keckley, P. H., & Jensen, G. L. (2008). School-based obesity prevention programs: An evidence-based review. *Obesity, 16*(5), 1009–1018.

Leef, K. H. (2006). Evidence-based review of oral sucrose administration to decrease the pain response in newborn infants. *Neonatal Network, 25*(4), 275–284.

O'Keefe-McCarthy, S., Santiago, C., & Lau, G. (2008). Ventilator-associated pneumonia bundled strategies: An evidence-based practice. *Worldviews on Evidence-Based Nursing, 5*(4), 193–204.

Sandelowski, M., Lambe, C., & Barroso, J. (2004). Stigma in HIV-positive women. *Journal of Nursing Scholarship, 36*(2), 122–128. [A metasynthesis]

Sherrington, C., Whitney, J. C., Lord, S. R., Herbert, R.D., & Cumming, R. G. (2008). Effective exercise for the prevention of falls: A systematic review and meta-analysis. *Journal of American Geriatric Society, 56,* 2234–2243. [Includes meta-analysis]

Vanderwee, K., Grypdonck, M., & Defloor, T. (2008). Alternating air pressure mattresses as prevention for pressure ulcers: A literature review. *International Journal of Nursing Studies, 45,* 784–801.

CHAPTER TEN
Evidence-Based Clinical Practice Guidelines

Early in the book, research findings were described as raw products that must be transformed into products that can be used in practice. Often, research findings are summarized in a systematic research review, and the conclusions of the systematic research review are used to produce an evidence-based clinical practice guideline (EbCPG). The recommendations of the evidence-based clinical practice guideline are subsequently translated into an agency-specific clinical protocol, which sets forth specific actions to guide nurses in giving care (these agency protocols are described in the next part of the book).

Thus, there is an often used, multi-phase process whereby research findings are transformed into the care standards of an agency clinical protocol (see Figure 10–1). The early steps can be performed by nurse-academics or clinical scholars, but the last step, development of an agency-specific clinical protocol, is always performed by a work group in the clinical agency. To effectively complete the development of a clinical protocol the panel developing it must:

- Agree on quality standards for evidence to be admitted
- Resolve differences of opinion about the quality of individual pieces of evidence
- Figure out how to deal with inconsistent findings from several studies
- Talk through differences of opinion about whether the evidence is conclusive enough to use as a basis for practice
- Decide whether to issue recommendations when no research evidence exists

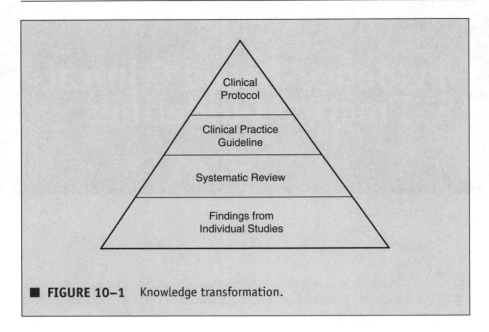

■ **FIGURE 10–1** Knowledge transformation.

Clarifications

When the recommendations of a clinical practice guideline are translated into practice standards for a particular agency or health system, we call it a clinical protocol. Having made a distinction between clinical practice guidelines and clinical protocols, we must recognize that some agencies and healthcare systems refer to protocols specific to their agency as clinical practice guidelines. However, for the purpose of clarity in this book, the term *clinical practice guideline* is used to refer to a set of generic recommendations, whereas clinical practice protocol, or more simply clinical protocol, refers to standards for care endorsed by a healthcare providing agency. The adjective *generic* conveys that clinical practice guidelines are designed for use across a variety of settings, thus the recommendations made are context-free.

There is another bit of confusion arising from the fact that any professional association, government agency, or health system can produce clinical practice guidelines using whatever process and standards they wish. Increasingly the standard in all healthcare professions is that clinical practice guidelines be research-based to the extent possible. Indeed, as I explain in just a bit, there is even considerable agreement in the healthcare professions regarding the production process for clinical practice guidelines. In this chapter, I use the abbreviation EbCPG to make it clear that the guidelines to which I refer are based on research evidence complemented by expert opinion when necessary.

A case could be made that expert opinion is evidence even though it is somewhat subjective; it is much like the testimony of a reliable eye-witness of an event—better than no witness but not as strong as physical evidence. The fact that expert opinion is the opinion of the whole panel, not just one individual, adds to its credibility.

Production Process

Multidisciplinary groups and professional associations in many countries provide manuals regarding the development of clinical practice guidelines (AGREE Collaboration, 2010; Marek, 1995; Scottish Intercollegiate Guidelines Network [SIGN], 2010). Perhaps, a good place to start in getting a sense for how EbCPGs are produced is with SIGN's description of its methodology:

> SIGN guidelines are developed using an explicit methodology based on three core principles:
>
> - Development is carried out by multidisciplinary groups
> - A systematic review is conducted to identify and critically appraise the evidence
> - Recommendations are explicitly linked to the supporting evidence (Scottish Intercollegiate Guidelines Network, 2008)

These principles capture in broad brush strokes most of the standards put forth by other groups, and thus they can serve as the structure for a description of EbCPGs.

Panel Composition and Expertise

The professional association or organization commissioning the development of a guideline typically provides specific goals for the development panel and decides on the composition of the development panel. Some groups such as SIGN design for an international audience, whereas others develop the guideline for a national audience or a discipline-specific audience. The important point is that all stakeholders, that is, those who will be affected by the EbCPG, should be represented on the development panel. Panel members are chosen to ensure that the needed expertise is at the table. That would include the following:

- Clinical expertise in the various issues the guideline will address
- Research expertise to help appraise study quality and interpret the study results
- Evidence-based practice expertise to ensure sound transfer of knowledge from science to clinical recommendations
- Information search and retrieval expertise to help locate research evidence
- Group process expertise to facilitate the development process, group dynamics, and consensus decision making

Evidence

Scope   Assuming clear and specific goals, the production process begins with a search for research evidence and other objective evidence related to the clinical issues that will be addressed in the guideline. The scope of this retrieval effort depends on whether the guideline is broad or focused. An example of a broad guideline is the American Society of PeriAnesthesia Nurses' (ASPAN) guideline on the prevention and management of postoperative nausea and vomiting (2006), which addressed many sub-issues including risk factor assessment, prevention, pharmacological management, complementary modalities, and post-discharge nausea and vomiting. To produce this guideline, the project directors recruited 16 experts from several healthcare disciplines with expertise in these sub-issues, and then searched and retrieved research articles on each of these issues. After the subgroups had read the reports related to their sub-issue, a consensus conference was held to critique and summarize the research evidence on each of the issues and to develop evidence-based recommendations.

In contrast, the National Association of Orthopaedic Nurses (NAON) commissioned a seven-member panel to produce a guideline on a much more focused topic, nursing management of skeletal pin sites (Baird Holmes & Brown, 2005). For various kinds of orthopaedic fractures and skeletal corrections, pins are inserted through the bone and attached to an external frame that stabilizes the bone pieces so they will heal. These pins come out through the skin and have the potential to develop infection at that point. Four advanced practice nurses, a staff nurse, a nurse researcher, and an orthopaedic surgeon comprised the panel. An extensive search of the literature produced only seven studies examining the relationship between pin site care and infection; two of these were randomized experiments. As a result of the limited number of studies, only three research-based and one expert opinion recommendations were offered.

I suggest that you look at the ASPAN or NAON articles (American Society of PeriAnesthesia Nurses, 2006; Holmes & Brown, 2005) because they provide a good sense of the production process as well as how recommendations are stated.

Types of Evidence   The evidence used to develop EbCPGs varies widely depending on how much research has been done on the various issues that make up the guideline. If a great deal of research has been done, it is likely that a published systematic review (or several of them) will be available; if this review is of high quality and is current, the guideline development panel can use it as the basis for their work. If the review is several years old, the panel will have to check out studies published since those that were included in the review. Increasingly, several relevant, evidence-based clinical practice guidelines are available and can be used in developing the new guideline, which may have a slightly different focus or just be an update.

If no systematic review or previous EbCPG can be located, the panel will have to locate relevant original (also called primary) studies, and conduct a systematic review before formulating recommendations. Depending on the topic, there may be sub-issues for which there is no research or very limited research, and the panel has to base their recommendations on the expert opinions of those on the panel. When this is the case, they often offer them as *practice points* or *practice pearls* to distinguish them from recommendations, which are research-based.

Level of Evidence?   A controversial question is, Are some types of evidence better than others? For evidence regarding the effectiveness of a nursing intervention or medical treatment, the answer is clearly yes. There is wide agreement that randomized experiments, and especially randomized controlled trials (RCTs), are the strongest study designs for evaluating the causal relationship between a clinical intervention and patient outcomes. As described in the previous chapter, if several randomized experiments of the same intervention have been conducted, a systematic review (SR) of them provides additional information about the consistency of findings across studies. Thus, if the experimental studies included in the SR were well conducted and if the SR itself was well done, the conclusions of a systematic review of experimental studies are considered better evidence than are the findings of a single or several experimental studies.

On the other hand, studies that do not use random assignment of participants to treatment groups are considered a weaker form of support for intervention effectiveness because confounding variables are not as well controlled. This deficit leads to a lower level of confidence in the results of observational studies of intervention effectiveness—observational studies being descriptive, correlational, and cohort studies. And lowest on the hierarchy of evidence regarding intervention effectiveness are surveys, case studies, and expert opinion.

The logic just described regarding evidence relevant to intervention effectiveness leads to evidence ranking systems that grade types of evidence from the strongest to the weakest. There are many such grading systems, also called evidence hierarchies. A typical one, used by the University of Iowa Gerontological Nursing Interventions Research Center (see Box 10–1), places a systematic review at the top of the ranking hierarchy followed by at least one randomized controlled trial. Also, note the use of the qualifiers such as "well-designed," "consistent results," and "high quality."

Role of Qualitative Studies   In most of the evidence grading systems pertaining to interventions, it is not clear how qualitative research studies should be ranked—most of the levels systems don't even mention them. That is unfortunate because qualitative studies often provide information about the following:

- The acceptability of an intervention to patients
- Problems patients have following a particular treatment regimen
- How following provider recommendations intrudes on daily living
- The extent to which patients consistently integrate treatment recommendations into their daily lives

Clearly, these are important considerations when evaluating the evidence in support of an intervention. They shed light on the use or adherence aspect of effectiveness, which may be different than effectiveness under the controlled circumstances of an experimental study. Real patient-world effectiveness of an intervention or treatment is most likely a combination of direct physiological or psychological action and patient-use factors.

Box 10–1   EVIDENCE GRADING

SCHEME FOR GRADING THE STRENGTH AND CONSISTENCY OF EVIDENCE IN THE GUIDELINE

A1 = Evidence from well-designed meta-analysis or well-done systematic review with results that consistently support a specific action (e.g., assessment, intervention, or treatment)

A2 = Evidence from one or more randomized controlled trials with consistent results

B1 = Evidence from high-quality evidence-based practice guideline

B2 = Evidence from one or more quasi-experimental studies with consistent results

C1 = Evidence from observational studies with consistent results (e.g., correlational, descriptive studies)

C2 = Evidence from observational studies or controlled trials with inconsistent results

D = Evidence from expert opinion, multiple case reports, or national consensus reports

Source: Courtesy of Research Translation & Dissemination Core. University of Iowa College of Nursing (NIH Grants P30NR03979, PI. Toni Tripp-Reimer). Used with permission.

Many nursing organizations that produce EbCPGs recognize the value of incorporating findings from qualitative research studies, and recently several medical organizations have become open to them. The following statement is from the Cochrane Collaboration (2010):

> Systematic reviews largely ignore the complexity of clinical problems and the social aspects of health care. The Cochrane Collaboration is working on how qualitative studies can be used to inform and add to the information obtained from controlled studies—where the outcomes are often measured in numerical terms (and so are termed quantitative studies). Qualitative measures include "quality of life" and lifestyle changes obtained from detailed questionnaires. Qualitative studies use narrative interviews where participants are asked to talk about their experiences around sets of semi-structured questions and prompts to explore particular issues that information is needed on for a study.

A similar statement has been issued by the Scottish Intercollegiate Guidelines Network (2008). So qualitative research is gaining respect for its unique contribution to intervention knowledge.

Evaluating a Body of Evidence   There is also increasing recognition that it is important to consider more than just the type of design used to produce evidence in support of a recommendation. Thus, systems are being developed to evaluate the body of evidence supporting guideline recommendations. These systems recognize the following features of a body of evidence:

- The aggregate quality of the individual studies
- The number of studies addressing the issue
- The consistency of the findings across studies (Agency for Healthcare Research and Quality, 2002)
- The precision of the estimate of the treatment effect in the population

Quality addresses whether the studies in the body of evidence were well conducted. *Consistency* addresses whether the body of evidence reveals treatment effect in the same direction (e.g., most studies found that a positive, clinically significant outcome resulted from the intervention). A precise estimate of the treatment effect in the population is afforded when confidence intervals around treatment effect measures are narrow (see Box 10–2).

Recommendation-Evidence Linkage

Ideally, for each recommendation of an EbCPG, there is a discussion of the relevant evidence, supporting references, and/or an evidence grade indicating the strength of the evidence supporting the recommendation. For instance, in a guideline on acute confusion/delirium in the elderly by the University of Iowa Gerontological Nursing Interventions Research Center, Research Translation

---

Box 10–2   EXAMPLE OF PRECISE POPULATION ESTIMATE

In a systematic research review of interventions for preventing falls in older people living in the community (Gillespie et al., 2009), it was reported that pooled data from 14 studies of group exercise involving several types of exercise showed a reduction in the rate of falls. The relative risk (RR) was 0.78, 95% CI = 0.71 to 0.82. This result means that the fall risk of those in exercise groups was 78% that of those in the usual activity groups; although in the population, persons who exercise would have 71% to 82% of the risk of those who do not exercise. (If the RR were 1, the risk of the two groups would be equal; a RR value less than 1 indicates lower risk and a value higher than 1 indicates greater risk.) This confidence interval is narrow (11% points), thus it provides the clinician-reader with a fairly precise estimate of the risk reduction that might be experienced from exercise programs in the population.

and Dissemination Core, the following recommendations were offered regarding assessment; each recommendation is followed by supporting references and the grade of the supporting evidence, which is based on the grading system in Box 10–1 (National Guideline Clearinghouse, 2010):

- Nurses should maintain a high index of suspicion for delirium in the older adult, specifically for those with more predisposing factors that increase risk for delirium (Inouye et al., 1993; Registered Nurses Association of Ontario [RNAO], 2003. *Evidence Grade = B1*).
- Nurses must recognize that delirium may be superimposed on dementia and differentiate baseline from more acute changes in cognitive function (Fick & Foreman, 2000; Fick, Agostini, & Inouye, 2002; RNAO, 2003; Royal College of Physicians, 2006. *Evidence Grade = A1*).
- Assessment for predisposing/vulnerability factors for delirium should occur on hospital admission and are the most powerful factors for identifying patients at greatest risk for developing delirium (Inouye & Charpentier, 1996; Inouye et al., 1993; Pompei et al., 1994; Schor et al., 1992; Williams-Russo et al., 1992. *Evidence Grade = C1*).

Other developers grade the recommendations instead of, or in addition to, rating the evidence. The U.S. Preventive Services Task Forces grading system (Box 10–3) includes both the strength of the recommendation and the likelihood of benefit if the recommendation is implemented. The system in Box 10–4 was used to grade the recommendations in a guideline regarding nonpharmacologic treatment of chronic insomnia in the elderly produced by the University of Texas School of Nursing Family Nurse Practitioner program (University of Texas School of Nursing, 2005). Note that it also links the recommendation to an underlying level of evidence.

As you can see, there is no standardized way of representing the supporting evidence for the recommendations in a clinical practice guideline. Neither is there a uniform standard for determining how strong the evidence should be to make a recommendation. Generally, the answer depends on the evidence available and on the consequences of causing harm by issuing a recommendation that is not supported by strong research evidence. In addition to grading systems, some authors summarize the research evidence regarding a recommendation or course of action with descriptive terms (see Appendix A). You should also note that all of these evidence grading systems recognize expert opinion as a backup form of evidence. In short, "opinion often fills in the gaps in the evidence base" (Steinberg & Luce, 2005, p. 84).

Box 10–3 EXAMPLE OF RECOMMENDATION GRADING

What the Grades Mean and Suggestions for Practice

The U.S. Preventive Services Task Force (USPSTF) has updated its definitions of the grades it assigns to recommendations and now includes "suggestions for practice" associated with each grade. The USPSTF has also defined levels of certainty regarding net benefit. These definitions apply to USPSTF recommendations voted on after May 2007.

Grade	Definition	Suggestions for practice
A	The USPSTF recommends the service. There is high certainty that the net benefit is substantial.	Offer or provide this service.
B	The USPSTF recommends the service. There is high certainty that the net benefit is moderate or there is moderate certainty that the net benefit is moderate to substantial.	Offer or provide this service.
C	The USPSTF recommends against routinely providing the service. There may be considerations that support providing the service in an individual patient. There is at least moderate certainty that the net benefit is small.	Offer or provide this service only if other considerations support offering or providing the service to an individual patient.
D	The USPSTF recommends against the service. There is moderate or high certainty that the service has no net benefit or that the harms outweigh the benefits.	Discourage the use of this service.
I Statement	The USPSTF concludes that the current evidence is insufficient to assess the balance of benefits and harms of the service. Evidence is lacking, conflicting, or of poor quality, and the balance of benefits and harms cannot be determined.	

Source: Agency for Healthcare Research and Quality. (2008). *Grade definitions after May 2007.* Retrieved from http://www.ahrq.gov/clinic/uspstf/gradespost.htm

> **Box 10–4   EXAMPLE OF LEVELS OF RECOMMENDATIONS**
>
> **Standard:** This is a generally accepted patient-care strategy that reflects a high degree of clinical certainty. The term *standard* generally implies the use of Level I evidence, which directly addresses the clinical issue, or overwhelming Level II evidence.
>
> **Guideline:** This is a patient-care strategy that reflects a moderate degree of clinical certainty. The term *guideline* implies the use of Level II evidence or a consensus of Level III evidence.
>
> **Option:** This is a patient-care strategy that reflects uncertain clinical use. The term *option* implies either inconclusive or conflicting evidence or conflicting expert opinion.
>
> *Source:* University of Texas School of Nursing, Family Nurse Practitioner Program. (2005). Practice parameters for the nonpharmacologic treatment of chronic primary insomnia in the elderly. Retrieved from http://www.guideline.gov/summary/summary.aspx?doc_id=7354&nbr=004352&string=elderly.

Formats

If you look on the National Guideline Clearinghouse website (http://www.guideline.gov) or the Registered Nurses' Association of Ontario website (http://www.rnao.org/Page.asp?PageID=861&SiteNodeID=133), you will notice that many of the guidelines are quite long. There are several reasons for this:

1. The broad nature of the guideline's purpose
2. The inclusion in the guideline of details about the research evidence
3. Inclusion of a description of the guideline production process
4. Recommendations are made for practice, education, and organizations

Although there is no standardized format for EbCPGs, the one that follows, which is used by the Registered Nurses' Association of Ontario, is typical:

    I. Title
   II. Producing Agency (Date)
 III. Table of Contents

To make guidelines more convenient and usable for clinicians, some EbCPG producers issue a quick reference guide separate from the full version of the guideline. Quick reference guides typically list the recommendations and indicate a level of support for each recommendation but do not present the supporting research evidence; the reader must go elsewhere to view a summary of the evidence. Importantly, the production process should be described in one of these documents or in an accompanying document because this is the only way clinicians can determine if the guideline was developed using sound methodology. Recently, the Registered Nurses' Association of Ontario (RNAO) began making available abbreviated versions of their guidelines for personal digital assistants (PDAs).

With this introduction under your belt, I highly recommend that you look at Appendix B, which contains a 22-step process for producing an evidence-based clinical practice guideline. I have used it in consulting with professional associations that want to produce an EbCPG. These are action steps, not abstract principles. Twenty-two steps may seem excessive, but the reality is that producing an EbCPG is a rigorous, demanding, and expensive undertaking. As you go over the steps, try to picture yourself as a member of a professional association panel that is creating an EbCPG.

Exemplar

📖 *Reading Tips*

The version of the EbCPG you are about to read is a reduction of the full guideline. The reprinted sections introduce the guideline, how it was produced, the full set of recommendations, and the evidence relative to exercise and lifestyle modification. Large sections about psychological therapies, self-help, alternative therapies, and herbal therapies are not included in the reprint.

To truly get a sense for this guideline, it is best to establish a link to the SIGN methodology website (http://www.sign.ac.uk/guidelines/fulltext/50/index.html) so you can refer to it as suggested in the guideline and in my commentary.

Note that the abbreviation CBT stands for cognitive behavioral therapy, and the ☑ symbol indicates a Good Practice Point, which is a non-research-based recommendation based on the clinical experience of the guideline development panel.

Non-pharmaceutical Management of Depression in Adults: A National Clinical Guideline

Scottish Intercollegiate Guidelines Network

(2010). Retrieved from http://www.sign.ac.uk/pdf/sign114.pdf

KEY TO EVIDENCE STATEMENTS AND GRADES OF RECOMMENDATIONS

LEVELS OF EVIDENCE

1++   High quality meta-analyses, systematic reviews of RCTs, or RCTs with a very low risk of bias

1+   Well conducted meta-analyses, systematic reviews, or RCTs with a low risk of bias

1-   Meta-analyses, systematic reviews, or RCTs with a high risk of bias

2++   High quality systematic reviews of case control or cohort studies

High quality case control or cohort studies with a very low risk of confounding or bias and a high probability that the relationship is causal

2+   Well conducted case control or cohort studies with a low risk of confounding or bias and a moderate probability that the relationship is causal

2-   Case control or cohort studies with a high risk of confounding or bias and a significant risk that the relationship is not causal

3   Non-analytic studies, e.g., case reports, case series

4   Expert opinion

GRADES OF RECOMMENDATION

Note: The grade of recommendation relates to the strength of the evidence on which the recommendation is based. It does not reflect the clinical importance of the recommendation.

A   At least one meta-analysis, systematic review, or RCT rated as 1^{++}, and directly applicable to the target population; *or*

A body of evidence consisting principally of studies rated as 1^{+}, directly applicable to the target population, and demonstrating overall consistency of results

B   A body of evidence including studies rated as 2^{++}, directly applicable to the target population, and demonstrating overall consistency of results; *or*

Extrapolated evidence from studies rated as 1^{++} or 1^{+}

C   A body of evidence including studies rated as 2^{+}, directly applicable to the target population and demonstrating overall consistency of results; *or*

Extrapolated evidence from studies rated as 2^{++}

D   Evidence level 3 or 4; *or*

Extrapolated evidence from studies rated as 2^{+}

GOOD PRACTICE POINTS

☑   Recommended best practice based on the clinical experience of the guideline development group.

NHS Quality Improvement Scotland (NHS QIS) is committed to equality and diversity and assesses all its publications for likely impact on the six equality groups defined by age, disability, gender, race, religion/belief and sexual orientation.

SIGN guidelines are produced using a standard methodology that has been **equality impact assessed** to ensure that these equality aims are addressed in every guideline. This methodology is set out in the current version of SIGN 50, our guideline manual, which can be found at **www.sign.ac.uk/guidelines/fulltext/50/index.html** The EQIA assessment of the manual can be seen at **www.sign.ac.uk/pdf/sign50eqia.pdf** The full report in paper form and/or alternative format is available on request from the NHS QIS Equality and Diversity Officer.

Every care is taken to ensure that this publication is correct in every detail at the time of publication. However, in the event of errors or omissions corrections will be published in the web version of this document, which is the definitive version at all times. This version can be found on our web site **www.sign.ac.uk**

Contents

1 Introduction

1.1 Background

Depression is a significant health problem. It affects men and women of all ages and social backgrounds. Around one in five of the population of Scotland will experience depression at some point in their lives.[1] Prevalence is higher in women than men.[1] It can range in severity from a mild disturbance to a severe illness with a high risk of suicide. The impact of the disorder will also be experienced by family, friends and colleagues.[2] In Scotland in 2006/07 there were around 500,000 general practitioner consultations with depression and other affective disorders.[3] Over half of those with depression do not seek formal treatment.[4]

As well as the personal and social consequences of depression there are also negative economic effects. Depression is associated with sickness absence and prevents many people seeking, maintaining or returning to employment. In an economic analysis the total loss of output due to depression and chronic anxiety in England in 2002/3 was estimated at £12 billion.[5]

The most common intervention for depression is prescribed antidepressant medication. A total of 3.65 million items of antidepressant medication were prescribed in Scotland during 2006/07 at a cost of £43.7m. It is estimated that 8.8% of the Scottish population aged 15 and over make daily use of antidepressant medication.[6]

1.2 The Need for a Guideline

Depression Alliance Scotland proposed the development of this guideline based on feedback from service users who were seeking information about interventions, other than prescribed antidepressants, which could be helpful in treating depression. This highlighted the need for accessible and robust information about the alternatives to prescribed antidepressants to be available to both GPs and service users.

The Scottish Integrated Care Pathway (ICP) for depression sets standards for appropriate care and treatment of people with depression. This includes a standard that requires an offer of matched self help and signposting to other services. It also states that for those who choose a non-pharmacological approach, or for whom medication is not effective, there should be the offer of a brief depression-focused psychological intervention.[7]

A small qualitative primary care study (n = 60) of patients with depression found that almost two thirds had attempted to use self chosen therapies, although few had discussed their use with health practitioners. A broad range of therapies was identified. The most commonly reported were

St John's wort, counselling, relaxation tapes and gym, walking or other leisure interests.[8]

1.3 Remit of the Guideline

The focus of the guideline is to examine the evidence for depression treatments which may be used as alternatives to prescribed pharmacological therapies. Interventions were prioritised for inclusion by the guideline development group if they were known to be delivered, or be under consideration for delivery, by NHS services in Scotland or if, based on the experience of group members, they were interventions which patients asked about or sought outside of the health service.

Depression is often a multifactorial illness with biological, social and psychological factors all contributing to the development, severity and length of a depressive episode. During a period of depression, people typically report symptoms in all three domains: at a biological level, e.g., sleep disruption, appetite changes; at a psychological level, e.g., impaired concentration and memory, increased negative thinking; and at a social level, e.g., loss of self confidence, withdrawal from social contact. Recovery in one of these domains may be reflected in concurrent improvement in the others; thus the interventions for depression examined in this guideline are wide ranging, covering both biological and psychosocial modes.

This guideline examines psychological therapies, exercise and lifestyle interventions, and complementary and alternative treatments, many of which are not routinely available within the NHS. This guideline provides an assessment of, and presents the evidence base for, the efficacy of these interventions for depression in adults aged 18 years and over. Therapies commonly available to patients without prescription in Scotland were selected for inclusion and are described in Annex 1. The key questions on which the guideline is based are outlined in Annex 2.

This guideline focuses on systematic review and randomised controlled trial (RCT) evidence of effectiveness, with searches extended to identify observational studies only where appropriate.

Unless otherwise stated, recommendations apply to adults aged 18 years and over with no upper age limit.

Depression in children and young people is a significant issue but is beyond the scope of this guideline development project.

1.4 Defining the Patient Group

The evidence base for depression presents several difficulties including the wide range of diagnostic and severity definitions and the heterogeneity and lack of equivalence between measures. The guideline development group adopted a pragmatic definition of depression. Given the nature of the treatment approaches studied, study populations tended to be patients with mild to moderate depression. Many studies either do not make clear the severity of depression studied and/or use diagnostic systems that do not include severity descriptors.

Studies were excluded where there was no formal diagnosis by International Classification of Disease (ICD) 9, ICD 10, Diagnostic Statistical Manual (DSM)-III or DSM-IV, or use of a recognised, validated and reliable measurement scale specifically for depressive symptoms.

Studies in patient groups with clear indicators of severe depression or with significant psychological comorbidities were excluded as below:

- psychotic depression
- depression in the perinatal period (which includes postnatal depression)
- bipolar disorder
- personality disorder
- dysthymia
- seasonal affective disorder
- primary addiction
- significant cognitive impairment (brain injury or dementia)
- learning disability.

Studies in patients with significant physical comorbidities were also excluded.

A large number of studies of depression had mixed patient groups, typically with anxiety disorders and personality disorders. Individual studies were excluded unless there was clear analysis of the depression subgroup. Where recommendations were based on systematic reviews which included studies with mixed patient groups this was taken into account when grading recommendations.

The guideline development group recognised the limitations of adopting such specific diagnostic criteria in terms of applicability to routine care populations, but required a clear remit to assure rigour in study selection and analysis.

1.5 Outcomes

The primary outcome of interest was reduction in depressive symptoms as measured by a recognised depression scale. Short term outcomes and longer term benefits were examined.

Where appropriate, secondary outcomes including illness duration, relapse, quality of life, and patient satisfaction were considered.

1.6 Target Audience

This guideline will be of particular interest to those developing mental health services, healthcare professionals in primary and secondary care, and patients with depression and their carers. It may also be helpful to voluntary organisations and exercise professionals working in exercise referral schemes, public or private fitness centres, and promotion of physical activity.

1.7 Statement of Intent

This guideline is not intended to be construed or to serve as a standard of care. Standards of care are determined on the basis of all clinical data available for an individual case and are subject to change as scientific knowledge and technology advance and patterns of care evolve. Adherence to guideline recommendations will not ensure a successful outcome in every case, nor should they be construed as including all proper methods of care or excluding other acceptable methods of care aimed at the same results. The ultimate judgement must be made by the appropriate healthcare professional(s) responsible for clinical decisions regarding a particular clinical procedure or treatment plan. This judgement should only be arrived at following discussion of the options with the patient, covering the diagnostic and treatment choices available. It is advised, however, that significant departures from the national guideline or any local guidelines derived from it should be fully documented in the patient's case notes at the time the relevant decision is taken.

1.7.1 Patient Version

A patient version of this guideline is available from the SIGN website, www.sign.ac.uk

1.7.2 Additional Advice to NHSScotland from NHS Quality Improvement Scotland and the Scottish Medicines Consortium

NHS QIS processes multiple technology appraisals (MTAs) for NHSScotland that have been produced by the National Institute for Health and Clinical Excellence (NICE) in England and Wales.

The Scottish Medicines Consortium (SMC) provides advice to NHS Boards and their Area Drug and Therapeutics Committees about the status of all newly licensed medicines and any major new indications for established products.

SMC advice and NHS QIS validated NICE MTAs relevant to this guideline are summarised in the section on implementation.

2 Summary of Recommendations

2.1 Psychological Therapies

A   Behavioural activation is recommended as a treatment option for patients with depression.

A   Individual CBT is recommended as a treatment option for patients with depression.

A   Interpersonal therapy is recommended as a treatment option for patients with depression.

B   Mindfulness based cognitive therapy in a group setting may be considered as a treatment option to reduce relapse in patients with depression who have had three or more episodes.

B   Problem solving therapy may be considered as a treatment option for patients with depression.

B   Short term psychodynamic psychotherapy may be considered as a treatment option for patients with depression.

2.2 Self Help

A   Guided self help based on CBT or behavioural principles is recommended as a treatment option for patients with depression.

A   Within the context of guided self help, computerised CBT is recommended as a treatment option for patients with depression.

2.3 Structured Exercise

B   Structured exercise may be considered as a treatment option for patients with depression.

5 Exercise and Lifestyle Modification

5.1 Exercise

Studies described relate to structured exercise interventions (*see Annex 1*).

The effects of both aerobic exercise (e.g., walking and jogging) and anaerobic exercise (e.g., weight training) have been examined in younger and older adults with depression, with a large variety of intervention types delivered across a range of settings.[45-58] There is a larger evidence base for aerobic exercise than for anaerobic exercise. Limitations of the evidence base include small sample sizes in many studies and the use of volunteer subjects who may be particularly motivated to adhere to an exercise programme.

A Cochrane meta-analysis of 23 trials from 1979–2007 (n = 907)   **1++**
found a large and statistically significant clinical effect of exercise
(measured post-treatment) when compared to no treatment or control intervention. The effect was moderate when the five trials with
long term follow up were analysed separately. Only three trials in
the Cochrane review were assessed as high quality with respect to
allocation concealment, intention to treat analysis and blinded outcome assessment. A meta-analysis of these trials (n = 216) found a
moderate clinical benefit which was not statistically significant
(standardised mean difference –0.42 (95% CI –0.88, 0.03).[59]

Those trials which systematically reported adverse events found   **1++**
that adverse events were low in both the exercise and control
groups. There was between 55% and 100% completion of exercise
interventions.[59]

In comparisons of effectiveness with antidepressant medication and   **1++**
CBT there was no difference between exercise and the established
interventions.[59]

The benefits of exercise have generally been shown to be inde-   **1+**
pendent of social group effect.[50-54]

A small number of studies were identified which examined the   **1+**
duration, frequency and intensity of physical activity required to
produce benefit.

The results of one study support the following minimum require-   **1++**
ments: three sessions per week; of 30-40 minutes duration each; and
a total energy expenditure of 17 kcal/kg per week. Similar effects
were also found for five sessions per week of 30 minutes at a lower
intensity with similar total energy expenditure.[50,60] Other studies
suggest a required intensity of exercise correlated to energy expenditure of 70-80% of heart rate reserve (*see Annex 1*).[45-47,49,56,61]

B   Structured exercise may be considered as a treatment option for
patients with depression.

☑   Individuals who are interested in using structured exercise as a treatment intervention for depression should be referred to appropriate
exercise counselling and activities in their local community that are
relevant to the type of exercise they feel they will enjoy. This may
include a range of community provision e.g., local gyms, swimming
pools, and voluntary walking groups. If there are doubts about the

individual's physical health they should be referred back to the GP for health/cardiovascular assessment.

☑   The physical activity readiness questionnaire (PAR-Q) provides a validated tool to determine whether individuals require screening investigations ahead of commencing a structured exercise programme. (www.csep.ca/CMFiles/publications/parq/par-q.pdf).

☑   Patients should be made aware of factors which may improve and help maintain motivation. For example: setting realistic goals may allow individuals to monitor their progress; exercising with others; and an exercise class or buddy system can increase enjoyment.

Annex 3 outlines resources related to physical activity for health.

5.2 Lifestyle Modification

5.2.1 Reducing Alcohol Consumption

No good quality evidence was identified on the effect of reducing alcohol consumption on depressive symptoms.

Examination of alcohol consumption as a causative factor in depression was outside the scope of the guideline.

Primary care interventions for patients with alcohol dependence, hazardous or harmful drinking are described in SIGN 74.[62]

5.2.2 Reducing Caffeine Intake

No good quality evidence was identified on the effects of reducing caffeine intake on depressive symptoms.

5.2.3 Return to Work

No evidence applicable to the UK employment and benefits systems was identified on the effectiveness of return to work programmes in reducing depressive symptoms.

5.2.4 Good Practice in Lifestyle Advice for Patients with Depression

☑   General advice on following a healthy lifestyle is relevant in the management of patients with depression. Advice should address:
  • alcohol and drug use
  • diet and eating behaviours
  • maintenance of social networks and personally meaningful activities
  • sleep problems.

10 The Evidence Base

10.1 Systematic Literature Review

The evidence base for this guideline was synthesised in accordance with SIGN methodology. A systematic review of the literature was carried out using an explicit search strategy devised by a SIGN Information Officer. Databases searched include Medline, Embase, Cinahl, PsycINFO, AMED, and the Cochrane Library. The year range covered was 1998-2008 with variations depending on topic. Internet searches were carried out on various websites including the US National Guidelines Clearinghouse. A complete search narrative, including search strategies and date ranges for each key question, is available on the SIGN website. The main searches were supplemented by material identified by individual members of the development group. Each of the selected papers was evaluated by two members of the group using standard SIGN methodological checklists before conclusions were considered as evidence.

10.2 Recommendations for Research

For many of the interventions described in this guideline there was little or no robust published evidence. This was particularly the case for complementary and alternative therapies, nutritional therapies, alcohol reduction and self help groups. In addition to a lack of primary studies on such interventions a number of wider research themes were identified:

- validity of trial designs for psychological therapies
- dose-response studies for effective psychological therapies
- factors which contribute to drop-out
- non-specific treatment factors including patient/therapist interaction
- patient selection for psychological therapies
- long term effectiveness of non-pharmaceutical interventions
- contribution of unstructured exercise to beneficial effects on mood
- optimum type of exercise (aerobic, mixed or strength)
- how exercise programmes can best be facilitated through primary care.

10.3 Review and Updating

This guideline was issued in 2010 and will be considered for review in three years. Any updates to the guideline in the interim period will be noted on the SIGN website: www.sign.ac.uk.

ANNEX 1: DEFINITIONS OF INTERVENTIONS

SECTION 4 SELF HELP

Computerised self help	Online or computer based packages of self help material.
Guided self help	Self help interventions which incorporate some form of therapist support.
Self help interventions	Self help interventions cover a range of interactive packages, paper or web-based written self help materials. Interventions supporting access to self help books may be termed bibliotherapy or books on prescription.

SECTION 5 EXERCISE AND LIFESTYLE INTERVENTIONS

Exercise	Exercise is a subset of physical activity, which is any movement of the body that results in energy expenditure rising above resting level, and includes activities of daily living, domestic chores, gardening and walking.
Structured exercise	Exercise that is undertaken three or more times a week for 30–40 minutes at an intensity sufficient to provide an energy expenditure of 70–80% of heart rate reserve; this equates to the public health dose of accumulating 30 minutes of moderate intensity physical activity on most days of the week. Walking at a level of moderate intensity, slightly out of breath, most days of the week can achieve the public health dose.
	Heart rate reserve is a term used to describe the difference between a person's measured or predicted maximum heart rate and resting heart rate. Some methods of measurement of exercise intensity measure percentage of heart rate reserve. As a person increases their cardiovascular fitness, their resting heart rate will drop, thus the heart rate reserve will increase.

SECTION 6 HERBAL REMEDIES AND NUTRITIONAL SUPPLEMENTS

Chromium	A mineral that humans require in trace amounts.
Folate	Folic acid and folate (the anionic form) are forms of the water soluble vitamin B_9. These occur naturally in food and can also be taken as supplements.
Ginseng	A perennial plant which grows in eastern Asia. The root extract is widely available as a herbal remedy.
Ginkgo biloba	*Ginkgo biloba*, also known as the Maidenhair tree, is a unique species of tree, the fruits and seeds of which are used in traditional Chinese medicine. Leaf extracts are available as supplements.
Glutamine	A naturally occurring, non-essential amino acid.
Hypericum extract (St John's wort)	A perennial herb of the genus *Hypericum*.
Inositol	An isomer of glucose. It is a naturally occuring compound which is widely available as a dietary supplement.
Polyunsaturated fatty acids (PUFAs)	"Essential fatty acids" that humans cannot synthesise de novo; intake is dependent on dietary sources such as fish and seafood. The examples most studied are the omega-3 fatty acids eicosapentaenoic acid (EPA) and docosahexaenoic acid (DHA).
S-adenosyl-L-methionine (SAMe)	A coenzyme involved in methyl group transfers. It is available as a nutritional supplement.
Selenium	A non-metallic element which rarely occurs in its elemental state in nature.

ANNEX 2: KEY QUESTIONS USED TO DEVELOP THE GUIDELINE

This guideline is based on a series of structured key questions that, where possible, define the population concerned, the intervention under investigation, the type of comparison group, and the outcomes used to measure the effectiveness of the interventions. These questions form the basis of the systematic literature search.

THE KEY QUESTIONS USED TO DEVELOP THE GUIDELINE

DELIVERY OF CARE/LIFESTYLE AND SELF DIRECTED INTERVENTIONS

Compare with psychological therapies, pharmacological therapies, placebo or waiting list control. Consider short term effects and any longer term benefits.

KEY QUESTION	SEE GUIDELINE SECTION
1. Do the following lifestyle changes reduce depressive symptoms, and are any reductions in symptoms sustained? • reducing caffeine intake • reducing alcohol consumption • increasing physical activity • return to work	5.2
2. What is the effectiveness of assisted return to work programmes in alleviating depression compared with no assistance? Include: • assisted return to employment/education/ meaningful activity • back-to-work treatment • condition management • recovery-based treatment • rehabilitation • REMPLOY	5.2
3. What is the evidence for the effectiveness of the following on depressive symptoms? • bibliotherapy • self help support groups • guided self help • psychoeducation	4.1, 4.2, 4.3
4. What is the evidence for the effectiveness of exercise (any structured physical activity) alone or in combination with psychological therapies, on depressive symptoms?	5.1

Profile & Commentary

The topic is clearly set forth in the guideline title. The Contents page gives you a sense for the various non-pharmaceutical therapies considered and the format of the guideline as a whole. The Key to Evidence Statement and Grades of Recommendations section links recommendations to the underlying strength of evidence. Together they take the following into consideration: methodological quality of individual studies, design type, control of bias and confounding, and directness of applicability to the target population. The levels and grades appear throughout the document.

Section 1, Introduction, sets the stage for the recommendations by providing a clinical context for non-pharmaceutical treatments of depression. Although the background statement cites data from Scotland and England, there is no reason why the evidence used is not applicable in many other countries. In Section 2, Summary of Recommendations, all the recommendations are set forth. Notice the wording of the recommendations; some say: "is recommended" while others say "may be considered." This difference in vigor of the recommendations reflects the confidence in the recommendation resulting from varying strength of the supporting evidence. In Section 5 a summary of the evidence relevant to exercise is provided.

Methods

In Annex 2, you see the key questions pertaining to lifestyle modifications and exercise that were addressed in the guideline; six other key questions are not shown in the reprint.

The methods used to produce the guideline are a bit difficult to get a handle on because they are not spelled out in the guideline itself. Instead, in Section 10.1 it says that they follow the SIGN methodology. I suggest you look at the *Guideline Development Handbook* at http://www.sign.ac.uk/guidelines/fulltext/50/index.html. Chapters 6 (Systematic literature review) and 7 (Forming guideline recommendations) are particularly important to understanding the guideline development process.

The databases, websites, and dates used in the search for evidence for this guideline are briefly described in Section 10.1, but are spelled out in great detail in the file *Search Narrative* for which there is a link on the guideline's website.

Recommendations and Evidence

In Section 5.1 Exercise, we first read a discussion of the evidence related to exercise, which is comprised of 1+ or 1++ level studies. (Note that the statements about the evidence also have references.) However, it is noted that just three studies were appraised as high quality. Further, a meta-analysis of those three studies showed only a modest clinical benefit, which was not statistically significant. These weak features of the research base led the panel to issue a rather tentative recommendation, "Structured exercise may be considered," and three Good Practice Points.

For Lifestyle Modification (Section 5.2), the research is almost nonexistent. This is extremely unfortunate because these are probably suggestions that are frequently given to patients by healthcare providers. This impression is confirmed by the fact that the reviewers' experience led them to issue a Good Practice Point about alcohol and drug use, diet, maintaining social activities, and sleep problems.

Wrap-Up

I realize going back and forth between print and online documents makes it difficult for some readers to put the whole picture together; however, this is today's reality. Most guidelines these days are quite long, ranging from 20 pages to a few hundred pages. The upside is they often contain a wealth of information for agency work groups that are developing a local protocol or standard of care. You might want to take a look at the Quick Reference Guide (http://www.sign.ac.uk/pdf/qrg114.pdf), which provides a one-page summary of the main recommendations of this guideline. A Patient Booklet is also available on the guideline's website.

REFERENCES

Agency for Healthcare Research and Quality. (2002). *Systems to rate the strength of scientific evidence: Summary*. Retrieved from http://www.ncbi.nlm.nih.gov/bookshelf/br.fcgi?book=erta47

AGREE Collaboration. (2010). Home page. Retrieved from www.agreecollaboration.org

American Society of PeriAnesthesia Nurses. (2006). ASPAN's evidence-based clinical practice guideline for the prevention and/or management of PONV/PDNV. *Journal of Perianesthesia Nurses, 21*(4), 230–250. Retrieved from http://www.aspan.org/Portals/6/docs/ClinicalPractice/Guidelines/ASPAN_Clinical Guideline_PONV_PDNV.pdf

Cochrane Collaboration. (2010). *Cochrane Consumer Network*. Retrieved from http://consumers.cochrane.org/

Holmes, S. B., & Brown, S. J. (2005). Skeletal pin site care, National Association of Orthopaedic Nurses Guidelines for orthopaedic nursing. *Orthopaedic Nursing, 24*(2), 99–107. Retrieved from http://www.orthonurse.org/portals/0/images/pdf/pincare2005.pdf

Marek, K. D. (for American Nurses Association). (1995). *Manual to develop guidelines*. Washington, DC: American Nurses Publishing.

National Guideline Clearinghouse. (2010). *Brief summary. Guideline title: Evidence-based practice guideline. Acute confusion/delirium*. Retrieved from http://www.guideline.gov/summary/summary.aspx?doc_id=14340&nbr=7208#s24

Registered Nurses Association of Ontario. (2010). Home page. Retrieved from http://www.rnao.org

Scottish Intercollegiate Guidelines Network. (2008). *A guideline developer's handbook*. Retrieved from http://www.sign.ac.uk/guidelines/fulltext/50/index.html

Scottish Intercollegiate Guidelines Network. (2010). *Non-pharmaceutical management of depression in adults: A national clinical guideline*. Retrieved from http://www.sign.ac.uk/guidelines/fulltext/114/index.html

Steinberg, E. P., & Luce, B. R. (2005). Evidence based? Caveat emptor. *Health Affairs, 24*(1), 80–92.

University of Texas School of Nursing, Family Nurse Practitioner Program. (2005). Practice parameters for the nonpharmacologic treatment of chronic primary insomnia in the elderly. Retrieved from http://www.guideline.gov/summary/summary.aspx?doc_id=7354&nbr=004352&string=insomnia#s24

OTHER EVIDENCE-BASED CLINICAL PRACTICE GUIDELINES*

Chasens, E. R., Williams, L. L., & Umlauf, M. G. (2008). *Excessive sleepiness*. Retrieved from http://www.guideline.gov/summary/summary.aspx?ss=15&doc_id=12263&nbr=006347&string=sleepiness

Brady, M., Kinn, S., Ness, V., O'Rourke, K., Randhawa, N., & Stuart, P. (2009). Preoperative fasting for preventing perioperative complications in children. *Cochrane Collaboration*. Retrieved from http://mrw.interscience.wiley.com/cochrane/clsysrev/articles/CD005285/pdf_

Registered Nurses' Association of Ontario. (2004). Best practice guidelines for the subcutaneous administration of insulin in adults with type 2 diabetes. Toronto, Canada: Registered Nurses Association of Ontario. Retrieved from http://www.rnao.org/Page.asp?PageID=924&ContentID=794 [Reprint with Profile & Commentary posted on the companion website for this book, which can be accessed at *go.jblearning.com/brown.*]

Rubenstein, E., Peterson, D. E., Schubert, M., Keefe, D., McGuire, D., Epstein, J., et al. (2004). Clinical practice guideline for the prevention and treatment of cancer therapy-induced oral and gastrointestinal mucositis. *Cancer, 100* (Suppl. 9), 2026–2046.

University of Texas (Austin), School of Nursing. (2006). Unintentional weight loss in the elderly. Retrieved from http://www.guideline.gov/summary/summary.aspx? doc_id=9435&nbr=005056&string=University+AND+Texas

*Note: Several professional nursing associations sell their clinical practice guidelines in book form. The extent to which they are evidence based varies.

Evidence-Based Practice

From Part I, hopefully you have acquired an appreciation of and basic knowledge about the different kinds of research studies that are used to study nursing phenomena—and the desirable features of each. You also have basic knowledge about how systematic reviews are done and how evidence-based clinical practice guidelines are produced. Figure P2–1 graphically portrays the ground that is covered in the first part of the book. This knowledge is essential to using research evidence in your own nursing practice and to participating in evidence-based practice (EBP) projects in your work setting.

However, research knowledge is not enough; you also need to be able to find research evidence, appraise it, and consider how to use it in practice—and that is what this part of the book addresses. To this point, the focus has been on research evidence, and that will continue to be the focus in the next nine chapters, albeit from the perspective of appraising its quality and applicability. In Chapter 17, the lens is opened up and you will learn how research evidence is used in combination with other types of evidence. As a result, evidence-based practice in a broader sense will come into view.

The Evidence-Based Practice Impact Model

The Evidence-Based Practice Impact Model shown on the next page depicts the major steps in achieving effective evidence-based practice. Importantly, each step should be carried out using explicit and rigorous methods.

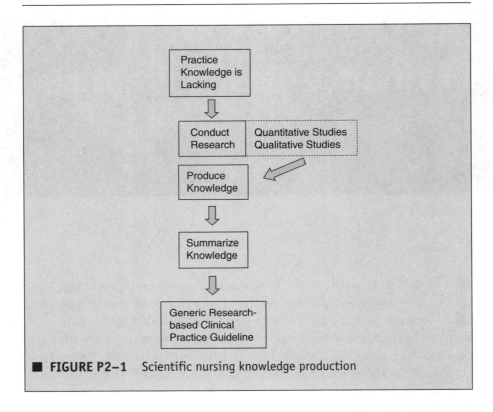

■ **FIGURE P2–1**　Scientific nursing knowledge production

Discipline in doing so ensures that the agency protocol produced is truly evidence-based and that the implementation of the protocol has the desired effect on patient outcomes. To achieve this level of transfer of evidence into practice, evidence-based practice projects are conducted by unit, service-line, or agency teams. The E-B Practice Impact Model portrays how evidence-based practice plays out in everyday activities and serves as a map for this part of the book. The activities described will enable you to contribute to EBP project work.

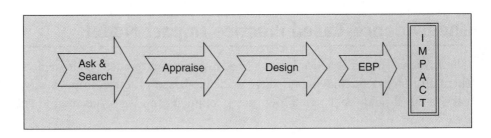

In Chapter 19, the individual nurse's use of research evidence, research-informed practice (RIP), is described. The steps individual nurses use to incorporate research evidence into clinical decision making for individual patients and to refine their own methods of practice are similar to those of EBP, albeit performed with less rigor (Eddy, 2005). I think a distinction between agency evidence-based practice and the individual's use of research evidence is important. The distinction retains high standards for translating research evidence into clinical protocols while recognizing the value of individual nurses seeking better information when agency protocols are lacking or are not applicable to a particular patient situation. The distinction also recognizes that EBP is an organizational activity, whereas RIP is the individual professional nurse's responsibility; maximally effective nursing care requires research utilization at both levels. I would add that this distinction is not universally used; some people use the term *evidence-based practice* more broadly to encompass both agency and individual activities aimed at using research evidence in practice.

The EBP Impact model serves to organize this part of the book. It is similar to several other models that are used as working frameworks for the evidence-based practice programs of healthcare agencies (Rycroft-Malone & Bucknall, 2010). If these more detailed and comprehensive models are of interest to you, see the paper *Evidence-Based Practice Models* on the companion website for this book, which can be accessed at ✍ *go.jblearning.com/brown.*

REFERENCES

Eddy, D. M. (2005). Evidence-based medicine: A unified approach. Two approaches to using evidence to solve clinical problems and how to unify them. *Health Affairs, 24*(1), 9–17.

Rycroft-Malone, J., & Bucknall, T. (Eds.). (2010). *Models and frameworks for implementing evidence-based practice: Linking evidence to action.* Hoboken, NJ: Wiley-Blackwell.

CHAPTER ELEVEN
Asking Clinical Questions

$$\boxed{\text{Ask} \longrightarrow}$$

The starting point for a clinical team embarking on a project to develop an evidence-based protocol is to formulate a clinical question in a way that will guide the search for research evidence and keep the project on mission. First, we need to consider how an issue might have risen to the level of the agency deciding to develop a care protocol regarding the issue. Clinical questions for which research evidence has a high probability of providing answers (or at least partial answers) arise while giving care, are revealed by agency quality data, or are brought to the forefront in professional exchanges. Sometimes they arise out of problematic patient care situations, such as a family complaint, an adverse event, or even a lawsuit. In the Iowa Model of Evidence-Based Practice these initiating situations are referred to as *triggers* (Titler et al., 2001).

Triggers

Clinical Practice

Care providers who are thoughtful and not robotic while giving care find themselves asking questions such as the following:

- What groups of people should we be screening in the emergency department for domestic violence?
- Should I recommend once-a-day vitamin supplements to my elderly patients?

- Should we be using bladder scans to determine urinary residual on all patients who have had an indwelling/Foley catheter removed?
- What nonpharmacological measures can we use to prevent and treat muscle spasms in persons who have had cervical fusion surgery?
- Is acetaminophen or ibuprofen more effective and safer in treating fever in young children?
- Why do some adolescent girls in poor, urban neighborhoods aspire to good diet, exercise, good grades, and sexual abstinence?
- What factors determine whether middle-aged men working in an industrial plant follow recommendations regarding how to avoid back injury?

These kinds of questions can be answered in part by examining the knowledge produced by research. Another part of the answer for some of them may require looking at the systems of care currently in place and how they could be made safer, more efficient, and more cost effective.

Quality Data

All healthcare agencies collect a great deal of information to prove to licensing boards, accrediting agencies, and the public that important aspects of care are being given consistently and that their patients are attaining the appropriate outcomes. For example, for people with ischemic stroke, the hospital might keep track of the following: mortality, global disability status at discharge, discharge destination, special after-hospital services required, and readmission within 30 days. Based on these outcomes, if the hospital's patients were not doing as well as patients in other hospitals, the clinical staff would be obliged to reevaluate their clinical care protocol, both in terms of the recommended actions and the staff's compliance with those recommendations. This might take them back to looking at research evidence regarding how this patient population should be managed. Nurses might be asked to examine how they are doing patient teaching regarding anti-clotting medications to assure that their approach is evidence based. If the current protocol is satisfactory, they might also collect quality data to determine the percentage of patients who are actually receiving this teaching in the ways set forth by the protocol.

Professional Standards

When national professional associations and organizations issue evidence-based guidelines, agencies are obligated to take notice and decide if they should change the way they are giving care. Similarly, when licensing and accrediting agencies, such as the Centers for Medicare and Medicaid Services (CMS) or The Joint Commission, set forth new standards of care, agencies have to decide how they will meet them, and this initiates a search for research evidence to help develop a new protocol. This was the case when The Joint Commission and the CMS required inpatient psychiatric settings to report data regarding their use of holding patients in seclusion rooms.

At a less formal level, a staff nurse might see an article or a research report in a clinical journal about a care approach that seems promising. Or he may learn about a new approach in a session at a conference or workshop. After thinking about the matter, he may come to the conclusion that this aspect of care as it is being done in his setting is of dubious effectiveness. Taking the concern and idea to a nurse leader, clinical nurse specialist, or case manager might lead to a search for research evidence about the alternative approach to care.

Questions Not Answerable by Research Evidence

Before looking at how to formulate a focused clinical question for an evidence-based project, it might be helpful to address the issue of the kinds of questions that cannot be answered by research evidence. A starting point is the ethical principle that each competent patient has the right to determine what happens to his or her person and body, and this principle must be respected regardless of what research evidence shows. Questions about what care should be given to an individual must be decided by the patient and his or her care providers (which providers depends on the care issue and the setting). Research evidence can provide useful information to consider in the discussion, but ultimately the decision is the patient's; there are exceptions to this, such as when the patient is not competent to make a decision or when the well-being of others is endangered, but that is not an issue for consideration here.

In light of the ethical principle just described, research evidence is of limited use in questions having to do with values or deciding what is a moral or ethical course of action. The question "Should we treat pneumonia in nursing home residents older than 90 years of age who have cognitive deficits?" is a moral question. Research may shed some light on the question by providing data regarding the proportion of this population that has an uncomplicated recovery and returns to their former functional status when treated with antibiotics, but research cannot answer the question. In fact, the question cannot be answered in general. It must be answered on a case-by-case basis because the answer depends on how cognitively compromised the person was prior to the onset of the pneumonia, whether intubation is a likely possibility, and what the patient's end-of-life wishes were when last expressed—again, the ethical principle of self-determination. These reminders are necessary to assure that research evidence is used for the purposes it inherently serves and not as a means of controlling individual lives.

Focus

To avoid spending a lot of time searching for, sifting through, and appraising research evidence, it helps to formulate a focused question—as opposed to a very broad or vague question. One of the previously listed questions asked about doing an ultrasound bladder scan on all patients who have an indwelling catheter removed. This is a legitimate question, but it is vague and requires more focus. Let's assume that a medical–surgical practice council decides to look into this issue and, if it has benefits to patients, develop an evidence-based protocol for its use.

The council might use an approach that many healthcare providers have found useful in focusing their evidence-based clinical projects; it is referred to by the acronym PICOT (Sackett, Straus, Richardson, Rosenberg, & Haynes, 2000; Stillwell, 2010). The PICOT format helps clinicians zero in on specific elements of a question that is of interest.

P   Patient population
I   Intervention
C   Comparison intervention
O   Outcomes
T   Timing

Generally, when using PICOT, the patient population can be characterized by attributes such as age, illness experience (e.g., shortness of breath), disease, risk, or living setting, to name a few. The intervention of interest can be specified by naming a clinical intervention, a particular approach, or a group of interventions (e.g., school-based programs regarding weight loss). A comparison of the intervention to another intervention or to usual care may be of interest; the effectiveness of just one intervention may be what is under consideration. Patient outcomes are almost always of interest; most often they should be outcomes that are important to patients, such as improved functional ability or fewer episodes of hypoglycemia. The timing, in terms of clinical status, duration, or frequency, may be relevant.

Getting back to the council developing a bladder scanning protocol, the PICOT question would be the following:

> In patients who have an indwelling bladder catheter removed (P),
> is bladder scanning (I)
> after the first voiding (T)
> useful in identifying those who have a large urine residual (O) and
>   require further monitoring of their urination?

A related question might pertain to the use of bladder scanning in patients who cannot void. That question would be the following:

> In patients who cannot void after having an indwelling catheter removed (P),
> is bladder scanning (I)
> after 8 hours (T)
> useful in avoiding patient discomfort by identifying the need for straight
>   catheterization (O)
> and in reducing urinary tract infections (O)?

In neither question is a comparison intervention suggested.

Another focused question could be as follows:

> What methods of pain control and comfort measures (I)
> should nurses use with full-term newborn infants (P)
> during, and after venipuncture and insertion of intravenous lines (T)?

Notice that in this question that the outcomes, pain control and comfort (O), are inferred by the way I is stated. Again, no comparison is explicitly specified in the question itself; however a comparison is implied because several methods are in use and the studies most likely compare these methods. The question could be made more specific by asking "Is oral sucrose pacifier or topical anesthesia more effective in controlling pain during and after venipuncture of newborns?" Note that the population specified is newborns, so the team looking into this issue would not retrieve or review studies done on premature infants or infants older than 28 days.

PICOT works best for questions about intervention effectiveness. Although not every clinical question about an intervention will have every element, it is useful to at least consider each one. Questions regarding patients' experiences, relationships among clinical variables, and risk require modification of the PICOT format. If a project team asking a non-intervention question realizes that their question is not focused, it sometimes helps to have several members spend a half hour muddling around in a database looking at various articles and studies about the issue. This muddling may help identify aspects of the issue and result in a more focused question.

Assuming the protocol development team has a focused question that is consistent with the agency's commitments and resources, the next step is to look for research evidence related to that question.

REFERENCES

Sackett, D. L., Straus, S. E., Richardson, W. S., Rosenberg, W., & Haynes, R. B. (2000). *Evidence-based medicine: How to practice and teach EBM* (2nd ed.). Edinburgh, Scotland: Churchill Livingstone.

Stillwell, S. (2010). Asking the clinical question: A key step in evidence-based practice. *American Journal of Nursing, 110*(3), 58–61.

Titler, M. G., Kleiber, C., Steelman, V. J., Rakel, B. A., Budreau, G., Everett L. Q., et al. (2001). The Iowa model of evidence-based practice to promote quality care. *Critical Nursing Clinics of North America, 13*(4), 497–509.

CHAPTER TWELVE

Searching for Research Evidence

Ellen F. Hall

> **Search** ➤

I n this chapter we will look first at how to locate systematic reviews (SRs) and evidence-based clinical practice guidelines (EbCPGs). We will not cover all possible sources, just those that are the most significant and widely recognized by clinicians, and broadly available. In the second half of this chapter we will cover techniques for finding quality research evidence when SRs and EbCPGs are not available for the clinical issue you wish to investigate. We will do this by looking at the major databases for the practice of nursing.

Searching for SRs and EbCPGs

The first step in your search is to have your population and intervention or issue in mind. The second step is to explore the various sources of EbCPGs and SRs. They save you time because finding, reading, evaluating and synthesizing the results has already been done. However, there are over 12,000 known diseases, most of these with several possible interventions. EbCPGs and SRs do not exist for each of these population-intervention combinations. SRs are most likely to have been developed for those conditions that have a high frequency or a high cost to third-party payers. Consider back pain. Seventy percent of workers in industrialized nations lose some days at work due to back pain. EbCPG and SRS are broadly available for this condition. However, when there is not a substantive body of original studies, there is no basis on which a team can develop an SR. For instance, there are few research reports on the use of diet therapy for migraine sufferers. Consequently, there is currently only one SR on this topic, and it is limited to a study of the effectiveness of feverfew.

Because reviews and guidelines do not exist for every issue you wish to investigate, it is critically important for you to know how to efficiently find original research studies. The second part of this chapter will help you develop the skills to do your own investigation for individual research studies.

Sources of EbCPGs and SRs

Following are descriptions of the major evidence-review organizations providing EbCPGs and/or SRs for use in nursing practice, along with where and how their reports are available.

Registered Nurses' Association of Ontario

The Registered Nurses' Association of Ontario (RNAO; www.rnao.org) sponsors a Nursing Best Practice Guidelines program. To date there are nearly 40 patient care guidelines. Examples of current guidelines include: Establishing Therapeutic Relationships, Management of Hypertension, Primary Prevention of Childhood Obesity, and Stroke Assessment.

These excellent guidelines are freely available at the RNAO website by clicking on the *Nursing Best Practice Guidelines* tab, then *Clinical Practice Guidelines*, then *Guidelines and Fact Sheets*.

Joanna Briggs Institute

The Joanna Briggs Institute (JBI; www.joannabriggs.edu.au) is a collaboration of nurses, medical and allied health researchers, clinicians, academics, and quality managers in 40 countries. JBI has a dual mission of promoting the use of peer-reviewed health research to identify best practice, as well as providing access to this information. Their nursing content enables nurses to see which nursing practices are supported by evidence. Besides evidence related to practice, they have a special interest as well in systematic reviews of economic, qualitative, and policy research.

To date the JBI has developed over 2,300 reports of three types.

- Systematic Reviews provide extensive summaries of all research on selected clinical topics.
- Evidence Summaries provide short extracts of research literature on selected clinical topics that are based on structured searches of the

literature and selected evidence-based healthcare databases. They focus on the characteristics of the evidence, the clinical bottom line, and best practice recommendations.

- Best Practice Information Sheets summarize the findings of systematic reviews of evidence.

Most JBI resources are available only by subscription, so nursing students typically access these resources through their library. Since 2008 JBI has also made their systematic reviews, evidence summaries and best practice information sheets available via subscriptions to the Proquest Nursing and Allied Health Source database. Many libraries subscribe to this database and thus have access to these JBI resources. Look for the JBI resources in your library's Proquest Nursing and Allied Health Source database, or ask your librarian about its availability at your school.

Cochrane Collaboration

The Cochrane Collaboration develops and distributes high quality systematic reviews of interventions for use by many healthcare professions. Their reviews integrate findings, pool data, and generate overall results. Most of these have been based on randomized controlled trials that investigate the effects of interventions. Increasingly, however, other kinds of study design are being included.

The Cochrane database contains over 3,000 reviews, many with relevance to nursing care. Happily, Cochrane is becoming an even more valuable resource for nursing practice with the 2009 establishment of the Cochrane Nursing Care Network (CNCN) within the Collaboration. The CNCN is specifically charged with supporting the conduct, dissemination and utilization of systematic reviews relevant to nursing.

Access to the full text of Cochrane's systematic reviews requires a subscription. Check with your librarian to see if your library subscribes to the Cochrane Collaboration. If your library doesn't subscribe to Cochrane, you may search for findings directly at their website (http://www.cochrane.org). This free access will enable you to read abstracts, and often plain language summaries, of the findings. Cochrane is also experimenting with delivery of reviews of therapeutic interventions by mobile devices. At this time, however, they make only several hundred reviews available for this mode of delivery.

National Guideline Clearinghouse

The National Guideline Clearinghouse (NGC; www.guideline.gov) is principally a database of thousands of clinical practice guidelines. An interactive search box allows the user to enter a disorder. The *Limit Search* tab allows one to limit the results in several ways, including: the gender and age range of the population group; the intended user group, for example, nurses, dieticians, occupational therapists, physicians, or social workers; and the methodology used to analyze the evidence, for instance, a systematic review.

The NGC is a part of U.S. Department of Health and Human Services. The guidelines are free at their website. It should be noted, however, that the guidelines in this database are of variable quality; some are excellent but others were developed using uncertain methods.

National Library of Guidelines

Similar to the U.S. National Guidelines Clearinghouse, the excellent National Library of Guidelines (www.library.nhs.uk/guidelinesfinder) collection is made available by the National Health Service in the United Kingdom.

Database of Abstracts of Reviews of Effects (DARE)

DARE (www.crd.york.ac.uk/crdweb) is one of several databases produced by the Centre for Reviews and Dissemination (CRD), an agency within the United Kingdom's National Institute for Health Research. This database focuses on the effects of health and social care interventions. While the search interface offers no feature to efficiently limit the database's 15,000 abstracts of systematic reviews to those addressing nursing practice, over 1,000 of the reviews do mention nurses. A useful feature of this database is the *Search History* link located on the right side of the screen. It records your search activity, and in fact it creates sets of abstracts for each of your search statements. These sets can be combined for highly targeted searching. There is no charge for searching this database online.

Centre for Evidence-Based Physiotherapy (CEPD)

The CEPD (www.pedro.org.au) sponsors the Physiotherapy Evidence Database, also known as PEDro. The database is of more value to nursing practice than the title at first might suggest. Certainly it's an excellent source of SRs and EbCPGs for use with any of the movement disorders. A surprisingly broad range of other medical conditions are included as well, such as COPD and asthma. The reviews and guidelines are available free online.

CINAHL

This database can be used to find systematic reviews as well as practice guidelines. A fuller introduction to the use of this database to find systematic reviews, and practice guidelines as well as original studies will follow later in this chapter.

CINAHL is available only by subscription and is the most broadly available database at universities or colleges with nursing programs. Many hospitals also subscribe to this database. Look for access via your library's website, or ask your librarian.

Specialty Nurses' Associations

Specialty nurses' associations (e.g., American Association of Critical-Care Nurses, American Psychiatric Nurses Association, Emergency Nurses Association, Oncology Nursing Society, etc.) are another excellent source for systematic reviews and practice guidelines. Many make these documents available through their websites, usually through a tab. You can also search for them by using their website's search box and typing in *practice guidelines*. Browse a list of over 80 specialty associations with links at the American Nurses Association website (www.nursingworld.org/EspeciallyForYou/Links/SpecialtyNursing.aspx).

Searching Databases

We now move on to discover how to find quality evidence when SRs or EbCPGs have not yet been developed for your chosen topic.

Databases are best understood as a tool for communication. I think of them as another form of what clinicians frequently refer to as the "hallway consult." Picture yourself in the hospital hallway saying to yourself, "I wonder why . . .?", or "I wonder if . . .?" Another clinician approaches, one whom you trust with your question. We all do this frequently in our everyday lives as well. The discourse can be as simple as asking a friend which website they used to get that low ticket price. In fact a study of clinicians found that they generate about three questions for every ten patients seen (Ely et al., 1999). Health sciences databases are constructed to facilitate this transfer of information from research to clinical practice. Unlike the hallway consult, in which you are limited to the expertise of your immediate associates, you can use a database to pose your question to a much more extensive group of experts. And, in a sense, you can even ask them how they came to their conclusion. For the most part, databases allow access to original research studies, although many include book chapters, letters to the editor and even cartoons as well. For the purposes of this chapter, we will focus on research studies published as articles in professional journals.

What's in a Database?

First, no database includes all studies. Even Google only provides access to about 10% of the information delivered over the Internet. Databases, such as Medline/PubMed, CINAHL and PsycINFO, provide access to the contents of a defined group of journals. For instance there are about 20,000 journals in the biomedical sciences. Medline indexes almost 5,000 of these, concentrating on those of greatest benefit to physicians, dentists, veterinarians and health planners. It includes some of the major nursing journals as well. CINAHL looks at slightly less than 3,000 journals in the fields of nursing and allied health. There is some overlap between journals these two databases include, but most of what you might find will be unique to that particular database. Similarly, PsycINFO, which covers articles from thousands of psychology journals, is often of value to nurses and has some overlap with Medline and CINAHL.

Before a database decides to include a particular journal they carefully consider the typical quality of the articles the journal accepts. The very fact that a journal, for instance *Cancer Nursing*, is included in CINAHL is an indicator of CINAHL's perception of that journal's quality. Once a journal is selected, a record is created for each article in that journal. This record is made up of searchable fields, including the author's name, the title of the article, the name of the journal, the words in the abstract, and the date of publication. An indexer also reads the article and tags it with at least five subject headings to describe the content of the article (e.g., asthma, therapeutic exercise) and the nature of the population under study (e.g., female, adolescent). These headings are searchable. Just how they enable very powerful, precision searches will be demonstrated in the sections on intermediate and advanced techniques.

Are All the Articles in a Database Available in Full Text?

Because of U.S. Copyright Law, databases cannot legally distribute the full text of all the articles in all the journals they index. They may include only those for which they have been able to negotiate access with the copyright owner, typically the journal's publisher. Libraries and hospitals, in turn, purchase access to these databases through a vendor, like Ovid or EBSCOhost. Many vendors work very hard to negotiate access to as much full text as possible knowing that clinicians usually prefer those databases providing the greatest amount of full text.

I Know How to Search Google. Can I Use Those Same Skills to Search CINAHL or Medline?

The short answer is yes. We search Google by using text words, otherwise known as "everyday" or natural language. If you searched Google for the common cold it would list over 2,000,000 websites containing the phrase "common cold." However, if an author used a different word to discuss the common cold, let's say rhinitis, Google would not retrieve these for you. Google is very good at giving you what you ask for, but not necessarily at giving you what you want.

You can also use text words to search CINAHL and Medline. When you enter the text words, the search engine will scan all titles, authors' names, and words in the abstract for those text words. If you type in the word *AIDS*, it will return all the articles with that word, including those that are not about the disease, such as the following: "Electronic Aids for Daily Living," "A Comparison of Hearing Aids," "Assessment Aids Learning," and "Pain Management Aids in Rapid Recovery." These are called false hits. They are examples of getting exactly what you asked for but not what you wanted.

A further challenge in looking for clinical information is that medical terminology is a rich mix of Greek, Latin, and Anglo Saxon terms. Consequently we often have three different words for the same organ. Consider eye, opti- and ophthalm-, as well as kidney, renal and nephr-.

Because Medline and CINAHL are meant to support efficient clinical decision making, they enable you to search by subject headings in addition to a specific text word. I'll show you how this works in the sections on intermediate and advanced searching. While these are more advanced techniques, in many ways they make your search so much easier. Certainly searching with subject headings helps avoid the pitfalls described above. But let's first concentrate on simple text word searching.

Just the Basics

CINAHL offers you several search boxes that you can use to start your search. It's best to first consider your question and its component parts. Let's try something simple like nursing assessment of children with cancer. Using PICOT terminology, the P element would be children with cancer and the I element would be assessment.

The first concept in our search is cancer, so we type that word in the first box. I'll show you how we focus on the pediatric segment of the cancer population further below. Our second concept is nursing assessment, so we type those words into the second box, and then hit the search command. We combine these sets with the Boolean operator *and*. This enables us to identify just those articles discussing both cancer and nursing assessment. The following schematic illustrates the process and resulting number of journal articles.

1. Cancer   85,476
2. Nursing assessment   33,374
3. 1 *and* 2   1,909

Now, let's take our search a few steps further. Let's say we are only interested in research studies from the last five years, and since the patient is in grade school we are specifically interested in the 6- to 12-year-old population. Locate *Refine your results* on the left side of the screen and click on *Show More*. Here we find that CINAHL offers options for limiting the results of our search. These options are developed with the needs of the clinician in mind. Google does not offer these options as it was never designed to serve as a clinical decision support tool.

4. Results limited to research studies   875
5. Results limited to last 5 years   320
6. Results limited to ages 6–12 years   22

You can see that as we begin to consider the specifics of our patient population, and our interest in current research, our group of articles on nursing assessment quickly shrinks to a modest size. Following are some sample titles from this group of 22 studies: "Measuring Physical Symptoms in Children," "Symptom Monitoring during Cancer Treatment in Children," "Assessing Procedural Pain in Children with Cancer," and "Exploration of Social Support Available to Mothers of Children with Cancer."

Intermediate Techniques

Now let's move on to some intermediate level skills and consider a slightly different clinical situation. This time we will look for recent research on supporting the patient with breast cancer. Using PICOT terminology, the P element would be people with breast cancer and the I element would be support.

If we type *breast cancer* in the search box, CINAHL will retrieve 22,000 articles. Each of these articles will contain both the word breast and the word cancer. If we enclose this phrase in quotation marks *"breast cancer"* it will find the 17,000 articles with that exact phrase. Let's look instead at what happens if we use a very powerful tool for precision searching, the *CINAHL Headings* tab. We can use this tool to search by concept, that is, by the headings assigned by the indexer, and to free ourselves from the constraints of text word searching. You'll spot this tab near the top of the search screen. By clicking on this tab a browse box will open and we can type in the words *breast cancer*. The database will then advise us that all the articles on breast cancer are identified with the heading Breast Neoplasms. If we now run this search using this subject heading, we find over 25,000 articles. How can using a subject heading find so many more articles than the 17,000 produced by our text word search? The answer is that not all articles about breast cancer use the words breast and cancer. The following three titles of articles in nursing journals are examples: "Barriers to Follow-Up of Abnormal Screening Mammograms," "Advances in Symptom Management: Lymphedema," and "Mastectomy and Lumpectomy Offer Equal Chances of a Cure."

We now return to the CINAHL Headings tab to type the word *support* into the browse box. CINAHL returns a list of possible headings, including Support, Psychosocial which is the one we decide to search. CINAHL identifies over 25,000 articles on this topic. When we combine these two sets we see the following results:

1. Breast neoplasms   25,780
2. Support, psychosocial   25,092
3. 1 *and* 2   823

Combining these two sets with the Boolean operator *and* means that each of the resulting articles discusses both breast neoplasms and psychological support.

Let's take our search a few steps further. You may recall from the first part of this chapter that the CINAHL database can be used to find EbCPGs and SRs. Once you have created a set of articles on a specific population and intervention, as we have with the above search, click on the *Show More* link. You may also see an *Edit* icon on the right side of the screen. Either of these will present a screen with a number of ways to limit your results. One of these is a drop-down menu called *Publication Type.* Among the various types listed under *Publication Type* are *Systematic Review* and *Practice Guidelines.* Selecting either or both of these will limit your results to just those articles which are systematic reviews or contain practice guidelines.

But this section of the chapter is not simply an introduction to the use of databases, but how to use databases in the absence of available SRs and EbCPS. This means we are interested in finding original research studies, and specifically those that include the outcomes of a process or an intervention. Let us consider our current PICOT search where P stands for breast cancer and I for support. Let's now try to determine if this intervention enables a reduction in the anxiety level of the patient. In other words, we are looking at anxiety reduction as the outcome, or the O element using PICOT terminology. Following the process above, we enter *anxiety* into the browse box available through the *CINAHL Headings* tab, and then combine this set of articles (set 4) with the previous set, set 3. Using either the *Show More* or *Edit* links, we further refine our results to research articles. And then, because we're interested in the psychosocial support provided by nurses, we finally narrow our results to articles in nursing journals.

4. Anxiety	9,989
5. 3 *and* 4	48
6. Results limited to research	38
7. Results limited to nursing journals	16

Our assumption in narrowing our results to nursing journals is that if the study is published in a nursing journal, the clinician most likely to be providing the psychological support would be a nurse. You can narrow your results to nursing journals by using the drop-down menu *Journal Subset,* then clicking on *Nursing.* Be sure to select *Nursing* rather than *Core Nursing,* as the latter is a much smaller group of nursing journals.

What we know about these remaining 16 articles is that each is a research study published in a nursing journal and addressing anxiety, psychosocial support, and breast neoplasms. A few titles from our resulting 16 articles are: "Effect of Supportive Care on the Anxiety of Women with Suspected Breast Cancer," "Coping with a Possible Breast Cancer Diagnosis," and "Identifying the Educational Needs and Concerns of Newly Diagnosed Patients with Breast Cancer after Surgery."

You may note that we have not tried to include the C or T elements of PICOT terminology in our search strategies. Finding comparative studies (C) involves additional techniques that are outside the scope of this volume, and there are numerous indexing inconsistencies in capturing the timing concept (T), so I generally do not recommend including it in a search strategy.

Advanced Techniques

In this section we look at three additional features available in both the CINAHL and Medline databases. These are the *Explode, Subheading* and *Citation* features and they deserve a bit of explanation first. To understand the *Explode* feature I'll share an example I use in class. Let's assume there is a subject heading Dogs, and, in addition, there are the following subject headings as well, Airedale, Basset Hound, and Cocker Spaniel. In fact, let's assume there is a separate subject heading for every major breed of dog. What if you were interested in finding studies researching the extent to which dogs reduce the level of loneliness in nursing home residents? It would be so much easier if you could use the subject heading Dogs and automatically retrieve all the articles about dogs, even if the articles were specific to a certain breed. The *Explode* feature allows you to do just that. Consider the following results in our dog search. Our search on the subject heading Airedale would retrieve just those articles about that breed. If we did a search on Dogs without using the *Explode* command we would retrieve only those articles about dogs in general, articles that aren't about a specific breed. But when we use the *Explode* command we retrieve all the articles about dogs, those that are specific to particular breeds that have their own subject headings and those that are about dogs in general.

Airedale	22
Basset	90
Cocker	230
Dogs	15,338
Explode dogs	262,232

Let's now apply the *Explode* command to our search on breast cancer. In the following image we have just completed a subject heading search for breast cancer and we see the preferred term Breast Neoplasms. If we click on the *Breast Neoplasm* link the following image appears.

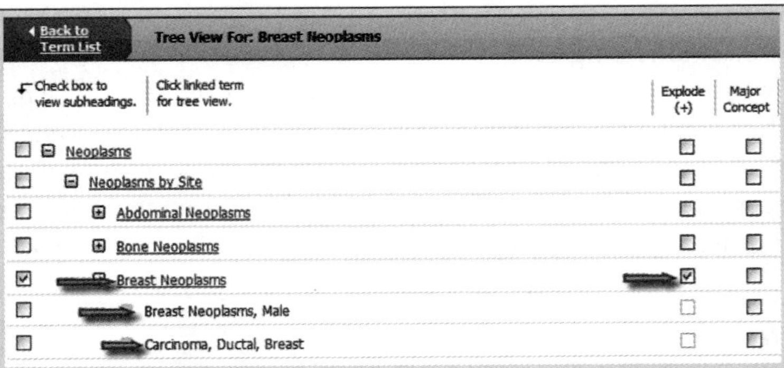

■ FIGURE 12-1 Using the *Explode* feature.
Source: Reproduced from CINAHL with Full Text database with permission from EBSCO Publishing.

As in our dog breed example we notice that there are several different kinds of breast cancer (male breast neoplasms and ductal carcinomas), each with its own subject heading. We know from our intermediate level example above that Breast Neoplasms will retrieve over 25,000 articles. But if we click on the *Explode* box on the right side of the screen, and then the *Search* box, we will get this group of articles plus all those about breast ductal carcinomas and male breast neoplasms. Thus a comparison of results looks like this.

Breast neoplasms   25,780
Explode breast neoplasms   25,982

If we repeat this process, exploding Support, Psychological and Anxiety we find the following differences in the number of resulting articles.

Support, psychological   25,092
Explode support, psychological   27,052
Anxiety   9,989
Explode anxiety   10,662

It should be noted that not all subject headings are explodable. For instance, there is no *Explode* box featured with the subject heading Patella. Using the *Explode* feature will increase the size of your sets and therefore may retrieve valuable results that you would have otherwise missed.

A second advanced technique is the use of the *Subheading* feature. While going through the *Explode* example above, you may have noticed the note in the upper left hand of the screen "Check box to view subheadings." Checking the box will produce a column of subheadings (Figure 12–2). Think of these as subgroups of your search. In the following image we see a subject heading search for Anxiety on the left and some of its associated subheadings in the column on the right. Clicking the box for Prevention and Control would narrow the search to articles about the prevention and control of anxiety.

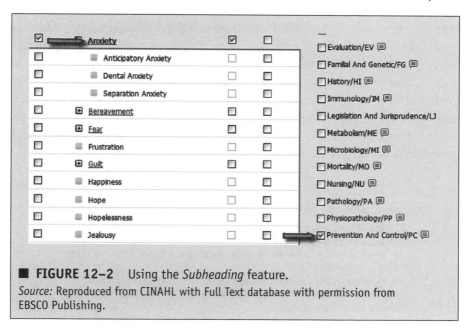

■ **FIGURE 12–2**   Using the *Subheading* feature.
Source: Reproduced from CINAHL with Full Text database with permission from EBSCO Publishing.

There are in fact over 1,300 articles on the prevention and control of anxiety. If we added in our set of breast neoplasm articles, we would then have over 30 resulting articles and our PICOT search would look like this: the P element for patients with breast neoplasms, the I element for prevention and control, and the O element for anxiety. We then use the *Show More* or *Edit* feature to further narrow our results to research articles and nursing journals. Titles of some of these research studies about control measures used by nurses include: "The Role of Education in Managing Fatigue, Anxiety, and Sleep Disorders in Women Undergoing Chemotherapy for Breast Cancer," "The Effectiveness of the Comprehensive Coping Strategy Program on Clinical Outcomes in Breast Cancer," and "Virtual Reality; a Distraction Intervention for Chemotherapy." Think of subheadings as another source for several interventions.

- The *Subheading* feature will always make your results smaller and more targeted.
- The use of the *Explode* feature will make your results larger.

The third feature allows one to track citations. What does this mean? You've all probably heard an instructor suggest that you look at the list of references at the end of an article to find more articles on the same topic. If we were to take our breast neoplasm and psychosocial support search from above and investigate the references at the end of any of the articles from our results we would be going back in time. That is, if an article is published in 2005 it is impossible for the author to cite work published in 2010. The author can only cite the older work he/she read while preparing to write the article. But what if you could go forward in time? What if you found an article that was very useful and you were able to find newer articles that referred to your useful article? Well, this in fact is possible. Consider the image below (Figure 12–3). It's a description of one of the three articles mentioned in our breast neoplasm search.

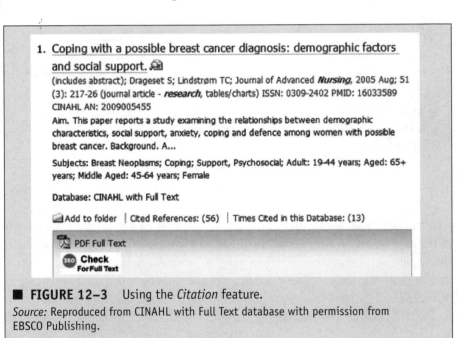

1. Coping with a possible breast cancer diagnosis: demographic factors and social support. 🗐

(includes abstract); Drageset S; Lindstrøm TC; Journal of Advanced *Nursing*, 2005 Aug; 51 (3): 217-26 (journal article - *research*, tables/charts) ISSN: 0309-2402 PMID: 16033589 CINAHL AN: 2009005455

Aim. This paper reports a study examining the relationships between demographic characteristics, social support, anxiety, coping and defence among women with possible breast cancer. Background. A...

Subjects: Breast Neoplasms; Coping; Support, Psychosocial; Adult: 19-44 years; Aged: 65+ years; Middle Aged: 45-64 years; Female

Database: CINAHL with Full Text

Add to folder   Cited References: (56)   Times Cited in this Database: (13)

PDF Full Text

Check ForFull Text

■ **FIGURE 12–3**   Using the *Citation* feature.
Source: Reproduced from CINAHL with Full Text database with permission from EBSCO Publishing.

Note the link *Times Cited in this Database*. This link will lead to 12 newer articles (i.e., newer than August 2005) that reference this article. The link *Cited References* takes you to 56 older articles (i.e., older than August 2005). These are the articles referenced at the end of "Coping with a Possible Breast Cancer Diagnosis."

What About Medline and PsycINFO?

While the results mentioned above all come from searches on the CINAHL database, Medline is used the same way. Recall that Medline is searching, for the most part, through a different set of journals. It also searches a greater number of journals. Some database vendors, like EBSCOhost, make it very easy to switch between databases, allowing you to use the same search strategy without having to type it in again. This seems quite tempting, but only works if Medline and CINAHL use exactly the same subject headings. For instance, both databases use Anxiety, Breast Neoplasms, and Patella, but where CINAHL uses Support, Psychological Medline uses Social Support. If either database encounters a subject heading it doesn't recognize in your search strategy, it will return zero results. This can be most misleading!

Because Medline is produced by a federal agency, the National Library of Medicine, it is also available for free through the Internet under the name PubMed (http://www.ncbi.nlm.nih.gov/pubmed). If you search it this way, that is, without going through your library's website, it is likely to come with significantly less full text attached. Nevertheless, using PubMed is a great way to begin a search and get a sense of the current research.

PsycINFO and its companion database, PsycArticles, are broadly available at college libraries, even at those schools with no health sciences programs. These databases are of value to nurses investigating psychological disorders as well as the psychosocial aspects of nursing practice. Patient self-image, treatment compliance, or the therapeutic relationship are examples of topics that are well covered in the psychological literature.

A Final Word and a Few Tips

Looking for research evidence is by its nature an iterative process. You may not find the answers to your question on your first try. Experimenting with different approaches is a normal part of the process. You may need to restructure your search strategy several times. Both Medline and CINAHL have a function which keeps track of your search formulations each time you hit the enter key. On CINAHL and some versions of Medline this is labeled *Search History*. It's a good idea to print out this history of your searches before exiting the database. It will help you remember what worked well and will keep you from a return trip up those blind alleys. Similarly, after clicking the *Search History* link you will find another feature, *Save Searches*. This feature allows you to set up a user profile whereby you can save your search strategy for easy rerunning at a later date. This is an especially valuable feature when you are using a library computer because the hard drives are generally not available for saving your work. Finally, most databases allow you to e-mail your results to yourself and others.

These databases have a number of powerful features and there is a learning curve in using them effectively. As with any other nursing skill, proficiency comes from practice! You can speed up the process by signing up for a searching class at your library or making an appointment with a nursing or health sciences librarian for an individual session. Many libraries are now creating their own online tutorials for CINAHL and Medline. Ask if these are available.

REFERENCE

Ely, J., Osheroff, J., Ebell, M., Bergus, G., Levy, B., Chambliss, M., et al. (1999). Analysis of questions asked by family doctors regarding patient care. *British Medical Journal, 319*(7206), 358–361.

CHAPTER THIRTEEN
Appraising Research Evidence

> Appraise ▶

Published guidelines, reviews, and individual study reports cannot be accepted on face value, even when they are published in respected journals. Reports of seriously flawed research do get published. Therefore, an organization or individual considering using research evidence as the basis for care must appraise it and decide whether it should be used as the basis for clinical decisions and actions.

Appraisal Systems

Numerous appraisal systems for rating the quality of studies, systematic reviews, and guidelines exist. The ones used in this book were developed specifically for students who are encountering evidence-based practice appraisal for the first time. They require a level of research knowledge appropriate to what a BSN nurse should possess. Therefore, you should be able to answer the questions in the appraisal guides with the knowledge you acquired in reading the first part of the book. Importantly, these appraisal guides will help you develop basic appraisal skills so that you can be a valued member of an evidence-based project team in the future.

Appraisal guides are provided in subsequent chapters for clinical practice guidelines (Figure 14–1), integrative research reviews (Figure 15–1), original qualitative studies (Figure 16–1), and original quantitative studies (Figure 16–2). The same template is used in all four guides although the specific questions are different from one guide to another.

Appraisal in General

The goal of critical appraisal of any type of research evidence is to judge whether the research evidence is

- Credible
- Clinically significant
- Applicable (Brown, 1999)

Appraising credibility requires an answer to the question: Was the guideline/review/study produced using methods that were sound enough that you can trust its recommendations/conclusions/findings? A judgment regarding the credibility of the guideline/review/study is primary. If it lacks credibility, then the clinical significance and applicability of its recommendations/conclusions/findings need not be appraised because they become moot. There is no sense in appraising the clinical significance and applicability of recommendations/conclusions/findings that were not soundly produced—they are not trustworthy and should not be considered as a basis for practice.

You will notice in the guides provided that some questions pertain to "the guideline," "the review," or "the study," whereas others pertain to the individual recommendation, conclusion, or finding. The rationale behind the differentiation between the piece of evidence as a whole and individual recommendations, conclusions, or findings (i.e., the end products) is that a sound development process or study design generally confers credibility on its end products. However, each recommendation of a guideline, each conclusion of an integrative review, and each finding of a study stands on its own and must be appraised separately. That is because one of these end products might be credible, clinically significant, and applicable, whereas another may come up short in one or more appraisal category. And ultimately, the recommendation, conclusion, or finding is what is incorporated into practice, not the study.

What follows is a brief introduction to each area of appraisal—synopsis, credibility, clinical significance, and applicability. In the following three chapters, each area will be discussed in greater detail—as it pertains to the particular form of research evidence.

Synopsis

The starting point for appraisal of all forms of research evidence is understanding how the guideline/review/study was produced and what was found.

Writing a synopsis not only ensures that you have this understanding, it also provides a brief to refer back to later. A synopsis contains just the facts, no judgments or interpretations. Typically, research articles are very "dense," meaning that every sentence contains important information—there is little fluff. Consequently, in addition to several readings, you may find that you have to refer back to the article several times to complete the synopsis.

Credibility

After getting a sense of the methods and recommendations/conclusions/findings of a piece of research evidence, the next goal is to make a judgment as to whether the evidence was rigorously enough produced to deem it *credible*. The criteria for credibility are different for each type of research evidence, and each is discussed in depth in the next three chapters. However, all the criteria are based on the premise that the methods of producing the guideline, review, or study determine the credibility of its end products. Therefore, the discerning reader (and potential user) of the recommendation/conclusion/finding has to appraise the production process critically, lest erroneous research evidence be used in the design of nursing care.

The credibility of findings is also judged by whether they are similar to findings from other studies conducted in the field of study. Findings that are different are not automatically assumed to be not credible; however, they are held to a high level of rigor, even skepticism. The researcher should acknowledge differences between the findings of the study being reported and findings from other studies; reasons why her findings might be different should be set forth.

> Credible findings are produced by sound methods.

Clinical Significance

Clinically significant findings are those that have enough impact or substance to make a difference in patients' experiences or outcomes should you use or implement them in your clinical setting. Appraising clinical significance would lead you to ask questions such as the following:

- Is the average increase in patients' coping abilities found in the study sizable enough to make practical differences in patients' everyday lives?

- Is a change in women's attitudes regarding osteoporosis prevention likely to produce a change in their dietary, exercise, or smoking behaviors?
- Are the insights offered about the process of living with a history of breast cancer after successful treatment informative enough to provide clinicians who see these women for follow-up with a fresh perspective?

In short, how strong are the findings from a clinical perspective? Is the treatment effect strong enough to make a difference on patient outcomes or well-being? Is the relationship between two variables strong enough that it can be built on in some way to make a difference in patient outcomes?

Often the clinical significance of research evidence is not explicitly discussed in the report. The clinical implications paragraph in the discussion section of the research report sometimes addresses the clinical significance of the findings, but other times it consists mainly of opinions about the ways the findings could be used—not descriptions about how clinically strong the findings were. As a result, you will often have to piece together your judgment about the clinical significance of the findings from bits and pieces of information in the report in combination with your clinical knowledge. The fact that clinical significance does not have several clear-cut criteria (like credibility) is not a reason to gloss over it in appraisal—it is an important consideration.

Applicability

If a recommendation/conclusion/finding is judged credible and clinically significant, you will then proceed to determine whether it is applicable to your setting, its patients, and its resources.

The applicability questions that should be asked will vary greatly depending on the nature of the evidence being translated into a clinical protocol and the nature of the change or changes that need to be made. Generally, the questions fall into four categories:

- Fit of the evidence to the setting (Stetler, 1994)
- Feasibility of incorporating the change
- Safety
- Expected benefit

The recommendations/conclusions/findings being considered as a basis for the protocol were derived from study samples. The fit question then is, "Were the persons who made up the samples of the studies similar to those in our setting?" If all the studies were done on white suburban women, the applicability to a multiethnic, inner-city group of women may be very limited. Sometimes, particularly with systematic reviews, the studies had diverse samples and the project team can focus on the results from the studies most similar to their setting and patients.

Feasibility has to do with the ability of the setting to implement the change in a way that is quite similar to the way it was tested in the studies. If major changes have to be made in the intervention from the way it was implemented in the studies, then the question could be raised as to whether the protocol will indeed be research-based. Assuming a faithful translation from the evidence to the protocol, the project team should still consider whether their setting has the professional skills, support services, equipment, financial resources, and support of key persons to make the change and sustain it over time. A change that has a high cost in terms of dollars or effort required by direct care providers or support services faces an uphill road to successful implementation.

Safety and expected benefit are important bottom-line considerations. If a protocol is likely to produce meaningful benefits to patients and has few associated risks, the other hurdles can usually be overcome. Both safety and expected benefit must be considered at length prior to deciding to introduce a new protocol or make a major change in practice. The expected benefit should actually be quantified. Let's say a new protocol for self-monitoring of blood sugar and administration of insulin is being introduced. The expected benefit might be stated as, "We expect an absolute decrease of 5% in the percentage of patients whose glycosylated hemoglobin (HbAC1c) values are above 7%." Such a specific organizational target allows the agency to determine the proportion of patients in the study that had met the target.

Applicability has four dimensions:

1. Is the research evidence based on patients similar to those for whom we provide care?
2. Can we effectively and safely incorporate the recommendations or evidence-based innovation into our setting?
3. What implementation strategies will assure adoption of the innovation by those whose work will be affected by it?
4. How will we know the innovation has resulted in improved patient care?

The applicability questions set forth in the guides are directed at making an organizational change in practice, that is, implementing a new care protocol. Making a change in individual practice would involve fewer issues; however, risk, resources needed, and people affected should be considered. The use of research evidence in individual practice is addressed in detail in Chapter 19.

The guides for individual studies do not include applicability questions. That is because the applicability of findings from any single study should always be undertaken with care, particularly when the current approach to care is not causing major problems and is thought to be at least somewhat effective. The assumption is that before a change in practice is made several studies will be considered and applicability will be appraised based on across-study conclusions, not on findings from just one original study. Across-study analysis of findings is addressed in Chapter 16.

In summary, four areas (synopsis, credibility, clinical significance, and applicability) serve as a template for the appraisal questions set forth for the recommendations of clinical practice guidelines, for the conclusions of integrative research reviews, and for the findings of original studies. The end point question of an appraisal is: Should we use the recommendation, conclusion, or findings to develop a unit or agency clinical protocol?

Appraisal Template

- Synopsis
- Credibility
- Clinical significance
- Applicability

Counsel

Even though appraisal of a piece of evidence is done using a set of objective criteria, appraisal inevitably involves judgment. Not infrequently, two appraisers using the same set of criteria will reach different judgments about the overall quality of a piece of evidence. The difference occurs for a variety of reasons, including the following:

- One appraiser may view a study or review as having a minor weakness, whereas the other appraiser may view it as having a critical methodological flaw.

- One appraiser may consider bias or failure to control confounding influences in the way a study was done to be a major detractor from its credibility, but the other appraiser may view the same circumstances as inevitable.

- One appraiser may conclude that the findings of several studies are similar, while the other appraiser may see an important difference in the findings.

For these reasons, and many more, most panels that produce an appraisal of a body of research require that two or more appraisers rate each piece of evidence and reach consensus about its quality.

In a related issue, in appraising research evidence, you have to strike a balance between identifying key study shortcomings and being overly critical. The judgments made as part of a critical appraisal are not directed at identifying every weakness in the guideline, review, or study because there is no such thing as a perfect piece of research. When researchers design guidelines, reviews, or studies, they often have to make trade-offs or conduct their work with limited resources. Thus, you should reject only guidelines, reviews, or studies that are seriously flawed, although you should note when a study had very sound methodology or very weak methodology. EBP teams that combine findings from several studies (discussed in Chapter 16) may want to weight studies with strong methodology more heavily than studies with weak but acceptable methodology.

REFERENCES

Brown, S. J. (1999). *Knowledge for health care practice: A guide to using research evidence*. Philadelphia, PA: Saunders.

Stetler, C. B. (1994). Refinement of the Stetler/Marram Model for application of research findings to practice. *Nursing Outlook, 42,* 15–25.

CHAPTER FOURTEEN

Appraising Recommendations of Clinical Practice Guidelines

> Appraise ⟩

The healthcare literature (electronic and paper) includes an abundance of clinical practice guidelines—produced by professional associations, healthcare systems, specialty centers, and government agencies. Most of these are research-based to the maximum extent possible. However, some were produced with little effort to systematically and widely examine the relevant research bases and use an unbiased production process. Even when a guideline carries a title indicating it is "evidence-based," a measure of skepticism is needed.

As described in Chapter 10, producing an evidence-based clinical practice guideline (EbCPG) involves quite a few steps, and each step has the potential for error or bias to creep in and distort the translation of the research evidence into clinical action recommendations. Thus, when considering using a clinical practice guideline as a basis for an agency protocol or as a guide for the care of an individual patient, the user should appraise the credibility, clinical significance, and applicability of the guideline's recommendations. In this chapter, you will be revisiting the clinical practice guideline about nonpharmaceutical management of depression in adults that you read in Chapter 10, appraising it, and then comparing your appraisal to one a colleague and I did. First, a bit of background.

AGREE and GRADE

The AGREE Collaboration is an international organization that produced and validated an evaluation instrument for appraising the process used to produce a the quality of clinical practice guidelines (AGREE Collaboration, 2001). The instrument consists of 23 criteria organized under six domains:

(1) scope and purpose, (2) stakeholder involvement, (3) **rigor** of development, (4) clarity, (5) applicability, and (6) editorial independence. A score for each domain and a total score are calculated; these can be compared to the maximum and minimum points possible to determine if a sound development process was used to produce it. The AGREE instrument and the process they recommend is quite useful for groups considering a guideline. However, the instrument does not grade the evidence base or the actual recommendations, other than to require that there be an explicit linkage between recommendations and supporting evidence.

Another system, the GRADE system, grades both the body of evidence and the strength of the recommendation (GRADE, 2010). The grading of the body of evidence takes into account the design of studies, quality of studies, and consistency of findings. The grading of recommendations takes into account nine different factors, including: certainty regarding the benefits, risks, and inconvenience; size of the benefit produced; importance of the benefit produced; precision of the benefit estimate; and cost. Several nursing organizations are represented in the GRADE working group; still, the applicability of the GRADE system to the appraisal of nursing guidelines remains to be seen.

The appraisal tool in Figure 14–1 includes criteria with elements from both the AGREE appraisal instrument and the GRADE system, but it is not as comprehensive or in-depth as either one.

Synopsis

The first step in the appraisal of a clinical practice guideline is to get a grasp of the issues addressed, the recommendations that were made, and how the recommendations were produced. You want to summarize this in brief so that you can refer to it throughout your project. At this point, I suggest you look at the Synopsis questions in the guideline appraisal tool (Figure 14–1).

Credibility

In broad terms, appraising the credibility of a guideline involves the following steps:

- Determine if the guideline indeed is evidence-based
- Determine if the organization and persons that produced the guideline had the credentials to do so
- Decide if the process used to produce the guideline was systematic and free of bias.

Citation:

Synopsis
What does the guideline address (clinical questions, issues, and subissues)?

What population of patients is the guideline intended for?

What process was used to develop the guideline?

What clinical outcomes were the guideline designed to achieve?

What group or groups produced it?

What is the date on it, and how recent are the cited research sources?

What are the main recommendations?

Credibility
Was the panel that developed the guideline made up of people with the necessary expertise?   Yes ___   No ___

Was a systematic and comprehensive search for research evidence conducted?   Yes ___   No ___

Are the criteria for selecting research evidence clearly described?
Yes ___ No ___

Is the evidence supporting each recommendation indicated and/or discussed?   Yes ___   No ___

Is it clear when research evidence was lacking and expert opinion became the basis of the recommendation?   Yes ___   No ___

Was the process for formulating the recommendations systematic and free of bias?
Yes ___   No ___   Can't tell ___

Are the guidelines current?   Yes ___   No ___

Was the guideline peer-reviewed or tested?   Yes ___   No ___

ARE THE RECOMMENDATIONS CREDIBLE?   YES___ NO___

Clinical Significance
Were all important decisions the nurse would have to make addressed by this guideline?   Yes ___   No ___

Were patient concerns and risks associated with the recommendations addressed?
Yes ___   No ___   Not clear ___

■ **FIGURE 14–1**   Appraisal Guide for a Clinical Practice Guideline's Recommendations

(continues)

Is there reasonable certainty (based on the research evidence) that the recommendations, if implemented, are likely to produce good patient outcomes?
Yes ___ No ___

Are the projected benefits of the guideline valued by patients?
Yes ___ No ___ Not clear ___

Is the intervention or action required by patients acceptable to them?
Yes ___ No ___ Uncertain ___ Not applicable ___

ARE THE RECOMMENDATIONS CLINICALLY SIGNIFICANT?
YES___ NO___

Applicability
Does the guideline address the problem, situation, or decision we are redesigning in our setting? Yes ___ No ___

Should we consider using the guideline in its entirely or just parts of it?
Yes ___ No ___

To implement the recommendations, what will we have to do differently?

Do we have the resources and capability to implement the recommendations safely and accurately? Yes ___ No ___

Which departments or other providers would be affected by this change and how can we bring them into the change process?

How will we know if our patients are benefiting from our new protocol?

ARE THE RECOMMENDATIONS (ALL OR IN PART) APPLICABLE TO OUR SETTING? YES___ NO___

SHOULD WE ADOPT ALL OR SOME OF THE RECOMMENDATIONS?
YES ___ NO ___

COMMENTS

■ **FIGURE 14–1** Continued

To be credible, it must be clear that the developers conducted comprehensive reviews of the research evidence relative to the issues the guideline addresses and used that evidence as the basis for the recommendations made. In addition, each recommendation set forth should be explicitly linked to specific supporting research evidence and the evidence relative to each issue should be presented. If these actions are evident in the guideline document, you can be reasonably confident that the recommendation is credible, that is, trustworthy (Sackett, Straus, Richardson, Rosenberg, & Haynes, 2000). Your confidence in the credibility of the recommendation is further bolstered if the group producing the guideline was made up of people with credentials and expertise related to the issues addressed by the guideline, and the process used to formulate the recommendations is adequately described.

Linkage to Evidence

Basing recommendations on research evidence is the major determinant of the credibility of a clinical practice guideline. Beyond whatever shorthand system was used to indicate the strength of the evidence supporting a recommendation, linkage between the recommendations and the research evidence should at the very least consist of references used to assign the strength of evidence indicator. Better yet is a discussion of the research evidence or a detailed table setting forth the evidence relevant to each recommendation. The relevant evidence may be included in the guideline itself or in an accompanying document.

Production Process

Explicit linkage between recommendation and relevant evidence allows a potential adopter of the guideline to determine if the recommendations are true to the research evidence. Description of the production process allows the potential adopter to determine if the search for evidence was extensive and if steps were taken to avoid bias during production. First, the composition of the panel that produced the guideline should be noted as well as the credentials of the persons on the panel. The composition of the panel should cover the issues addressed by the guideline. For instance, if the guideline makes reference to medications, a pharmacist, nurse practitioner, or physician in the field of practice should be included on the panel.

Then, the production process should be described in some detail. Unfortunately, some guidelines do not include any description at all of the development process. Omission of information about the development process makes appraising the credibility of a guideline almost impossible. The important steps of the process that should be described are: (1) how the search for evidence was conducted, (2) inclusion and exclusion criteria that were applied to what was found, (3) how decisions were made regarding whether or not to include a recommendation, and (4) how differences of opinion were resolved (AGREE, 2001). Although the rigor of the process used to produce the guidelines is extremely important in appraising their quality, other issues such as its clarity, its freedom from influence by vested interests, and the degree to which it has been field tested also need to be considered.

Current Status

If a guideline was produced four years or longer ago, it certainly would be advisable to search for more recent research evidence that might update the recommendations of the guideline. In 2001, a study of clinical practice guidelines produced by the U.S. Agency for Healthcare Research and Quality found that half of their 17 guidelines were outdated in 5.8 years (Shekelle et al., 2001). Research on some clinical topics is being done at a fairly fast rate, for example, management of the blood sugar levels of diabetics; thus, a guideline or review done even two years earlier could be out-of-date. In contrast, other clinical topics receive much less research attention so that a guideline is stable for quite a few years.

Clinical Significance

Evaluating the clinical significance of a guideline recommendation requires consideration of the following:

- Importance of the health benefits expected
- Likelihood of health benefits
- Side effects and risks
- Practicality and acceptability to patients

Consideration of these issues helps decide whether the recommendation would make a difference in patient outcomes. In addition, to be clinically significant, the set of recommendations that make up the guideline should address all the issues that are important to patients as well as all the important decisions nurses make while delivering the care. Some guideline producers pilot test their guidelines prior to releasing them. If this is done, it addresses the clinical significance issue by providing future users with information about how patients and providers view the value and practicality of the recommendations and whether following the guidelines actually resulted in the presumed outcomes.

Applicability

In the final section of the appraisal tool, *Applicability*, you will be asked to make a judgment regarding the fit between the recommendations and the setting in which you intend to implement them. If you are familiar with one agency or hospital, you should try to envision what would be involved in making the changes in practice that a new care protocol requires. The *Applicability* questions will help you think through some of those requirements. At the very least, you should consider the applicability questions and appreciate what is involved in making an organizational change in care practice. The issue of implementation of a research-based change in practice receives more attention in Chapter 16.

A guideline can be soundly produced and make clinically significant recommendations, but it may not be feasible for the setting in which a protocol project team intends to use it. Perhaps the population of patients or providers in the setting is not similar to those for whom the guideline was intended. Perhaps implementation of the protocol would require expenditure for training that is beyond what the setting can afford. Thus, one possible bottom line judgment resulting from appraisal of a guideline may be, "The guideline's recommendations are credible and clinically significant but are not applicable to our setting." Alternatively, some recommendations may be applicable but others may not be.

Your Turn

After you have read through the appraisal questions in the Appraisal Guide for a Clinical Practice Guideline's Recommendations (Figure 14–1), reread the SIGN clinical practice guideline, *Nonpharmaceutical Management of*

Depression in Adults, in Chapter 10. Then complete an appraisal of this guideline using the criteria in the appraisal guide. Although some questions on the appraisal guide ask for a yes/no answer, for most purposes, but particularly for student learning, a one- to three-sentence rationale for the yes/no answer should be given. To get various perspectives, you might want to do the appraisal with one or several classmates. Afterwards, look at how a colleague and I appraised the guideline (Appendix C) and compare our judgments to yours.

As noted when you first read this guideline, the reprint contains only part of the guideline. In doing the appraisal, you really will benefit from moving between the full SIGN guideline (http://www.sign.ac.uk/pdf/sign114.pdf) and the SIGN 50 Guideline Developer's Handbook (http://www.sign.ac.uk/guidelines/fulltext/50/index.html).

REFERENCES

AGREE Collaboration. (2001). *Appraisal guidelines for research and evaluation instrument*. Retrieved from http://www.agreecollaboration.org/instrument

GRADE Working Group. (2010). *Welcome*. Retrieved from http://www.gradeworking group.org/index.htm

Sackett, D. L., Straus, S. E., Richardson, W., Rosenberg, W., & Haynes, R. B. (2000). *Evidence-based medicine: How to practice and teach EBM*. Edinburgh, Scotland: Churchill Livingstone.

Shekelle, P. G., Ortiz, E., Rhodes, S., Morton, S. C., Eccles, M. P., Grimshaw, J. M., & Woolf, S. H. (2001). Validity of the Agency for Healthcare research and quality clinical practice guidelines: How quickly do guidelines become outdated? *Journal of the American Medical Association, 286*(12), 1461–1467.

ADDITIONAL RESOURCE

A completed appraisal of the EbCPG posted on the companion website for Chapter 10 (RNAO, 2004) is available on the companion website page for this chapter, which can be accessed at ***go.jblearning.com/brown***.

CHAPTER FIFTEEN

Appraising Conclusions of Integrative Research Reviews

> **Appraise**

A systematic review (SR) is an important resource when designing an evidence-based care innovation. The comprehensive and systematic synthesis SRs provide is essential to a complete understanding of clinical topics. However, research evidence in the form of the conclusions of SRs, like the recommendations of clinical practice guidelines, must be critically appraised before using them as the basis for nursing care protocols or care of an individual patient. SR conclusions are a bit easier to appraise than are guideline recommendations because the translation of evidence into recommendations is not an issue. Still, there is much to consider because the move from individual findings to across-studies conclusions is complex and open to bias.

The appraisal framework discussed in this chapter uses the template introduced in Chapter 13: synopsis, credibility, clinical significance, applicability. The questions in the guide provided are specific to integrative research reviews (IRRs), the most common type of SRs seen in clinical nursing journals. The IRR from Chapter 9 about heart attack patients' delay in getting to emergency departments is used to demonstrate appraisal of an IRR.

There are many appraisal guides for systematic research but none as widely recognized as those for clinical practice guidelines. However, several premier review organizations have spelled out their methods of conducting systematic reviews (Cochrane Collaboration, 2010; Joanna Briggs Institute, 2008), and those methods have become standards for appraising them. The set of appraisal questions for IRRs presented in this chapter (see Figure 15–1) is representative of, albeit more basic than, the criteria of the premier

Citation:

Synopsis
What topic or question did the integrative research review address?

How were potential individual research reports identified?

What determined if a study was included in the analysis?

How many studies were included in the review?

What research designs were used in the studies?

What were the consistent and important across-studies conclusions?

Credibility
Was the topic clearly defined?   Yes ___ No___

Is there a description of the methods used to conduct the review?
   Yes ___ No___

   1. Was the search for study reports comprehensive and unbiased?
      Yes ___ No___

   2. Were the included studies assessed for quality?   Yes ___ No___

Were the design characteristics and the findings of the studies displayed or discussed in sufficient detail?   Yes ___ No___

Was there truly an integration (i.e., a synthesis) of findings—not merely reporting of findings from each study?   Yes ___ No___

Did the reviewers explore why differences in findings might have occurred?
   Yes ___ No___

Did the reviewers distinguish between conclusions based on consistent findings from a sufficient number of studies and those based on inferior evidence?
   Yes ___ No___ Varies ____

Which conclusions were supported by consistent findings from two or more studies?

ARE THE CONCLUSIONS CREDIBLE?   YES___   NO___   VARIES _____

■ **FIGURE 15–1**   Appraisal Guide for Conclusions of an Integrative Research Review

Clinical Significance
Which conclusions are likely to make a difference in patient safety, comfort, or outcomes?

Are the conclusions relevant to the care nurses give?
   Yes ___ No___ Varies ____

ARE THE CONCLUSIONS CLINICALLY SIGNIFICANT?
   YES___ NO___ VARIES ____ NOT SURE _____

Applicability
Does the integrative review address the problem, situation, or decision we are addressing in our setting?   Yes ___ No____

Are the patients in the studies similar to those we see, either overall or in a subgroup of studies?   Yes ___ No___ To a limited extent ____

Are there any reasons why the conclusions might not apply to our setting and patients?   Yes ___ No___

Are there any organizational, logistical, cost, or time barriers to incorporating into practice a protocol based on these conclusions? Could they be overcome?
Barriers: Yes ___ No___ Could be overcome: Yes ___ No___

What changes, additions, training, or purchases would be needed to implement and sustain a clinical protocol based on these conclusions?

How will we know if our patients are benefiting from our new protocol?

SHOULD WE PROCEED TO DESIGN A PROTOCOL INCORPORATING SOME OR ALL OF THESE CONCLUSIONS? YES___ NO___

■ **FIGURE 15–1**   Continued

producers and others who have written about critical appraisal of systematic research reviews (Sackett, Straus, Richardson, Rosenberg, & Haynes, 2000; Stetler et al., 1998). Nevertheless, staff nurses have found it helpful.

Synopsis

The purpose of doing a synopsis is to acquire an understanding of the scope of the review, how it was conducted, and what conclusions were reached. Completing a synopsis also allows you to become reacquainted quickly with the IRR when you have been away from it for a while. I would suggest looking at the synopsis questions in the appraisal tool (Figure 15–1).

Credibility

IRRs bring the findings of individual studies together to produce overall conclusions that reflect the body of findings. The conclusions are produced by the analytical and logical reasoning of those who conduct it. To produce across-studies conclusions, the reviewers must move from the findings of the original studies to conclusions that incorporate the whole body of findings. The conclusions are new products, more than the sum of the parts, hence the term synthesis. IRR synthesis is complex and prone to bias because it is all too easy for the reviewers to introduce their own predilections and beliefs into the review and synthesis process (Oxman & Guyatt, 1988). For this reason, the standards for IRRs include the requirements that the reviewers: (1) set out the evidence from the individual studies—to the degree that is possible in a published report; and (2) be explicit about how important steps in the review were done (Steinberg & Luce, 2005). This requires that IRR reports include the following elements:

- A clear objectives statement
- A description of how the search for relevant study reports was performed
- A description of the criteria for including or excluding studies
- A description of how the quality of individual studies was appraised and considered in the analysis
- Tables, or narrative, that describe the population, methods, and findings of the individual studies
- For each conclusion, the evidence that led to it should be clear, including the quality of studies, the quantity of studies, and the consistency of findings across the supporting studies (AHRQ, 2002).

When the research reviewers include these elements in their report, the reader is provided with information that can be used to decide if the conclusions are indeed derived from the individual studies and are unbiased. If the reviewers do not provide this information, the reader is placed in the position of having to trust the reviewers' interpretation of the evidence, which is not in keeping with the explicit nature of scientific decision making.

The reviewers should be careful not to reach conclusions that are beyond what the evidence shows. This would be the case if the conclusions were applied to "elders," but the studies had been done mainly with elders living in nursing homes. For many issues, the findings would not, or may not, apply to seniors living in their own homes or apartments, in assisted living facilities, or with family. Another example of going beyond the findings would be overstating the importance of the findings from several weak studies.

Importantly, when the evidence is inconclusive, that is, inconsistent across studies, the reviewers should not conclude that there is no effect, no difference, or no association. Rather, the conclusion should be that definitive evidence for or against an effect is lacking. A conclusion of *no effect* or *no association* assumes a clear finding of no effect based on consistent evidence, whereas a conclusion of *inconclusive evidence* or *insufficient evidence* recognizes that the evidence does not provide a clear and consistent answer regarding effect—two very different conclusions.

Clear connectivity between findings of the individual studies and the conclusions is established when the reviewers demonstrate a deep analysis of the data. The reviewers should convince you that they looked for patterns and similarities in findings and reasons for the differences. Reasons for different findings from one study to others would include differences in the samples studied, the form of an intervention, the outcomes studied, how the variables were measured, different measurement intervals, or length of follow-up. In short, conclusions based on a deep analysis would give you confidence in their credibility.

The reader has confidence that the conclusions are credible when:

- A comprehensive search was conducted
- Explicit inclusion criteria were used
- Findings are consistent across studies
- There is clear connectivity between the findings of the individual studies and the conclusions

Clinical Significance

To be clinically significant, the conclusions of a review should reflect issues that are important in everyday practice and that if incorporated into practice would make a difference in patient safety, comfort, or health outcomes. For reviews of interventions, this would include a conclusion that the treatment effect is large enough to be of benefit given costs and any burden to patients or staffs, as reflected in absolute benefit improvement (ABI), numbers needed to treat (NNT) findings, and economic analysis (if available). Clinical significance is more difficult to appraise in IRRs of issues other than intervention effectiveness, although the consistency of the findings across the studies, the strength of the relationship between variables across the studies, and the informativeness of the conclusions can be considered.

Applicability

The decision regarding whether the conclusions of a review are applicable to a particular setting is determined in part by the setting and patients that were included in the original studies reviewed. If they are similar, or the reporting is such that you can identify a subset of studies that were conducted in a setting similar to yours, then the results of that subset would be applicable to your setting. For instance, an emergency department in a rural hospital would have to consider whether the conclusions of a review about triage systems is applicable to their setting if all the studies included in the review were from inner-city or suburban emergency departments. The issues for the rural emergency department are very different—for instance, no option to close to admissions and divert ambulances elsewhere, and fewer clinical services available 24/7. Beyond the settings and patients studied, the feasibility of implementing, resources required, and costs of implementing should also be taken into account.

Your Turn

I suggest that you reread the Khraim and Carey (2008) article that is reprinted in Chapter 9 and complete an appraisal of it using the tool provided (Figure 15–1). Afterward, look at the completed appraisal in Appendix D. You could further practice appraisal of IRRs by appraising one of the systematic reviews listed at the end of Chapter 9. I strongly suggest that you not attempt appraisal of the meta-analysis or meta-synthesis at this point.

REFERENCES

Agency for Healthcare Research and Quality. (2002). *Systems to rate the strength of scientific evidence: Summary.* Retrieved from http://www.ncbi.nlm.nih.gov/bookshelf/br.fcgi?book=erta47

Cochrane Collaboration. (2010). *For authors and MEs. Review production resources for authors and managing editors.* Retrieved from http://www.cochrane.org/training/authors-mes

Joanna Briggs Institute. (2008). *2008 JBI Reviewers Manual.* Retrieved from http://www.joannabriggs.edu.au/about/system_review.php

Oxman, A. D., & Guyatt, G. H. (1988). Guidelines for reading literature reviews. *Canadian Medical Association Journal, 138,* 697–703.

Sackett, D. L., Straus, S. E., Richardson, W., Rosenberg, W., & Haynes, R. B. (2000). *Evidence-based medicine: How to practice and teach EBM.* Edinburgh, Scotland: Churchill Livingstone.

Steinberg, E. P., & Luce, B. R. (2005). Evidence based? Caveat emptor. *Health Affairs, 24*(1), 80–92.

Stetler, C. B., Morsi, D., Rucki, S., Broughton, S., Corrigan, B., Fitzgerald, J., et al. (1998). Utilization-focused integrative reviews in a nursing service. *Applied Nursing Research, 11*(4), 195–206.

ADDITIONAL RESOURCE

A completed appraisal of the IRR posted on the website for Chapter 9 (Hart, 2005) is available on the companion website page for this chapter. The companion website for this book can be accessed at ***go.jblearning.com/brown.***

CHAPTER SIXTEEN
Appraising Findings of Original Studies

> **Appraise** ➤

I f your project group cannot find a sound and recent research-based clinical practice guideline or systematic review, you may decide to locate and appraise the findings of individual studies—first one study at a time and then as a group of findings from several studies (assuming more than one study was located). As pointed out way back in Chapter 1, a finding of a single research study is like a block or stone in a wall—it is one piece contributing to knowledge about a topic. At some point there may be findings from only one or two studies about an issue, but gradually more studies are done and the knowledge about the topic becomes a more complete structure. Therefore, this chapter starts with a description of how to appraise the findings of individual studies and ends with a description of how to appraise findings from a group of studies.

Two appraisal guides are offered for the findings of individual studies: one for qualitative studies and one for quantitative studies. Of course, this differentiation requires that you be able to determine which type of study you are appraising. Often, the research report will inform you, but you should be able to make the determination on your own. Most often, determining if you are reading a qualitative study report or a quantitative one is quite straightforward. However, if you are not sure, the questions in Box 16–1 should help you decide what kind of study you are reading.

After you have determined the type of study you are reading, you will know which appraisal guide to use. If the study used a mixed design, you should consider using a combination of the two guides.

Box 16-1   DECIDING WHAT TYPE OF RESEARCH ARTICLE YOU ARE READING

Is the study qualitative, quantitative, or was a mixed approach used?

- If the data consists of words, quotes, verbal descriptions, and/or themes, the study is a qualitative study.
- If the data consists of scores, scales, numerical data, percentages, graphs, and/or statistics, the study is a quantitative study.
- If both quantitative and qualitative data was presented, the study has a mixed design.

Broad Credibility Issues

Appropriateness of Design

The credibility of findings of both qualitative and quantitative studies depends on the researcher having used study methods that were appropriate to answer the research questions. So far, you have read about five different research designs but were not asked to challenge whether the researcher used the right design. Short of obtaining a doctoral degree, you may not be able to do this with 100% accuracy; however, there are a few things you should know. The study design used is determined by the question being asked—for some questions there is not a "best" design, but rather several that would be good although providing a slightly different perspective on the question.

If the question has to do with understanding the decision-making process used by parents of a child with severe mental retardation when deciding whether to keep the child at home or place the child in residential care, a study using qualitative methods would get at the complexities of the decision process and how that thinking evolves over time.

A related but different question, "What are the characteristics of families that keep a child with severe mental retardation at home over at least a 5-year period?" could be studied using research methodology that quantifies characteristics such as number and ages of other children, ages of the parents, size of the extended family, social support, income, educational level, community services available, and housing situation. Such a study could produce a descriptive, quantitative profile of families who keep children with severe retardation at home.

If, instead of just quantifying family and community variables, the researcher also wanted to look for relationships among the variables, a correlation design could be used. This would be the case if the researcher looked for relationships between quantifiable family characteristics and the coping level of families who kept children with severe mental retardation at home. A more complex correlational design would examine a group of family and community variables to determine which ones are the best predictors of successfully keeping a child at home.

If the question was, "Does a day care service for children with mental retardation result in fewer children being placed in residential care than if families are paid to take care of their child 24/7 with periodic paid respite?" neither a qualitative study, a descriptive study, or a correlational study would get at the effectiveness of one intervention vis-à-vis the other. An experimental study would be best. Having said that, random assignment may not always be possible, and a quasi-experimental design may have to be used.

Peer Review

You will note that the first question under credibility of both appraisal guides asks whether the research report was published in a journal requiring that all published articles be reviewed by peers. In asking this, the assumption is that research reports published in peer-reviewed journals are of higher quality than are those published in journals that do not require review by peers prior to acceptance. Actually, opinions vary about whether this fact should affect judgment regarding the credibility of the findings. However, peer review does assure the nonresearcher reader that the report has been reviewed by two or three other persons in the field and was deemed worthy of publication.

Unfortunately, it is not always easy to determine if a journal requires peer review. If you cannot find a statement regarding peer review in the front material of the journal, you could check the journal's website—most have them. Research articles published on electronic sites are equally difficult to evaluate. In general, the absence of a statement on the website indicating that articles are peer reviewed should raise the possibility that they are not, which should cause you to be particularly careful in your appraisal of the study's credibility.

Appraisal of the Findings of a Qualitative Study

Credibility

When considering the credibility of the findings of a qualitative study, the main consideration is the rigor of the study's methods. Yet, the criteria for rigor of qualitative studies are diverse, numerous, and not widely agreed upon (Mackey, 2007; Sandelowski & Barroso, 2002). Given the many criteria of rigor, several frequently mentioned ones were incorporated into the qualitative appraisal guide of this chapter. In general, the findings and interpretations of qualitative studies are considered credible if:

- The sampling of participants and observations served the purposes of the study (Fossey, Harvey, McDermott, & Davidson, 2002)
- Observation and/or interviewing were adequately prolonged and persistent (Lincoln & Guba, 1985)
- There was interaction between data collection and data analysis (Morse, Barrett, Mayan, Olson, & Spiers, 2002)
- The findings were rooted in the data (Stiles, 1999)

The findings of qualitative studies tend to be cohesive, that is, they hang together as a group rather than stand separately as findings of quantitative studies often do. Therefore, the findings of qualitative studies can be appraised as a group, although sometimes you might want to consider them separately.

Clinical Significance

Kearney (2001) made a strong case for evaluating the usefulness of findings from qualitative findings based on their richness and informativeness. Richness pertains to the demonstrated linking of findings into a web of connections and the creation of a truly new perspective on the phenomenon under study (Kearney, 2001, p. 146). Thus, the findings are informative to clinicians because they go beyond previous ways of thinking about the situation or experience. Vivid portrayal of the experience or situation and description of how context or events produce variations to the experience add to the usefulness of the findings to the clinician. As you read more qualitative studies you will see that some studies penetrate the experience or situation and produce new insights, whereas others fail to get much beyond what most clinicians in the field of practice already know. In brief, the clinical significance of qualitative findings pertains to their usefulness to clinicians. I suggest that now you look at the appraisal guide for findings of qualitative studies (Figure 16–1) and note how the issues just discussed were incorporated into the guide.

Citation:

Synopsis
What experience, situation, or subculture does the researcher want to understand?

Does the researcher want to produce a description of an experience, a social process, or an event, or is the goal to generate a theory?

How was data collected?

How did the researcher control his or her biases and preconceptions?

Are specific pieces of data (e.g., direct quotes) and more generalized statements (themes, theories) included in the report?

What are the main findings of the study?

Credibility
Is the study published in a source that required that it be peer reviewed?
    Yes ___ No___

Were the methods used appropriate to the study purpose?

Was the sampling of observations and interviews persistent and varied enough to serve the purposes of the study?   Yes___ No___

Were collection methods effective in getting in-depth data?   Yes ___ No ___

Were data collection and analysis intermingled in a dynamic way?

Could the data collection methods have resulted in oversight, underrepresentation, or overrepresentation from certain types of sources?
    Yes ___ No___

■ **FIGURE 16–1**   Appraisal Guide for Findings of a Qualitative Study

---

(continues)

Was the data presented in ways that provide a rich portrayal of what was experienced or happening and its context?   Yes ___   No___

Does the data provided justify generalized statements, themes, or theories? Yes___   No___

How do the findings fit with the findings of other studies regarding this issue?

ARE THE FINDINGS CREDIBLE?   YES ___   NO___

Clinical Significance
Are the findings rich and informative? Yes___   No___

Is the perspective provided potentially useful in providing insight, support, or guidance in assessing patient status and/or progress?   Yes___ No___

ARE THE FINDINGS CLINICALLY SIGNIFICANT? YES___   NO___

Applicability
Were the findings discovered in patients similar to those for whom we provide care?   Yes ___   No ___

Will incorporation of the findings into a protocol enhance the guidance provided to nurses?   Yes ___ No ___

■ **FIGURE 16–1**   Continued

Appraisal of the Findings of a Quantitative Study

Credibility

In quantitative studies, the end products of the study are several, related findings, which are the researchers' data-based conclusions. Like all human conclusions, they can be right or wrong. In correlational and experimental studies, there are two possible correct conclusions and two possible erroneous conclusions.

The correct conclusions are the following:

1. Concluding that a relationship or difference exists in the population when in reality it actually does exist

Table 16–1   REACHING CORRECT CONCLUSIONS

		Is the difference real?	
		Yes	No
	Real difference	Correct	Type 1 error
Researcher's conclusion			
	No difference	Type 2 error	Correct

2. Concluding that no relationship or difference exists in the population when in reality it does not exist

The two types of **conclusion errors** are the following:

1. Concluding that a relationship or difference exists in the population when in reality it does not exist (Type 1 conclusion error)
2. Concluding that no relationship or difference exists in the population when in reality it does exist (Type 2 conclusion error)

For a graphic of these possibilities, see Table 16–1.

Avoiding Conclusion Error   The researcher is obviously aiming for correct conclusions and trying to avoid making conclusion errors. The ways in which she does this are as follows:

- Eliminate chance variation as an explanation
- Avoid low statistical power
- Control extraneous variables
- Control bias

Chance variation, which is always present to some degree when data is collected, can affect the statistical results of a study and lead to wrong conclusions. As you learned in Chapter 7, the researcher controls the role of chance variation by defining its limits. This is what is done when the researcher sets the maximal acceptable decision point *p*-level for significance at .05 or .01. In so doing, she is in essence saying, "I will accept only a low probability that my conclusion that there is a difference is due to chance variation." This in effect reduces the likelihood of a Type 1 conclusion error.

Studies with small sample sizes can have statistical results indicating no relationship or effect when in fact the problem is that the sample size was not large enough (Type 2 conclusion error). A too small sample size results in insufficient statistical power to detect a significant difference, that is, the microscope was too weak, to use a metaphor employed in Chapter 7. The problem is that there was insufficient data to allow the statistics to detect a relationship or a difference amid the chance variation that is inevitably present. The statistical result could lead the researcher to conclude that there is no relationship or difference, when in fact the problem is the low power of the study resulting from the too-small sample size. Using power analysis to determine sample size protects against Type 2 conclusion errors. Remember that from Chapter 7?

Other aspects of the study also determine whether a conclusion is right or wrong. As you learned earlier, researchers use inclusion/exclusion criteria, random assignment, adherence to study protocols, and awareness of what is going on in the research setting to eliminate or isolate the influence of the extraneous variables. However, it may not be possible to control all extraneous variables, or the researcher may not have thought to control a particular influence. Some extraneous variables enter a study without the researcher's awareness in the form of an event or change in the research setting, whereas still others are introduced by the research activities themselves.

Uncontrolled extraneous variables distort study results by mixing with the study variables and producing a statistical result that is an illusion. For example, a statistical result of a study may indicate that there is a significant difference in the outcomes of two treatment groups but reality is that two treatments have equal effects. The statistical result leads the researcher to make a Type 1 conclusion error. The reason underlying the misleading statistical result could be an uncontrolled extraneous variable, such as one treatment group had more persons with multiple co-morbidities than the other group did. The higher level of co-morbidities in one group could have caused that group to have a lower average score on the outcome than the other group, thereby producing a statistically significant difference. If the researcher does not recognize that a difference in co-morbidity levels is present, she could wrongly conclude that one treatment is more effective than the other. Extraneous variables can also produce an illusion of no relationship or no effect when indeed there would have been one had a confounding variable not been at work (Type 2 conclusion error). In short, when evaluating the credibility of findings, you want to ask, "Was anything else going on that could have produced the results obtained, other than what the researcher concluded?"

Bias, which can enter a study at various points in the form of preconceived ideas about what the results will be or unconscious preference for one treatment over another, is also a potential source of erroneous conclusions. In quantitative studies, bias is controlled by research methods such as random sampling, random assignment, checks on adherence to research protocols, blinding of study observers and/or staff, and use of placebo treatments. Generally, researchers will not speak to bias in their reports; rather, you as the reader have to be alert to the possibility of it and decide whether adequate means were taken to prevent bias from affecting study results, findings, and conclusions. Bias can produce either Type 1 or Type 2 conclusion errors.

Credible Versus Valid   The appraisal questions in the guide should assist you in identifying possible sources of wrong conclusions. When the researcher's conclusions are trusted as the best explanation for the results, not chance, extraneous variables, low statistical power, or bias, the findings are deemed credible (Stoddard & Ring, 1993). Although the appraisal guides provided use the term credible to convey that the researcher's conclusions are likely to be trustworthy, other appraisal guides ask, "Are the findings valid?" When used to characterize findings from a study, *valid* means that the findings are judged to be trustworthy reflections of reality and not the result of how the study was conducted or the result of an extraneous variable at work. Note that this usage of the word *valid* is different from the way in which it was used to characterize measurement instruments (in Chapter 5). The term *valid* is more technical and more complex than the word credible. However, the word credible has more commonsense resonance and is an adequate substitute. I suggest that now you look at the credibility questions of the Appraisal Guide for Findings of a Quantitative Study (Figure 16–2) to see how the issues you just read about are incorporated into appraisal.

Citation:

Synopsis
What was the purpose of the study (research questions, purposes, and hypotheses)?

Who participated or contributed data (e.g., target population, how sample was obtained, inclusion criteria, demographic or clinical profile, and dropout rate)?

What methods were used to collect data (e.g., sequence, timing, types of data, and measures)?

Was an intervention tested?   Yes ___ No___

    1. How was the sample size determined?

    2. Were patients randomly assigned to treatment groups?
       Yes ___ No___ Not sure___

What are the main findings?

Credibility
Is the study published in a source that required peer review?
   Yes ___ No___ Not sure___

Was the design used appropriate to the research questions?
   Yes ___ No___ Not sure___

Did the data obtained and the analysis conducted answer the research questions?
   Yes ___ No___ Some but not others ___

Was there anything about the way the participants were chosen or their characteristics that could have influenced the findings?   Yes ___ No___

Were the measuring instruments valid and reliable?   Yes ___ No___

Were important extraneous variables and bias controlled?   Yes ___ No___

Was there anything about the way the study was done that could have influenced the finding(s)?   Yes ___ No___

■ **FIGURE 16–2**   Appraisal Guide for Findings of a Quantitative Study

If an intervention was tested, answer the following five questions:

1. Were participants randomly assigned to groups and were the two groups similar at the start (before an intervention)?   Yes ___ No___ Can't be sure ____

2. Were the interventions well defined and consistently delivered?
   Yes ___ No___

3. Were the groups treated equally other than the difference in the intervention?
   Yes ___ No___ Can't be sure ___

4. If no difference was found, was the sample size large enough to find a difference, if one existed?   Yes ___ No___ Not sure ___

5. If a difference was found, are you confident that it was due to differences in the intervention?   Yes ___ No___

Is each finding consistent with or different from previous findings in this area of study?   Yes ___ No___ Not sure ___

FOR EACH MAIN FINDING, IS IT CREDIBLE?   YES ___ NO _____

Clinical Significance
Note any difference in means, r^2s, or measures of clinical effect (ABI, NNT, RR, OR).

Is the frequency, association, or treatment effect impressive enough to be confident that the finding would make a clinical difference if used as the basis for a care protocol?   Yes ___ No___

IS THE FINDING CLINICALLY SIGNIFICANT?   YES___ NO___

■ **FIGURE 16–2** Continued

Clinical Significance

As discussed in Chapters 6, 7, and 13, the clinical significance of the findings of an individual quantitative study is determined by the strength of the relationship between variables in correlational studies or the size of the difference in the outcomes of the two treatment groups in experimental or quasi-experimental studies. In a correlational study, one would consider the size of the r^2s, whereas in a study comparing interventions, one would consider: (1) the difference in the means of the two groups, (2) the absolute benefit increase (ABI), (3) the numbers needed to treat (NNT), or (4) the relative risk (RR). Therefore, in intervention studies, the clinical significance question is: Is the treatment effect found in the study large enough to make a clinical difference in patient outcomes or well-being?

Applicability

As mentioned earlier, no applicability questions are provided for single, original studies because the assumption is that *generally* a change in practice will not be made based on one study. Having stated the general principle that findings from a single study should not be used as the basis for a change in practice, two exceptions should be noted. One exception would be when a diligent search did not come up with another study and when the basis for current practice is clearly not effective. Of course, the study should have been soundly conducted. In the rare case when the findings of a single study will be used as the basis for practice, the applicability questions from the integrative research review (IRR) guide can be used.

The second exception to not using the findings from a single study as a basis for change might be the findings from a soundly conducted qualitative study. Some would assert that findings from even a single qualitative study make unique contributions to health care in that they "humanize" it (Zuzelo, 2007, p. 497). Findings from single qualitative studies provide understandings of patients' experiences that are useful for assessment, anticipatory guidance, and coaching (Kearney, 2001)—and this information can be incorporated into clinical protocols as well as individual practice. The usefulness of the findings from single qualitative studies is derived from the fact that most qualitative researchers provide considerable detail about the study participants' thoughts and feelings, their experiences, and the contexts of their lives. Thus, it is often quite clear with whom the findings might be used.

Your Turn

At this point, I suggest you appraise the Evangelista et al. (2008) study in Chapter 6 using the study guide of Figure 16–2, then read the critical appraisal a colleague and I did, which is Appendix E.

You also should consider completing an appraisal of the Jacobson et al. (2008) study in Chapter 4 or one of the qualitative studies listed at the end of that chapter to get some practice appraising qualitative studies. Alternatively, your instructor may ask you to appraise one of the articles in Chapters 5, 7, or 8. The more appraisals you do, the better you will get at using the questions to make a judgment regarding the credibility and clinical significance of study findings.

Across-Studies Analysis

Now that you have some skill in appraising individual studies, you need to at least be aware of what is involved in appraising several studies regarding a question or issue. This would have to be done when an agency team could not locate an evidence-based clinical practice guideline or systematic review, but did find several relevant studies. In addition to appraising each study separately, the several studies should be appraised as a body of studies; doing so is called **across-studies analysis** (Brown, 1999). In essence, the team has to do their own integrative research review before translating the evidence into an agency protocol (Stetler et al., 1998). This will require identifying, retrieving, and appraising studies, then bringing together the findings from all relevant and sound studies.

Doing an across-studies review and summary is not something an individual would be expected to do. It is an advanced skill and is best done by a group in which the individual members' interpretations and thinking regarding the findings of the various studies can complement and correct one another. Generally, project teams who do across-studies analysis have a few members with master's or doctoral education. You may, however, be asked to be a member of an evidence-based practice (EBP) project team, in which case you will learn by direct observation how across-studies analysis is done. To prepare you for that, I offer a brief description of what across-studies analysis involves.

The goal in looking at a body of evidence is to answer the question, "What findings earn our confidence because they are well supported by one or more sound studies?" To answer this question, the protocol development team must determine the following:

- How many studies addressed the issue?
- Were the studies of good quality?

■ Was the finding consistently produced by several well-conducted studies?

■ If an intervention was studied, was the size of the treatment effect or the relationship of similar magnitude across the studies?

■ Can inconsistencies regarding a finding be explained by study differences in patient populations or research methods?

Thus, the essential across-studies issues are the quality, quantity, and consistency of evidence across studies. If the project team is appraising two or more studies, they may work with a findings table (see Table 16–2). If the clinical issue has several sub-issues, such as prevention and management, the team might use separate findings tables for each sub-issue. As mentioned earlier, the team may decide to weight studies with strong methodology or samples similar to their own population of patients more heavily than studies with weak methodology or samples that are very different.

Unlike the findings of single studies, for which the general recommendation was made that they not be used as the basis for clinical protocols, whenever clear conclusions are produced by across-studies analysis, the conclusions can be used as the basis for practice. The applicability questions in the IRR guide (Figure 15–1) will assist in planning implementation of across-studies conclusions.

Appraisal of findings from several or many studies involves decisions about the credibility, clinical significance, and applicability of the body of evidence. Ideally, these decisions should be reached in a deliberative way by the consensus of the EBP project team (Lomas, Culyer, McCutcheon, McAuley, & Law, 2005). A deliberative process requires the following:

■ Clear objectives
■ Clear criteria for appraising the evidence
■ Clear rules regarding how to handle studies of poor quality
■ Good analytical thinking
■ Broad participatory dialogue
■ Formal polling to resolve differences of opinion
■ Skillful chairing

Appendix F is a completed findings table pertaining to fatigue in patients with congestive heart failure. Information from the study you read in Chapter 7 is extracted onto this table along with several other studies about the issue. Be advised that this findings table is not inclusive of all studies on this topic; rather the studies are representative of what might be found.

Table 16–2   FINDINGS TABLE

Topic _____   Date _____

Author(s) and date	Questions, variables, objectives, hypotheses	Design, sample, setting	Findings	Notes

Wrap-Up

Evaluating a body of evidence is definitely the long and labor-intensive way of establishing the state-of-the-science regarding an issue. However, sometimes a project group will have to do it; when necessary, it is important that the group include a person with knowledge of research methodology—be it an in-house person or a consultant.

REFERENCES

Brown, S. J. (1999). *Knowledge for health care practice: A guide to using research evidence.* Philadelphia, PA: Saunders.

Evangelista, L. S., Moser, D. K., Westlake, C., Pike, N., Ter-Galstanyan, A., & Dracup, K. (2008). Correlates of fatigue in patients with heart failure. *Progress in Cardiovascular Nursing, 23*(1), 12–17.

Fossey, E., Harvey, C., McDermott, F., & Davidson, L. (2002). Understanding and evaluating qualitative research. *Australian and New Zealand Journal of Psychiatry, 36,* 717–732.

Kearney, M. H. (2001). Levels and application of qualitative research evidence. *Research in Nursing and Health, 24,* 145–153.

Lincoln, Y. S., & Guba, E. G. (1985). *Naturalistic inquiry.* Beverly Hills, CA: Sage.

Lomas, J., Culyer, T., McCutcheon, C., McAuley, L., & Law, S. (2005). *Conceptualizing and combining evidence for health system guidance.* Canadian Health Services Research Foundation. Retrieved from http://www.chsrf.ca/kte_docs/Conceptualizing%20and%20combining%20evidence.pdf

Mackey, M. C. (2007). Evaluation of qualitative research. In P. L. Munhall (Ed.), *Nursing research: A qualitative perspective* (4th ed., pp. 555–568). Sudbury, MA: Jones and Bartlett.

Morse, J. M., Barrett, M., Mayan, M., Olson, K., & Spiers, J. (2002). Verification strategies for establishing reliability and validity in qualitative research. International Journal of Qualitative Methods 1(2), article 2. Retrieved from http://www.ualberta.ca/~iiqm/backissues/1_2Final/html/morse.html

Sandelowski, M., & Barroso, J. (2002). Reading qualitative studies. *International Journal of Qualitative Methods, 1*(1), article 5. Retrieved from http://ejournals.library.ualberta.ca/index.php/IJQM/issue/view/385

Stetler, C. B., Morsi, D., Rucki, S., Broughton, S., Corrigan, B., Fitzgerald, J., et al. (1998). Utilization-focused integrative reviews in a nursing service. *Applied Nursing Research, 11*(4), 196–206.

Stiles, W. B. (1999). Evaluating qualitative research. *Evidence-Based Mental Health, 2,* 99–101.

Stoddard, G. J., & Ring, W. H. (1993). How to evaluate study methodology in published clinical research. *Journal of Intravenous Nursing, 16*(2), 110–117.

Zuzelo, P. R. (2007). Evidence-based nursing and qualitative research: A partnership imperative for real-world practice. In P. L. Munhall (Ed.), *Nursing research: A qualitative perspective* (4th ed., pp. 481–499). Sudbury, MA: Jones and Bartlett.

ADDITIONAL RESOURCE

A completed appraisal of the correlational study posted on the website for Chapter 6 (Mentes et al., 2007) is available on the companion website page for this chapter. The companion website for this book can be accessed at *go.jblearning.com/brown.*

CHAPTER SEVENTEEN
Evidence-Based Practice

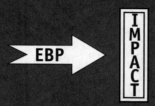

Now that you have some knowledge about how research is conducted and how to appraise research evidence for use as the basis of clinical practice, you need to learn how research evidence is translated into action. In this and the next two chapters, the research–practice connection is explored in greater depth than it was early in the book.

Professional Action

In an insightful book about the nature of professional practice (Schon, 1983), this very useful quote was offered, "All professional practice is centrally concerned with *design*, that is, with the process of changing existing situations into preferred ones" (Simon, 1969, p. 55). This is a potentially powerful description of nursing. The image of a bridge is useful. One can visualize professional actions as spans of a bridge that link two sides of a river. On one side: a problematic or potentially problematic patient situation; on the other side: a better situation. Effective professional actions, which include acts of physical care and treatment, self-care teaching, and encouragement, help the patient get to a better state of health or wellness.

> ▓ In the hospital, when the patient is uncomfortable, the nurse repositions him or gives pain medication to make him comfortable; pain is the existing situation, and comfort the preferred situation (discomfort → comfort).

343

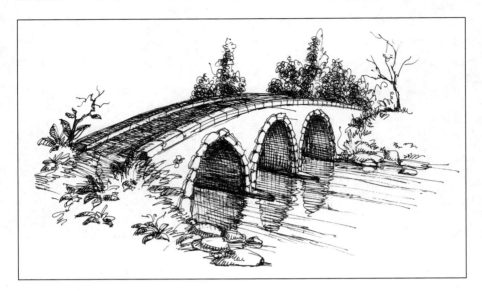

Source: © Danussa/ShutterStock, Inc.

- In the clinic, when a patient is at risk of hypertension, the nurse practitioner makes recommendations for lowering her blood pressure (existing level of risk → lower level of risk).
- At home, when the patient is not taking medications correctly, the nurse devises a system to promote more accurate medication taking (medication mistakes → fewer mistakes).
- In the ICU, when the patient has low oxygen saturation, the nurse suctions or repositions the patient to improve air exchange (low oxygenation → better oxygenation).

In all these situations, nurses help change problematic existing situations into preferred ones. Clearly, the ultimate goal of nursing, and indeed all of health care, is impact on patient outcomes.

Evidence-Based Care Design

The image of a bridge is applicable for another reason: A bridge is a designed structure. Bridges are not just put together at the site on a work-it-out-as-you-go basis. Rather, modern bridges are thoughtfully and carefully designed in advance using engineering knowledge that has been developed through research over the years. The same is true of professional nursing action—care should be designed in advance, to the degree possible, using scientific nursing knowledge.

Many providers work in clinical areas where most patients have health conditions that are seen over and over again. Thus, many aspects of care can be designed in advance of a particular patient. This is what is done when project teams develop clinical protocols for specific patient populations. Protocol development can be thought of as **prespecification design** in that the project team brings together knowledge about the issue and uses it as the basis for the protocol. Then, at the point-of-care,

> clinicians combine the recommendation of the pre-specification plan with all they know about the individual patient. Based on their understanding of the patient and their own past experience dealing with similar patients, they make judgments about whether and how to alter the protocol. They decide how and when to deliver the pre-specified protocol and develop plans for clinical problems and issues not addressed by the protocol. (Brown, 2001, p. 5)

In brief, effective nursing care for individual patients requires sound prespecification design in the form of evidence-based clinical protocols and astute **point-of-care design** in the form of adapting clinical protocols to the individual patient.

Care Design

Prespecification Design + Point-of-Care Design

Prespecification: Evidence-Based Care Protocols

There is general agreement that answers to the following kinds of questions should be based on the best scientific knowledge available (Institute of Medicine, 2001).

- Does preoxygenation before endotracheal suctioning reduce hypoxemia during and after suctioning?
- How should we carry out tight glucose control therapy with surgical patients?
- What is the best way to screen for domestic violence in the emergency department?

▪ Does "this" way of teaching self-catheterization of the bladder result in a low incidence of urinary tract infections and minimal patient and family distress?

▪ How can we differentiate between delirium, dementia, and depression in the elderly?

The practical hurdle to evidence-based practice is that practitioners engage in thousands of clinical actions each day. Obtaining and evaluating the research evidence for each action and each decision would be overwhelming for the individual practitioner. This is where agency-endorsed, clinical care protocols enter the picture—to support practitioners in their care planning and decision making. Clinical protocols serve two purposes:

▪ They set forth standards of care to guide clinicians in giving care.

▪ They promote consistency of patient care, that is, the care given by all providers to all patients in the population is similar.

Protocols can take many forms: comprehensive plans of care for specified patient populations, procedures for performing clinical actions, care bundles, standardized order sets, decision algorithms, care maps, and clinical pathways (for examples, see the websites listed at end of this chapter). By way of definition, "a **care bundle** is a group of e-b interventions related to a disease process that, when executed together, result in better outcomes than when implemented individually" (Institute for Healthcare Improvement, 2007). A widely used care bundle is the *prevention-of-ventilator-associated-pneumonia* bundle; nursing interventions that are part of this bundle include elevation of the head of the bed, oral care, meticulous hand washing, suctioning secretions above the endotracheal cuff, and interruption of sedation (Lawson, 2005). A review of six studies found that when used together, these practices decrease ventilator-associated pneumonia (O'Keefe-McCarthy, Santiago, & Lau, 2008).

Decision algorithms are step-by-step instructions for reaching a decision or solving a problem; they are often formatted as trees consisting of a series of yes/no questions leading to one of several possible decisions or actions. A clinical pathway is a multidisciplinary specification of patient management for a well defined group of patients over a specified period of time (DeBleser et al., 2006). A pathway explicitly sets forth time-based goals, key actions, and sequences of care.

Point-of-Care Design: Individualized Care

Care protocols help incorporate scientifically supported care actions into actual care and promote consistency of care. However, as noted earlier, most scientific evidence is based on what works best *on average*. Thus, even when the research evidence is strong in support of a care approach, we cannot expect everyone to benefit from it. Most certainly, scientifically based care has a high probability of benefiting patients in specified ways, but it is not a guarantee of effectiveness. Additionally, even though it is effective, the care approach may not be acceptable to some persons. For these reasons, a person's care ultimately should be individualized based on whether the care being offered is effective and acceptable to him or her. When care is adapted or modified to individual preferences and responses, it is considered individualized, personalized, or tailored to the individual.

Consider this example. A nurse sees a patient in a diabetes mellitus clinic. Noticing that he has some shortness of breath at rest, the nurse looks into his healthcare record to determine how his persistent asthma is being managed. He has a prescribed steroid inhaler (with a spacer) and a PRN inhaler for relief of shortness of breath. The nurse then asks the patient about how often he uses the inhalers; he admits that he doesn't use the steroid inhaler very often because "it has a bad taste, it dries out my mouth, and it ruins the taste of good food." He says he'd rather use the PRN inhaler. The nurse explains the value of the steroid medication in preventing asthma symptoms and explains why it should be taken regularly, not when he "needs more air." He says, "Yeah, I know." She also suggests gargling with warm water after using the steroid inhaler.

Two months later when the nurse sees the patient in the clinic, he is still noticeably short of breath. She asks about his use of the steroid inhaler. Again, he admits that he is not using it very much. The nurse talks with him more and finds out that he doesn't mind taking pills; she says she will talk with his physician about his medications and try to come up with an alternative approach for managing his asthma. Thus, even though the asthma protocol recommends inhaled steroid as a first-line treatment, his plan of care needs to be adjusted to take into account his rather strong aversion to using the inhaled steroid. This is individualized care. The nurse was attuned to how the patient was responding to protocol-recommended care and tried to help the patient get comfortable with it, but eventually she had to seek a different approach.

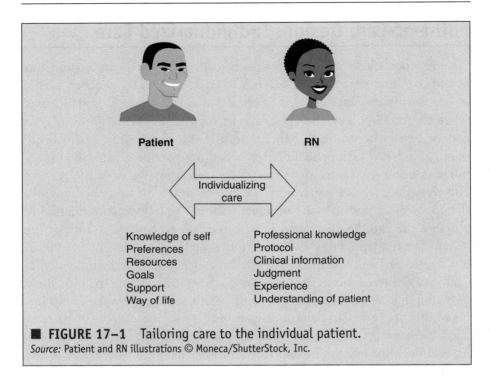

■ FIGURE 17–1   Tailoring care to the individual patient.
Source: Patient and RN illustrations © Moneca/ShutterStock, Inc.

As shown in Figure 17–1, at the point of care, the clinician and the patient together (whenever possible) decide if the evidence-based protocol endorsed by the agency or health system is appropriate, acceptable, and effective. The patient brings to this discussion responses, preferences, experiences, life goals, family support, and resources. The clinician brings clinical knowledge, prior experience with similar cases, and professional judgment. Through such an exchange, evidence-based protocols are tailored to the individual patient (Brown, 2001; Flynn & Sinclair, 2005).

Evidence-Based Quality Management

Clinical protocols are one component of larger programs aimed at achieving good patient outcomes by making sure that the most effective clinical interventions are consistently provided to patients. These larger programs go under a variety of names: *performance improvement, clinical improvement,* and *total quality management.* Each of these programs has a slightly different perspective on how to achieve quality health care, but they

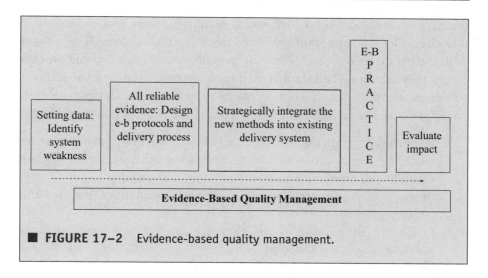

■ FIGURE 17–2   Evidence-based quality management.

have a great deal of commonality of purpose and overlap of methods (Oleson, 1999). Rather than distinguish among them, which would be a diversion from the purposes of the book, I am going to use the term **evidence-based quality management** (EBQM) to refer to these programs (see Figure 17–2). I choose this term because it conveys the following program characteristics:

- Quality of care as the goal
- The use of various sources of information, that is, evidence
- Active management as the process used to achieve and maintain quality care

Sources of Evidence

These programs use a combination of research evidence, expert opinion, benchmarking data, and setting-specific data to design effective practice methods and systems of care. Research evidence is essential to designing effective protocols; however, scientifically based protocols are not sufficient by themselves—they must be embedded in care delivery systems that are safe, patient-centered, efficient, and timely (Institute for Healthcare Improvement, 2007). All healthcare systems collect a great deal of information to help evaluate the performance of their systems of care. For hospital systems, this information profiles the patient stay, including information such as admission and discharge diagnoses, surgical procedures done, complications, length of stay, discharge destination, total cost, and re-hospitalizations within 30 days of discharge. Other information, extracted from the medical records of patients with specific diagnoses, reveals the care patients actually received and the outcomes they attained. This data is used to detect weaknesses in the setting's processes of care and creates opportunities to improve care. Setting performance data typically provides information about the following aspects of care:

- Proportion of patients who received an assessment or intervention required by agency protocol (for example, smoking cessation counseling offered to patients with acute myocardial infarction)
- Proportion of patients who achieved specific outcomes (positive and negative)
- Frequency of adverse events that occurred during care (such as hospital-acquired infections)
- Patients' level of satisfaction with care
- Cost (often as cost per case)

Many hospitals and agencies collect this kind of data in conjunction with various quality monitoring programs. Many also use benchmarking to compare their performance to that of other similar agencies and to get a sense of what level of quality is achievable. For instance, an agency might determine that their patient fall level is 4.6 falls per 1,000 patient-days, whereas other similar agencies in their benchmarking network have a fall rate of 1.9 falls per 1,000 patient-days. This information is evidence in support of the need for a new approach to fall prevention in the agency.

I would suggest that you go to the website of several hospitals and look at their quality reports—many hospitals post them. Alternatively, go to the United States Department of Health and Human Services' *Hospital Compare* website, http://www.hospitalcompare.hhs.gov and obtain quality information about several hospitals familiar to you. The reality is that a great deal of hospital performance information is publicly available.

Research data and setting performance data are a natural twosome (Ingersoll, 2005; Levin et al., 2010). Setting performance data and benchmarking help identify and pinpoint quality problems in the delivery system, whereas research evidence provides a scientific basis for new care protocols. Conclusive research evidence may not be available for all major clinical actions and decisions the agency team wants to include in the protocol, thus a protocol development team may have to rely on expert opinion at the table to develop some parts of the protocol—much like guideline development panels do.

Project Scope

Evidence-based quality management (EBQM) projects are initiated when:

1. Care in general or a care method in particular has been recognized as less effective than it could be; or
2. A new component of care is going to be introduced (e.g., perioperative blood salvage and administration during and after surgery).

Both situations require that clinical care or an aspect of care, for a certain population of patients be specified or specified anew. EBQM projects can range from narrow to very broad in scope. A narrow EBQM project involves redesigning just one aspect of care, whereas a broad project could involve redesigning a whole system of care. An EBQM project of narrow scope was undertaken by a nursing staff when the issue of whether patients had to lie flat to get accurate hemodynamic parameters came up in a staff meeting. They decided to redesign their hemodynamic monitoring protocol based on research evidence and redo their staff orientation module about the protocol. Another narrow-scope project would be redesigning a new plan for how to convey essential information preoperatively to persons having same-day surgery, whereas redesigning same-day surgery care from the time a surgery is scheduled through patient discharge would be a very broad project.

Although commitment to quality improvement is an organizational commitment, actual quality improvement projects are increasingly carried out at the microsystem level, that is, by the people who work together in delivering care to a population of patients. This may be the unit, such as the medical intensive care unit, or a service line, such as those providing care to patients with pulmonary diseases. For example, one inpatient medical unit team "decided to focus on the environment of care and how physical space, clutter, noise and light affect the patient experience, communication patterns, efficiency and staff satisfaction" (http://dms.dartmouth.edu/cms/materials/workbooks/inpatient.doc).

Project Team

The EBQM project requires a team with skills in the following areas:

- Database searching for relevant research articles (especially guidelines, summaries)
- Critically appraising guidelines, summaries, and individual research reports

- Analyzing and summarizing setting performance data
- Designing evidence-based protocols and systems of care
- Knowledge of how the unit or service line works logistically
- Implementing organizational change

To achieve the full complement of skills, the team may be comprised of direct care providers, advanced practice nurses, managers, a health science librarian, quality improvement staff persons, and an evidence-based practice specialist (e.g., nurse researcher).

To recap, **evidence-based care design** is the immediate antecedent of evidence-based nursing practice (EBN). It takes place away from the direct care setting when project teams meet to develop clinical protocols that become the standards of care for their agency. The protocols, which are mainly based on research evidence and agency performance data, serve as evidence-based (e-b) guides for clinicians regarding what care should be given to individual patients and how it should be given.

Evidence-Based Care

Ideally, once an e-b protocol has been developed and explained to the staff, they will begin to change their practice to bring it into alignment with the protocol. The reality is that this is not always the case. Even when clinicians value research evidence and strive to practice in an evidence-based way, a new protocol may be difficult to incorporate into a busy day. There are many reasons why staff may not fall in line with an evidence-based protocol. The needed supplies may not be readily available, the protocol may not fit in with the work flow, or a learning curve may be associated with some aspect of the new protocol. Thus, clinical protocols have to be strategically introduced and promoted to ensure uptake of the protocol actions by clinicians.

Organizational Characteristics

In some hospitals and healthcare agencies, evidence-based practice (EBP) is thriving—the place is alive with care improvement projects and ideas for projects—whereas in others EBP is struggling. Organizational characteristics contributing to EBP have been identified in the following areas:

- Culture
- Capacity

- ○ EBP knowledge and skills
- ○ Skill in making organization change

- ▦ Organizational structure
- ▦ Computer systems

Culture   Organizations in which EBP is the established way of designing care value e-b protocols as important tools in their unrelenting quest for quality (Cullen, Greiner, Greiner, Bombei, & Comried, 2005; Estabrooks et al., 2008; Rycroft-Malone, 2004; Stetler et al., 2009). Quality monitoring and bringing up new ideas for care are encouraged as ways to identify weaknesses and provide opportunities for care improvement. In a quality-oriented environment, nurse executives, managers, and unit leaders encourage EBP projects and applaud staff members who participate in them.

Importantly, initiation of EBP projects is not only a top-down responsibility. Every professional nurse has the responsibility to identify problems in care and bring them to the attention of nursing leaders. As an example, a staff RN in the operating room noticed that patients arriving in the post-anesthesia area had low body temperatures, and he was concerned that the methods of keeping patients warm in the operating room were not adequate. He knew there was research evidence showing that improved temperature control in surgical patients resulted in fewer surgical site infections, so he talked with his nurse manager and the infection control nurse. They decided to collect data from patients' records about their temperature before surgery and when arriving in the anesthesia recovery area. Eventually, this nurse's observations about patients' conditions and the data collected resulted in launching an evidence-based, care redesign project regarding maintenance of body temperature during the peri-operative period (Central Vermont Hospital, Barre, VT). Thus, EBQM began with a staff nurse making observations about patients.

I have a question . . .

I've noticed that . . .

I read this research article that says . . .

Capacity   Valuing EBP is a starting point, but to be successful an organization must also develop a capacity for EBP (Cullen et al., 2005; Melnyk, 2005; Stetler, 2009). Capacity for EBP requires: (1) persons on staff who have EBP knowledge and skills, (2) skills in managing organizational change, and (3) an organizational structure that facilitates the use of research and agency performance evidence in all decisions regarding nursing care.

EBP Knowledge and Skills   Some advanced practice nurses and nurse managers with master's degrees acquired EBP and quality improvement knowledge and skills during their graduate education. Others attended courses or workshops to acquire the knowledge. Consequently, advanced practice nurses and/or nurse managers often provide leadership for EBQM projects. By involving staff nurses in projects, the number of persons who understand EBP and quality improvement grows. All staff nurses should participate in EBQM projects in some way—by identifying problems in care, participating in protocol development, helping to implement new e-b protocols, or just making an effort to use them.

Several medical centers develop EBP knowledge and skill in their staff by offering in-depth workshops and mentored experiences:

- UCLA medical center offers evidence-based practice fellowships (Gawlinksi, 2008).
- Maine Medical Center has a clinical scholars program (http://www. mmc.org/nursing_body.cfm?id=4658).
- University of Iowa Hospital and Clinics has EBP internships (http:// www.uihealthcare.com/depts/nursing/rqom/evidencebasedpractice/ internship.html).

Participants in these programs attend workshops about EBP, develop skills in examining research evidence regarding a clinical issue, and are mentored in making an evidence-based change in practice.

Skill in Making Organizational Change   As mentioned earlier, e-b innovations and protocols cannot just be dropped into a care system; rather they must be strategically introduced, promoted, and maintained (Pearson, Field, & Jordan, 2007; Solberg et al., 2000). The issue of making organizational change is a huge topic unto itself, so only a few pointers are provided here. Most importantly, introducing a new protocol into an organization's workflow can be a make-or-break point for an EBP project. The evidence can be strong and clear and the protocol can be carefully developed; however, it will not fly if its introduction is not carefully planned and executed. In a sense, a care system is like an oceanliner in that quite a bit has to be done to make even a small change in course.

When developing a protocol, early on it is wise to involve major stakeholders, that is, departments and persons whose work will be directly affected by the protocol. Then, at the time of planning the implementation, it may be smart to involve others, such as the unit teacher or a home care nurse. A nursing research council that was revising the protocol for assessment of patients who were receiving blood transfusions involved a laboratory technician from the blood bank early in the project. This person provided valuable data about transfusion reactions that had occurred in the hospital and had good suggestions when the protocol was being developed and implemented. The evidence-based assessment protocol eventually became part of a larger policy on the administration of blood and blood components (Rutland Regional Medical Center, 2007).

Protocol intervention is also facilitated if highly respected persons in the work setting are recruited to be "champions" for the protocol. Champions are not persons with organizational status, rather they are peers that other people go to for answers—they are the informal leaders. These persons may be part of the project team right from the beginning or brought in during the discussion of implementation. Champions help with introduction of the protocol by modeling it, by discussing it with others, and by helping troubleshoot problems in implementation.

The logistics of implementing the protocol need to be worked out in detail so as to make adoption of the protocol easy for direct care providers. This might require increasing the floor stock of a certain item, changing a standardized order set, adding a space on a documentation form or dialogue box, providing a pocket quick guide, or holding classes on how to perform a new clinical skill. The champions can talk to other staff and learn if there are any snags or barriers to following the protocol—often these can be overcome, which will increase the likelihood that the protocol will be adopted.

Making a change in practice typically encounters both enthusiasm and resistance. Cullen et al. (2005) described the tag-flag-nag approach to supporting EBP innovation. Tagging involves identifying and visibly recognizing staff nurses who adopt the practice change. Flagging involves identifying less compliant staff and discussing with them how they can incorporate the change into their care. Nagging is the way of dealing with persistent noncompliers; it involves recruiting opinion leaders on the unit to talk with the noncompliers about their failure to adopt the new standard of care, and, if necessary, more firm ways of dealing with their resistance to change. Thus, leaders use a variety of carrot and stick strategies to convey that quality of care is the goal and that persons who detract from that goal will be held accountable for their failure to meet unit standards.

In short, EBP cannot be just an espoused value; it must also be an enacted value that permeates the thinking and decision making of the organization (Cullen et al., 2005). Organizational change is a way of life; healthcare systems must constantly change in responses to new knowledge, new technology, and shifting healthcare policies. A department that lacks the ability to skillfully introduce and sustain change will struggle achieving EBP. Articles describing in detail the development and implementation of an e-b protocol are provided at the end of the chapter.

Organizational Structure   The organizational structure of successful EBP nursing departments are quite clear about which councils or committees have responsibilities for EBQM, and about how various roles contribute to it (Cullen et al., 2005; Gawlinksi, 2008). Importantly, EBQM is not done by one council, but rather it requires collaboration among councils because all councils have the same objective: quality of care—and achieving that objective requires various approaches and programs. A nursing practice council should not revise nursing procedures and policies without referring to the research base relevant to the issue. A quality management council should not develop a needlestick injury prevention program without knowledge of the research evidence about what has worked elsewhere. A research committee in a home care agency should not develop an evidence-based program for managing polypharmacy in their elderly patients without understanding exactly what kinds of problems are actually occurring, which would require collecting some data. In summary, the overlapping and multifaceted nature of quality improvement efforts makes it wise to structure an organization in a way that creates dynamic linkages between the councils or committees (Cullen et al., 2005).

Computer Systems   Nursing practice runs on knowledge and information. They fuel care design and clinical decision making. Fortunately, making knowledge and information available to clinicians in formats usable in real time is an area that is expanding rapidly. Information systems increasingly link clinicians to a full range of information sources in an integrated and practical manner (Porter-O'Grady, 2006). Clinical information systems that integrate agency protocols into plans of care for individual patients and remind nurses of care actions required by protocol foster adoption of changes in practice. Further, access to healthcare evidence on the Internet promotes clinical curiosity and information seeking by staff confronted by care dilemmas. There is more discussion about computer support at the point-of-care in the next chapter.

EBP Organizational Profile

- Evidence-oriented culture
- Capacity for using evidence

  - EBP knowledge and skill
  - Skill in making organizational change

- Integrative organizational structure
- Facilitating computer system

Impact

The Ultimate Goal   Assume that an e-b protocol has been skillfully introduced and a significant part of the staff are following it. Evidence-based nursing (EBN) is a reality. The quest for quality has achieved its goal—right? Yes—and no. In fact, EBN has been achieved; however, EBN is not the ultimate goal. The ultimate goal is patients achieving good clinical and life outcomes as a result of the care they receive (Goode, 1995). EBN is the process of care, whereas patients' achieving desired outcomes is the endpoint of care. We cannot assume that because care actions are evidence-based, good patient outcomes are resulting (Landon et al., 2007; American Nurses Credentialing Center, 2010; Wimpenny, Johnson, Walter, & Wilkinson, 2008). What worked in research studies, what experts recommended, and changes made in agency workflow or methods may not have accomplished what everyone thought they would.

It must be objectively demonstrated that when the e-b protocol is used as the standard for care in the setting, good patient outcomes result—outcomes such as lower rates of adverse events and better functional status at discharge. Then, and only then, can clinicians say with confidence that the care they are providing is the very best possible, given what is known at the time. In brief, evidence-based nursing practice has a high probability of producing good patient outcomes; however, the protocol's actual impact must be evaluated.

Evaluation   Generally, the evaluation of a protocol's impact consists of measuring delivery system performance and patient outcomes (Goode, 1995; Kirchhoff & Rakel, 1999). Patient outcomes are typically measured through audits of patients' healthcare records or by extraction from the quality measures datasets required by federal, state, and accrediting agencies. These sources allow the EBQM team to determine the proportion of patients that experienced a particular outcome—good or bad. Examples of nursing sensitive patient outcome measures are skin integrity, symptom control, quality of life, self-care ability, and absence of pneumonia.

Measuring delivery system performance involves determining whether the system is meeting the process of care standards it set for itself; for example:

- Were all the aspects of assessment required by the protocol completed?
- Were the appropriate fall prevention interventions put into place?
- Did all patients in the protocol population receive a home care referral with the recommended information in a timely manner?

Sometimes system performance is difficult to get at because patients' health records do not always include documentation of every action that was performed. Often, however, data can be collected from existing work documents; other times a documentation form may need to be changed to provide for the documentation of a key step in care, such as a dedicated space for documenting that diabetic foot examination was done. When data cannot be obtained from work documents, a special data collection may need to be done, such as random observations of staff compliance with a positioning protocol for patients on ventilators. Or by conducting short, random interviews of patients, such as patients' views regarding the helpfulness of patient teaching about anticoagulants.

This evaluation of protocol impact need not be burdensome to the unit or agency. Collecting data for evaluation of a protocol's impact should involve a few easy-to-obtain measures—it need not be extensive and in-depth (Nelson, Splaine, Batalden, & Plume, 1998). Measurement of the patient outcomes of actual care delivery is not research (Ingersoll, 2005). It is like taking vital signs to get a general sense of a person's condition. Changes in the data over time measure the ongoing success or failure of the protocol or of its implementation—which are sometimes difficult to sepa-rate. If the system's performance data indicate that the key steps of care are *not* being performed, then the assumption must be made that the problem is in implementation, not in the protocol itself. In contrast, if the key steps are being carried out but patients are not achieving the desired outcomes, then the protocol itself may not be effective. An ineffective protocol must be revisited to determine why it is not working:

- Was the evidence not interpreted correctly?
- Was the translation of the evidence into the agency protocol faulty?

And so the quest for quality begins anew.

The appraisal guides for clinical practice guidelines and integrative research reviews (IRRs) include a question about how the protocol innova-tion will be evaluated. This question is included because the impact evalua-tion should be planned at the time the protocol is developed, not as an afterthought. Such an evaluation is critical to knowing whether the evidence-based practice has indeed produced good patient outcomes.

Recap

At this point, I want to ask you to pause and consider all that has been pre-sented to this point in the book. Figure 17–3 portrays the "really big pic-ture" beginning with recognition that knowledge for practice is not adequate, proceeding through the steps of knowledge production and EBP, and finally to confidence that patients are being given the best care possible at this point in time. It is a long path, culminating in patients benefiting from the care provided by professional nurses.

Full Disclosure

Having advocated EBP throughout the book, I must be completely up front about an important issue. The fact is that, although there is a widely held assumption that adoption of evidence-based practices results in better patient outcomes, there is not a great deal of research evidence to back this assumption (Bahtsevani, Uden, & Willman, 2004; Grimshaw et al., 2006). It's not that the research shows that EBP does not have a positive impact on patients' outcomes; rather, credible research linking EBP and patient outcomes is sparse. Importantly, this lack of demonstrated influence does

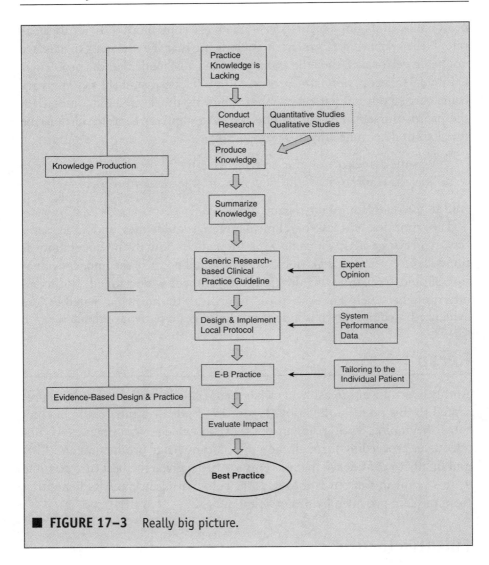

■ **FIGURE 17–3**   Really big picture.

not mean that the original research about the effectiveness of the interventions was wrong, rather that we have very little evidence indicating that research-based actions are effective when translated into local protocols and incorporated into diverse delivery systems.

Evidence regarding the benefits is lacking because direct, controlled studies of the impact of e-b nursing care are logistically and ethically very difficult to conduct (DiCenso, Ciliska, & Guyatt, 2005). Logistically, it is difficult to separate the effect of the recommendations from the effect of how the guideline was introduced, adopted, and sustained. Many e-b changes in practice are complex, affecting the actions of many people; this makes it difficult to evaluate the impact of a change in one part of the delivery system.

Quite a bit of research is underway in the field of implementation science, also called translation science. This is a field of study aimed at producing evidence about evidence-based practice implementation. At this point, the majority of completed studies focus on the personal, organizational, and health system factors that affect incorporation of recommended e-b actions into practice. Building knowledge about the impact on patient outcomes will be possible only after the incorporation of e-b recommendations into actual practice is better understood. However, evidence in support of better patient outcomes resulting from implementation of evidence-based practices is accumulating, albeit slowly (Medves et al., 2009).

Ethical issues also affect the study of EBP on patient outcomes. Once research establishes that a certain care action produced good patient outcomes, in actual care it is difficult to justify providing some patients with the research-based care and others with care that has not been research-tested. Consequently, at this time the evidence consists of numerous evaluation reports of better outcomes resulting from implementation of e-b protocols (e.g., Haycock et al., 2005; Lund et al., 2001; O'Keefe-McCarthy et al., 2008).

To summarize, when you follow an evidence-based protocol, you are engaging in evidence-based practice. You have the rigor of the evidence-based care design process behind your actions. However, there are times when the protocol is not effective or important aspects of nursing care are not guided by agency protocol. When you become aware of these gaps in care, you should bring them to the attention of the practice council or nurse leader of your unit. Other ways in which you might participate in and contribute to evidence-based nursing projects are described in the next chapter.

References

American Nurses Credentialing Center. (2010). Announcing a new model for ANCC's Magnet recognition program. Retrieved from http://www.nursecredentialing.org/Magnet/NewMagnetModel.aspx

Bahtsevani, C., Uden, G., & Willman, A. (2004). Outcomes of evidence-based practice guidelines: A systematic review. *International Journal of Technology in Health Care, 20*(4), 427–433.

Brown, S. J. (2001). Managing the complexity of best practice health care. *Journal of Nursing Care Quality, 15*(2), 1–8.

Cullen, L., Greiner, J., Greiner, J., Bombei, C., & Comried, L. (2005). Excellence in evidence-based practice: Organizational and unit exemplars. *Critical Care Nursing Clinics of North America, 17*, 127–142.

DeBleser, L., Depreitere, R., De Waele, K., VanHaecht, K., Vlayen, J., Sermeus, W. (2006). Defining pathways. *Journal of Nursing Management, 14*(7), 553–563.

DiCenso, A., Ciliska, D., & Guyatt, G. (2005). Introduction to evidence-based nursing. In A. DiCenso, G. Guyatt, & D. Ciliska (Eds.), *Evidence-based nursing: A guide to clinical practice* (pp. 14–19). Orlando, FL: Elsevier Mosby.

Estabrooks, C. A., Scott, S., Squires, J., Stevens, B., O-Brien-Pallas, L., Profetto-McGrath, J., et al. (2008). Patterns of research utilization on patient care units. *Implementations Science, 3*, 31. doi:10.1186/1748-5908-3-31

Flynn, A. V., & Sinclair, M. (2005). Exploring the relationship between nursing protocols and nursing practice in an Irish intensive care unit. *International Journal of Nursing Practice, 11*, 142–149.

Gawlinski, A. (2008). The power of clinical nursing research: Engage clinicians, improve patients' lives, and forge a professional legacy. *American Journal of Critical Care, 17*(4), 315–327.

Goode, C. J. (1995). Evaluation of research-based nursing practice. *Nursing Clinics of North America, 30*(3), 421–428.

Grimshaw, J., Eccles, M., Thomas, R., MacLennan, G., Ramsay, C., Fraser, C., et al. (2006). Toward evidence-based quality improvement. Evidence (and its limitations) of the effectiveness of guideline dissemination and implementation strategies 1966–1998. *Journal of General Internal Medicine*, February 21 (Suppl. 2), S14–S20.

Haycock, C., Laser, C., Keuth, J., Montefour, K., Wilson, M., Austin, K., et al. (2005). Implementing evidence-based practice findings to decrease postoperative sternal wound infections following open heart surgery. *Journal of Cardiovascular Nursing, 20*(5), 299–305.

Ingersoll, G. L. (2005). Generating evidence through outcomes management. In B. M. Melnyk & E. Fineout-Overholt (Eds.), *Evidence-based practice in nursing and healthcare: A guide to best practice* (pp. 299–332). Philadelphia, PA: Lippincott.

Institute for Healthcare Improvement. (2007). *What is a bundle?* Retrieved from http://www.ihi.org/IHI/Topics/CriticalCare/IntensiveCare/ImprovementStories/WhatIsaBundle.htm

Institute of Medicine. (2001). *Crossing the quality chasm: A new health system for the 21st century*. Washington, DC: National Academy of Sciences.

Kirchhoff, K. T., & Rakel, B. A. (1999). Outcomes evaluation. In M. A. Mateo & K. A. Kirchhoff (Eds.), *Using and conducting nursing research in the clinical setting* (2nd ed., pp. 76–89). Philadelphia, PA: Saunders.

Landon, B. E., Hicks, L. S., Malley, A. J., Keegan, T., McNeil, B. J., & Guadagnoli, E. (2007). Improving the management of chronic disease at community health centers. *New England Journal of Medicine, 356*, 921–934.

Lawson, P. (2005). Zapping VAP with evidence-based practice. *Nursing, 35*(3), 66–67.

Levin, R. F., Keefer, J. M., Marren, J., Vetter, M., Lauder, B., & Sobolewski, S. (2010). Evidence-based practice improvement: Merging 2 paradigms. *Journal of Nursing Care Quality, 25*(2), 117–126.

Lund, C. H., Osborne, J. W., Kuller, J., Lane, A. T., Lott, J. W., & Raines, D. A. (2001). Neonatal skin care: Clinical outcomes of the AWHONN/NANN evidence-based clinical practice guidelines. *Journal of Obstetrical, Gynecological, and Neonatal Nursing, 30*(1), 41–51.

Medves, J., Godfrey, C., Turner, C., Paterson, M., Harrison, M., MacKenzie, L. et al. (2009). Practice guideline dissemination and implementation strategies for healthcare team and team-based practice: A systematic review. *Joanna Briggs Institute Library of Systematic Reviews, 7*(12), 450–491. Retrieved from http://www.joannabriggs.edu.au/pdf/SRLib_2009_7_12.pdf

Melnyk, B. M. (2005). Creating a vision: Motivating a change to evidence-based practice in individuals and organizations. In B. M. Melnyk & E. Fineout-Overholt (Eds.), *Evidence-based practice in nursing and healthcare: A guide to best practice* (pp. 443–455). Philadelphia, PA: Lippincott.

Nelson, E. C., Splaine, M. E., Batalden, P. B., & Plume, S. K. (1998). Building measurement and data collection into medical practice. *Annals of Internal Medicine, 128*, 460–466.

O'Keefe-McCarthy, S., Santiago, C., & Lau, G. (2008). Ventilator-associated pneumonia bundled strategies: An evidence-based practice. *Worldviews on Evidence-Based Nursing, 5*(4), 193–204.

Oleson, K. J. (1999). Continuous quality improvement/total quality management, and the relationship of research. In M. A. Mateo & K. A. Kirchhoff (Eds.), *Using and conducting nursing research in the clinical setting* (2nd ed., pp. 13–30). Philadelphia, PA: Saunders.

Pearson, A., Field, J., & Jordan, Z. (2007). *Evidence-based clinical practice in nursing and health care*. London, England: Blackwell.

Porter-O'Grady, T. (2006). A new age for practice: Creating the framework for evidence. In K. Malloch & T. Porter-O'Grady (Eds.), *Introduction to evidence-based practice in nursing and health care* (pp. 1–29). Sudbury, MA: Jones and Bartlett.

Rutland Regional Medical Center, Nursing Practice Committee. (2007). [Administration of blood and blood components.] Unpublished protocol. Rutland, VT: Author.

Rycroft-Malone, J. (2004). The PARIHS framework—a framework for guiding the implementation of evidence-based practice. *Journal of Nursing Care Quality, 19*(4), 297–304.

Schon, D. A. (1983). *The reflective practitioner: How professionals think in action.* New York, NY: Basic Books.

Simon, H. (1969). *The sciences of the artificial.* Cambridge, MA: MIT Press.

Solberg, L., Brekke, M., Fazio, C. J., Fowles, J., Jacobsen, D. N., Kottke, T. E., et al. (2000). Lessons from experienced guideline implementers: Attend to many factors and use multiple strategies. *Joint Commission Journal on Quality Improvement, 26*(4), 171–188.

Stetler, C. B., Ritchi, J. A., Rycroft-Malone, J., Schultz, A. A., & Charns, M. P. (2009). Institutionalizing evidence-based practice: An organizational case study using a model of strategic change. *Implementation Science, 4,* 78. doi:10.1186/1748-5908-4-78

Wimpenny, P., Johnson, N., Walter, I., & Wilkinson, J. A. (2008). Tracing and identifying the impact of evidence—use of a modified pipeline model. *Worldviews on Evidence-Based Nursing, 5*(1), 3–12.

ARTICLES DESCRIBING IMPLEMENTATION OF AN EVIDENCE-BASED PROTOCOL

Boyer, D. R., & Steltzer, N. (2009). Implementation of an evidence-based bladder scanner protocol. *Journal of Nursing Care Quality, 24*(1), 10–16.

Dufault, M., Duquette, C. E., Ehmann, J., Hehl, R., Lavin, M., & Martin, V., et al. (2010). Translating an evidence-based protocol for nurse-to-nurse shift handoffs. *Worldviews on Evidence-Based Nursing, 7*(2), 59–75. Epub 2010 Mar 22.

Kenney, D. J., & Goodman, P. (2010). Care of the patient with enteral tube feeding: An evidence-based practice protocol. *Nursing Research, 59* (1S), S22–S31.

Lyerla, F., LeRouge, C., Cooke, D. A., Turpin, D., & Wilson, L. (2010). A nursing clinical decision support system and potential predictors of head-of-bed position for patients receiving mechanical ventilation. *American Journal of Critical Care Nurses, 19*(1), 39–47.

Madsen, D., Sebolt, T., Cullen, L., Folkedahl, B., Mueller, T., Richardson, C., & Titler, M. (2005). Listening to bowel sounds: An evidence-based practice project. *American Journal of Nursing, 105*(12), 40–49.

Robinson, S., Allen, L., Barnes, M. R., Berry, T. A., Foster, T. A., Friedrich, L. A., et al. (2007). Development of an evidence-based protocol for reduction of indwelling urinary catheter usage. *MEDSURG Nursing, 16*(3), 157–161.

Selig, P. M., Popek, V., & Peebles, K. M. (2010). Minimizing hypoglycemia in the wake of a tight glycemic control protocol in hospitalized patients. *Journal of Nursing Care Quality.* Advance online publication.

Van der Helm, J., Goossens, A., & Bossuyt, P. (2006). When implementation fails: The case of a nursing guideline for fall prevention. *Joint Commission Journal of Quality and Patient Safety, 32*(3), 152–160.

van Gaal, B. B., Schoonhoven, L., Julscher, M. E., Mintjes, J. A., Borm, G. F., Keepmans, R. T., et al. (2009). The design of the SAFE and SORRY? study:

A clustered randomized trial on the development and testing of an evidence-based inpatient safety program for the prevention of adverse events. *BMC Health Services Research, 9,* 58.

INTERESTING AND USEFUL WEBSITES

Institute for Clinical Systems Improvement. (2009). Health care protocol: *Rapid response team.* Retrieved from http://www.icsi.org/rapid_response_team__protocol_/rapid_response_team__protocol_with_order_set___pdf_.html

Institute for Clinical Systems Improvement. (2010). *Order sets.* Retrieved from http://www.icsi.org/guidelines_and_more/order_sets

Tools for safe medication administration: Institute for Healthcare Improvement: http://www.ihi.org/IHI/Topics/PatientSafety/MedicationSystems/Tools

CHAPTER EIGHTEEN

Evidence-Based Practice Participation Scenarios

> **EBP** ➤

There are several scenarios in which you might volunteer or be asked to participate in an evidence-based practice project. I thought I could provide a bit of guidance in this regard. Four scenarios will be described, and suggestions will be made regarding participation:

- As a member of a project team, you are asked to appraise one or several pieces of research evidence and give a short oral presentation about it.
- You decide to submit an evidence-based poster to be displayed at an association congress.
- You want to present an evidence-based clinical idea or concern to your nurse leader, clinical nurse specialist, or nurse manager.
- As a participant in a patient care planning conference, you present research evidence relevant to the care of a patient with complex issues.

In all the scenarios, you want to be organized and carefully select what you present, so you need to do your homework.

Present an Appraisal

First, let's imagine a context for this scenario. You work as a staff nurse on an orthopaedic unit. The unit is looking at its use of special beds and bed surfaces for patients at risk of skin breakdown. The work group is charged with developing a decision algorithm or decision tree regarding the use of special beds and surfaces. The unit already uses a risk assessment scale to quantify patients' risk for skin breakdown. In PICOT terms, this question would be outlined as follows:

P: Patients with orthopaedic injuries and/or recovering from orthopaedic surgery who are at risk for skin breakdown

I: Special beds and mattress overlays

C: Effectiveness of each and when to use one rather than another

O: Prevention of skin breakdown

T: Before breakdown occurs

The group decides to start by examining the effectiveness of various support surfaces aimed at preventing ulcers and then proceed to link risk assessment to the surfaces. At the second meeting of this group, you are asked to appraise a systematic review regarding alternating air mattresses (Vanderweek, Grypdonck, & Defloor, 2008). The expectation is that you will extract information from the SR onto a findings table and at the next meeting give a less than 5 minute summary and appraisal of the SR.

You could organize your talk in the following way:

- Give a summary of the SR along the same lines as the information in the synopsis part of the SR appraisal guide.
- State your overall impression of the credibility of the conclusions along with your reasons for confidence or concerns.
- State your opinion regarding the clinical significance of the conclusions.
- Address the applicability of the findings and conclusions to the patients seen on your unit and the resources that will be available.

Make a Poster

Professional conferences and congresses often issue calls for oral presentations or posters of research studies and EBP projects. A summary of evidence regarding a clinical question often makes a relevant and interesting poster. Posters are usually mounted on boards in specified areas at congresses, and people walk around and read them. Most congresses require that a person be present with the poster at specified times so people can ask questions.

When making a poster, you have to be very selective about the information included. If it has too much information or if the information is presented in a disorganized way, people will avoid stopping to read it or will read part of it and walk away. The idea of a poster is to present the main ideas—it's like an abstract. If the person looking at the poster is interested in knowing more, she will ask you some questions. You (the person explaining the poster) are the real resource; the poster is mostly just a lure.

There are no ironclad rules for how to design a poster, but many posters these days are created using PowerPoint or similar presentation software. Generally, information should be grouped in some logical way with a header for each block and three to five points under each header. You can use some abbreviations if you define them the first time you use them; of course this is not necessary if they are very common ones. You might want to have a list of the EbCPGs and SRs that are referenced in the poster for people who ask for them, or you could have interested persons write down their e-mail address, and after the congress you can send a list of references to them.

Continuing the first scenario, let's say the bed surface-skin breakdown group's work is moving along well when you notice a call from the National Association of Orthopaedic Nurses (NAON) for posters at their spring congress. Because your work group has not finished its work on the algorithm/protocol, you decide to submit a poster regarding just the evidence used to produce the algorithm. Most associations allow submission of work-in-progress posters. You would first submit to NAON an abstract of your poster's content. Then, if it is accepted, you would proceed to produce the poster.

The poster could look like Figure 18–1. This is a low-budget poster, produced with only gray tones. Color would spruce it up considerably but would add to the cost. Note that the poster in the figure is fabricated—it does not represent an actual project or literature search.

Having a poster at a congress is a fun and informative experience. A lot of people will talk with you, and you'll learn a lot. It's definitely a recommended step in your professional growth and development.

Present an Idea or Concern

Let's say while you were at the congress, you went to a session about preventing and managing mental confusion in elderly patients with hip fractures. You went to the session because this issue has recently been a challenge in caring for several patients on your unit. You decide to see what research evidence is available on the topic and to talk with the clinical nurse specialist for your unit. A 15-minute search on CINAHL—using the terms *delirium*, *hip fracture*, and *interventions*, with the *research only* and *evidence-based practice* filters on—turns up two EbCPGs, an SR, and

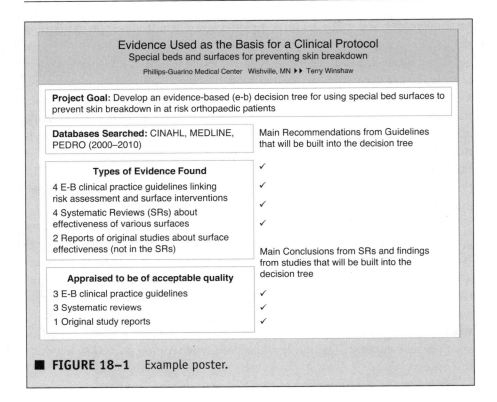

■ FIGURE 18-1 Example poster.

several research articles about preventing and managing delirium in patients with hip fracture; they indicate that pain relief is clearly important.

To talk to the clinical nurse specialist or nurse leader, it is best to make an appointment. Catch-as-catch-can in the hallway usually doesn't work; interruptions are bound to occur, or you may catch him when he has something else on his mind. Here are some suggestions for preparing for your appointment:

- Be able to give some recent examples of why you think delirium prevention and management is a problem on your unit. Specific patient examples would support your claim that delirium care is not as good as it could be.
- Briefly describe the research evidence you found on your quick search. It might be good to give him a copy of several of the research abstracts or URLs you found.
- If your unit already has a protocol about this topic, look at it before your appointment. If the protocol is evidence-based and well written,

maybe the appropriate action would be to bring it anew to the staff's attention along with any new research. If the protocol is not helpful, up to date, or consistent with newer research, point out its shortcomings.

- Ask his opinion about how to get things moving to make a change, but have an idea or two in mind beforehand.

There's no guarantee you will get a positive response and good follow-through, but the chances are good and the cause is a good one.

Contribute to a Patient Care Conference

Care design is not done just by organizational teams for populations of patients. It is also done in multidisciplinary patient care conferences. When a patient's care presents difficult problems or requires complex discharge arrangements, a patient care planning conference will often be called. The goal of such a conference is to bring together all the information about the patient's situation (from the chart, from the family, or from the various disciplines working with the patient) and develop a specific plan of care.

These planning sessions design more effective strategies when someone is assigned to spend an hour looking for research evidence relative to a key issue or issues in the management of the patient's problems. Perhaps there is an evidence-based guideline that is relevant to the patient's sleeping problem. Maybe a systematic review that addresses the issue of whether a teenager can take a shower even though he has external skeletal pins in place can be identified. Increasingly, evidence-based information is being brought to the table at patient care planning conferences.

If a conference is called and you will be involved, you should give some thought to the problems or issues that may be, or should be, discussed. There may be one or two issues for which it would be helpful for all participants to understand effective approaches that are supported by research evidence. If the person who leads the conference doesn't assign anyone to look at the research evidence about the problem, you might lead the way by doing so.

At the conference, you could bring what you found in your brief search to the table—not in a lecturing way, but in a contributing way. In that regard, I warn against the overused and vague phrase, "research shows." Instead, say something like, "I found one systematic review that looked at five studies about sleeping problems in hospitalized adolescents. The reviewers reached the conclusion that . . ." Have the article with you so anyone who chooses to can look at it. The inclusion of research-based information into the discussion will most likely be valued and will serve to take the exchange beyond opinions to more objective knowledge as the basis for care planning.

REFERENCE

Vanderweek, K., Grypdonck, M., Defloor, T. (2008). Alternating pressure air mattresses as prevention for pressure ulcers: A literature review. *International Journal of Nursing Studies, 45*(5), 784–801.

CHAPTER NINETEEN
Research-Informed Practice

Point-of-care design occurs when an individual nurse seeks out research evidence to use in her or his own care of patients. In fact, a great deal of care is designed at the point of care by direct-care providers. Generally speaking, this happens in one of two ways: (1) in the case of a patient who has perplexing or unusual nursing care needs or (2) in the nurse's approach to care of all patients with a particular problem or need.

Many aspects of care are not spelled out in detail in clinical protocols, and this provides an opportunity to use research evidence in individual practice. For instance, many protocols in hospitals, rehabilitation facilities, and home care agencies require that patients with asthma be taught how to take their aerosol medications using an inhaler. However, the type of inhaler used and the method of teaching the patient are left to the discretion of clinicians working with the particular patient—and there is research evidence relative to these issues (Dolovich et al., 2005; Brocklebank et al., 2001; Vincken, Dekhuijzen, Barnes, & ADMIT Group, 2010). The nurse who seeks out this research evidence or becomes aware of it at a specialty congress or workshop can enhance the care she delivers by incorporating that research evidence into her individual patient teaching.

Use of research evidence by the individual nurse is not as rigorous as the way evidence-based quality management (EBQM) teams use several forms of evidence to develop care protocols (Eddy, 2005). It just cannot be because the individual does not have the time, access to data, or skill that the team has. Usually, the individual nurse uses a care design process that is less comprehensive and systematic. The search for research evidence is not as sweeping, the appraisal is quicker, and the integration across a body of evidence is less systematic (see Table 19–1). Thus, an individual nurse's use

Table 19-1   EBP VIS-À-VIS RIP

CHARACTERISTIC	EVIDENCE-BASED PRACTICE	RESEARCH-INFORMED PRACTICE
Who does it?	Project group with skills and resources	Individual clinician
Question/issue	Well framed, often guided by organizational data	Arises in an individual's practice
Search	Extensive, librarian-assisted	Quick Broad or limited
Appraisal and summary	Systematic, criteria-based	Varies widely, typically not systematic
Translation	Methodical, consensus of group	Informal, often just one clinician
Evaluation	Planned and analytical	Often not planned, anecdotal

of research evidence to design care is informed by the research evidence available but not really based on it—hence the term **research-informed practice (RIP)**. Importantly the rigor of the process used to incorporate research into individual practice can be enhanced considerably by relying mainly on evidence-based clinical practice guidelines (EbCPGs) and systematic reviews (SRs) rather than individual study findings.

RIP Opportunities

Opportunities for research-informed practice occur when during the course of actually giving care a nurse recognizes she needs additional knowledge regarding management of a patient problem—and needs it immediately. Searching and retrieval of research-based information from the point-of-care can often help the nurse make a research-informed decision about care in real time. In some clinical settings, she also could search healthcare databases and evidence-based practice Internet sites for relevant sources from a wireless computer terminal or personal digital assistant (PDA). If there is any doubt about using the research-informed approach, it would be best to discuss it with the most experienced nurse available at the time.

- Know what you don't know
- Seek the information you need

Another RIP opportunity presents when a nurse reads an integrative research review article in his specialty journal that provides solid research evidence in support of a particular approach to care or method of care, but the method is not used in his setting. Either there is no protocol addressing that issue or the protocol does not specify the actions that the review addresses. In either case, this nurse should discuss using the research-based method with the unit's clinical leader to be certain it would not confuse or create a problem for other care providers. It may be a method he can use in care of patients without any official approval, or it may be something that an authoritative clinical leader should endorse. This action may also lead to a unit-wide consideration of the method.

When a nurse uses research evidence in the ways just described, she or he is engaging in research-informed practice. It is a different process from the use of research findings by a team developing an evidence-based clinical protocol, which spells out important and critical actions for a patient population. Because the protocol addresses the most important aspects of care and will affect so many patients, it is important that the team use a rigorous process to produce it. Locating and summarizing all the relevant evidence on an issue and then using it to design a clinical guideline or protocol is a very demanding undertaking in terms of the knowledge, skills, discipline, and time required—and is beyond what an individual nurse can do on her or his own. Still, research evidence can be incorporated into an individual's practice.

Specific RIP Activities

Consider further how an individual might engage in RIP:

- Reflect on the effectiveness of the clinical actions you perform
- When care dilemmas, new issues, or poor outcomes occur in your practice, make the effort to search the healthcare databases and professional Internet sites for a relevant evidence-based guideline or research summary
- Participate in a journal club where research articles are discussed

- Regularly read research summaries and report articles that are published in clinical journals
- Conduct a basic level appraisal to determine if a summary, study, or guideline that comes to your attention was soundly produced
- Conduct a basic level appraisal of whether the conclusions, findings, or recommendations would be applicable to the patients you care for and to the setting in which you practice
- Adjust or fine-tune your own practice based on credible findings—within the context of what is possible or changeable in your setting
- Regularly check websites that post evidence-based information related to your area of clinical practice

The Information Intersection

In a very real sense, the point-of-care is an information intersection (Porter-O'Grady, 2010). It is the point at which scientific knowledge, patient-specific information, e-b clinical protocols, available clinical services, and personal expertise converge as the basis for care design (see Figure 19–1). At present, electronic patient records, clinical decision support systems, bibliographic databases, electronic scheduling systems, and e-mail help clinicians access various sources of information. In the future, Porter-O'Grady (2010) sees healthcare information systems as providing clinicians with a

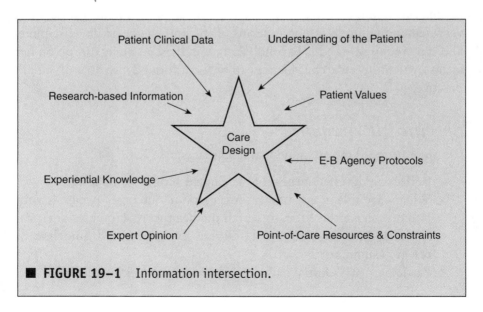

■ FIGURE 19–1   Information intersection.

"seamless intersection of data" on which to decide and act (p. 22). Such an information system would make patient data, agency standards, research evidence, assessment guides, and decision support tools available at the point-of-care in easily searched and quick-to-read formats. Wireless and mobile devices will increase access to information and provide decision-making support. However, only the human decider can synthesize all the information to make a decision about what care should be given to a particular patient.

Concise EBP Formats

As you have seen in this part of the book, evidence-based clinical practice guidelines, systematic reviews, and individual study reports can be quite lengthy. At the point of care, nurses need shorter versions of these documents. For that reason, many organizations are producing concise format summaries that can be downloaded onto personal data assistants (PDAs) and tablet personal computers (Doran, 2009; Hong, Kim, Lee, & Ki, 2009). The following organizations provide short versions of their EbCPGs:

- The Registered Nurses' Association of Ontario provides PDA versions of their guidelines (http://www.rnao.org/Page.asp?PageID=829&Content ID=2491&SiteNodeID=133&BL_ExpandID=).
- The Joanna Briggs Institute's JBI COnNect, Best Practice Information Sheets and Evidence Summaries are also available in concise formats (http://www.jbiconnect.org/agedcare/ebhc/summarise/search-form.php).
- Summaries and abstracts of the Cochrane Collaboration's SRs are available at no charge from their website (http://www2.cochrane.org/reviews).

Preappraised Research Evidence

Another time-saver is preappraised evidence. There is no reason why appraisal of credibility and clinical significance has to be done by every agency separately. These parts of appraisals can be done once by a respected organization, leaving only the appraisal of applicability to be done by the local agency. Summaries of EbCPGs, SRs, and individual studies that have been filtered for quality are being published electronically. Preappraisal is especially valuable for clinicians who are seeking evidence-based guidance from the point of care where they don't have time to do an appraisal.

Box 19–1   TYPES OF EVIDENCE TO ACCESS AT THE POINT OF CARE (ALL SHOULD
BE FROM RESPECTED ORGANIZATIONS)

- EbCPG condensed versions
- Synopses (ideally with appraisals) of SRs
- Synopses (ideally with appraisals) of individual studies

There are several sources for synopses of SRs. These synopses are one- to two-page summaries of SR conclusions, often with short commentaries regarding the soundness of the methodology. These sources include:

- Evidence-Based Nursing (http://ebn.bmj.com) provides citations for SRs and study reports with links to the original abstracts. An accompanying commentary provides a methodological and results perspective. This is a subscription resource.
- Centre for Reviews and Dissemination, University of York *DARE* database (http://www.crd.york.ac.uk/crdweb/Home.aspx?DB=DARE&SessionID =&SearchID=&E=0&D=0&H=0&SearchFor=) contains 15,000 abstracts of systematic reviews, including more than 6,000 quality-assessed reviews and details of all Cochrane reviews and protocols. A methodological commentary accompanies the abstracts.

The medical field already has commercial information retrieval services that provide preappraised EBP resources for physicians. Two of them are InfoPOEMs and Evidence Matters. They are subscription services that provide filtered, evidence-based information that can be accessed from handheld computers. They also offer alert services regarding topics of interest to the subscriber. These kinds of products are increasingly becoming available for nurses.

Clinical Decision Support

The clinical information systems (CIS) that are used to order and document patient care and store patients' clinical information are being designed to also guide clinical staff members regarding the care they should give patients. This feature of CIS is called clinical decision support. In general, it works by integrating individual patient data with evidence-based information resources and agency protocols in the computer's knowledge base (DiCenso, Bayley, & Haynes, 2009). When patient data is entered, the CIS generates recommendations for care and knowledge sources that the clinicians should consider when planning and giving care to the patient. Thus, the clinician does not have to look to see if there is a relevant protocol; rather, based on the data input, the CIS automatically brings up or provides a link to the protocol. CIS can also generate alerts, reminders, assessment guides, decision algorithms, and relevant professional papers. These features should enhance the degree to which care provided to individual patients is evidence-based and consistent with agency standards, as well as reduce errors and omissions of care.

Access to research-based knowledge to care for patients is quickly developing. Preappraised, easy-to-access, and easy-to-read formats of evidence-based sources will become increasingly available—stay tuned!

Box 19–2   PROFESSIONAL EVIDENCE-BASED PRACTICE BEHAVIORS FOR THE BSN NURSE

1. Deliver care using your unit's or agency's evidence-based protocols.
2. Constantly monitor the effectiveness of the care you are providing.
3. Be curious about the knowledge bases on which key actions rest; keep a list of issues and questions you want to pursue further.
4. When you identify a care dilemma or shortcoming, consult with a nurse leader.
5. Actively support implementation of evidence-based protocols in your unit, service, or agency.
6. Participate in the development of evidence-based protocols involving your clinical unit.
7. Be aware of quality improvement activities in your agency; actively participate as possible.
8. Read research articles published in clinical journals for your area of practice.
9. Bring credible research evidence to the attention of your peers and unit leaders.
10. Develop and maintain your EBP skills by appraising one research article per month.
11. Develop and maintain your EBP skills by conducting a monthly search for research evidence in an electronic database and at key association or government websites (particularly clinical practice guidelines and research summaries).

My Ending, Your Beginning

Having come to the end of this book, I would like to bring together in one place the specific EBP and RIP professional behaviors that have been recommended throughout this part of the book. In Box 19–2, notice the value placed on individual nurses being observant and curious about their daily delivery of care. Other behaviors pertain to participating in the quality management activities of your unit, clinical service, or agency. Still others relate to continuing to develop EBP and RIP skills.

Hopefully you have gotten my not-too-subtle message that *evidence-based practice is not a spectator sport.* It's an intellectually challenging, rewarding, and ethically-required professional activity. I hope you will take up the challenge as a way of contributing to better patient care and to the health and well-being of patients and their families.

REFERENCES

Brocklebank, D., Ram, F., Wright, J., Barry, P., Cates, C., Davies, L., et al. (2001). Comparison of the effectiveness of inhaler devices in asthma and chronic obstructive airway diseases: A systematic review of the literature. *Health Technology Assessment, 5*(26), 1–149.

DiCenso, A., Bayley, L., & Haynes, R. B. (2009). Accessing pre-appraised evidence: Fine-tuning the 5S model into a 6S model. *Evidence Based Nursing, 12,* 99–101.

Dolovich, M. B., Ahrens, R. C., Hess, D. R., Anderson, P., Dhand, R., Rau, J. L., et al. (2005). Device selection and outcomes of aerosol therapy: Evidence-based guidelines: American College of Chest Physicians/American College of Asthma, Allergy, and Immunology. *Chest, 127*(1), 335–371.

Doran, D. (2009). The emerging role of PDAs in information use and clinical decision making. *Evidence Based Nursing, 12,* 35–38.

Eddy, D. (2005). Evidence-based medicine: A unified approach: Two approaches to using evidence to solve clinical problems, and how to unify them. *Health Affairs, 24*(1), 9–17.

Hong, H. S., Kim, I. K., Lee, S. H., & Ki, H. S. (2009). Adoption of a PDA-based home hospice care system for cancer patients. *Computers, Informatics, and Nursing, 27*(6), 365–371.

Porter-O'Grady, T. (2010). A new age for practice: Creating the framework for evidence. In K. Malloch & T. Porter-O'Grady (Eds.), *Introduction to evidence-based practice in nursing and health care* (2nd ed., pp. 1–30). Sudbury, MA: Jones and Bartlett.

Vincken, W., Dekhuijzen, P. R., Barnes, P., & ADMIT Group (2010). The ADMIT series—Issues in inhalation therapy. (4) How to choose inhaler devices for the treatment of COPD. *Primary Care Respiratory Journal, 19*(1), 10–20.

Terms Used to Describe Bodies of Scientific Evidence Regarding Interventions

These terms are used in clinical practice guidelines documents to indicate the level of support for the recommendations; however, the authors rarely define them. The following definitions are what I have gleaned from those who do define their terms and from the ways they used the terms. Remember that for determining the effectiveness of interventions, the gold standard is the randomized experiment.

Terms Used When Sufficient Research Is Available

Supportive: Consistent study findings from adequately designed randomized studies show that the intervention is effective.

Suggestive: Consistent study findings from adequately designed observational studies or a trend in findings from adequately designed randomized studies can be interpreted as indicating that the intervention is effective.

Equivocal: Study findings are mixed with some finding effectiveness and others finding weak or no effectiveness; the result is that no conclusion can be reached regarding intervention effectiveness.

Terms Used When No, Very Few,
or Only Studies of Limited Quality Are Available

Insufficient: There are too few published studies of adequate design to determine intervention effectiveness.

Inconclusive: There are published studies, but their quality does not provide an adequate basis for determining intervention effectiveness.

Silent: There are no published studies examining the effectiveness of the intervention.

Source: Adapted from The American Society of Anesthesiologists Task Force on Sedation and Analgesia by Non-Anesthesiologists. (2002). Practice guidelines for sedation and analgesia by non-anesthesiologists. *Anesthesiology, 96*(4), 1004–1017.

APPENDIX B

22-Step Process for Producing an Evidence-Based Clinical Practice Guideline

Sarah Jo Brown, PhD, RN

☐ **1.** Agree on the clinical management issue or question the guideline will address; the issue should have a clear focus and should state the patients to whom the guideline is meant to apply and the target users. List specific clinical considerations and decision points (subissues or questions) for which the panel would like to make recommendations. For example, risk, prevention, and management; or pharmacological management, psychosocial management, and patient education.

☐ **2.** Decide whether all project work will be done via electronic communication or whether conference calls and/or meetings also will be held.

☐ **3.** Decide whether consumer input will be sought.

☐ **4.** Decide whether the guideline will be (a) externally validated by experts, (b) pilot tested, or (c) application tools/kit will be developed.

☐ **5.** Develop a timeline and a budget for the project; secure resources/funding.

☐ **6.** Appoint an expert panel and project coordinators. The panel should have expertise regarding the full breadth of the guideline's scope.

☐ **7.** Agree on a system to rate the strength of scientific evidence; the rating systems should consider number of supporting studies, quality of supporting studies, design of supporting studies, consistency of findings from study to study. In choosing or adapting a rating system, the panel should discuss and decide whether evaluation data from quality improvement projects and expert opinion (consensus opinion of the project panel and/or opinion of other expert panels) will be considered as evidence.

☐ 8. If you are going to issue recommendations based on expert opinion, agree on a process for polling the panel and reaching a consensus decision.

☐ 9. Conduct database and Internet searches for relevant evidence guidelines, systematic research reviews, meta-analyses, original studies, project reports, quality improvement reports, and expert opinion.

☐10. Retrieve all articles; keep notes regarding articles that were not available or that might have been missed.

☐11. Read abstracts of all articles

☐12. Group articles by subissues/questions.

☐13. Read and appraise each article.

☐14. Review reference lists for missed articles and retrieve for inclusion.

☐15. Working with the list of subissues/questions, identify those issues for which there is no study or too few adequate studies on which to base a recommendation; set these aside for now.

☐16. Complete findings table for each subissue/question; consider separate tables for randomized studies, observational studies, projects, and expert opinion.

☐17. Working with the findings tables of the subissues for which there are studies, identify statements that are supported by one or more studies. For each statement, note how many studies support it and the characteristics of the supporting studies (study design, quality of the study, sample size, sample profile).

☐18. Formulate recommendations that are derived from the statements with research support.

☐19. Develop expert consensus-based recommendations on the issues that lack research support—if that is the plan.

☐20. Using the system for rating scientific evidence on which the panel agreed earlier, assign a rating number, letter, or term to the evidence supporting each recommendation.

☐**21.** Assemble the recommendations and determine if they address all the issues that you think should be addressed.

☐**22.** Produce a document that includes the following information:

- A clear statement of the clinical issue the guideline addresses

- A statement regarding the importance and/or prevalence of the problem

- A description of the process used to produce the guideline, including the method used to reach consensus among the panel

- The recommendations and the level of support for each (including expert consensus if that was used); indicate why the recommendation was made rather than alternative actions

- An explicit indication of the studies on which each recommendation was based either with tables or footnotes

- A discussion of the strength and characteristics of the research base for each subissue in brief narrative form

---

Proceed to external validation and/or pilot testing if that is the plan. Proceed to develop application tools/kit if that is the plan.

The process outlined here reflects the author's experience, various evidence-based practice sources, the AGREE Research Trust Instrument for Appraisal of Guidelines, and Stetler et al., 1998.

REFERENCES

AGREE Research Trust. (2008). *Welcome to the AGREE website.* Retrieved from www.agreetrust.org

Stetler, C. B., et al. (1998). Utilization-focused integrative reviews in a nursing service. *Applied Nursing Research, 11*(4), 195–206.

Completed Appraisal of a Clinical Practice Guideline's Recommendations

Citation: Scottish Intercollegiate Guidelines Network. (2010). *Non-pharmaceutical management of depression in adults: A national guideline.* Retrieved from http://www.sign.ac.uk/pdf/sign114.pdf

Synopsis

What does the guideline address (clinical questions, issues, and subissues)?
Non-pharmaceutical treatments of depression in adults, including: psychological therapies, self-help, exercise and lifestyle changes, meditation, herbal remedies and nutritional supplements, and complementary and alternative therapies as "alternatives to prescribed pharmacological therapies."

What population of patients is the guideline intended for?
Adults with mild to moderate depression.

What process was used to develop the guideline?
The SIGN methodology, which requires an extensive search, conducting a SR, and a specified decision-making process; all this is spelled out on the SIGN website.

What clinical outcomes were the guideline designed to achieve?
Reduction in depressive symptoms as measured by a recognized depression scale, illness duration, quality of life, or patient satisfaction.

What group or groups produced it?
A 22-member panel of clinical and academic mental health experts from various disciplines and Scottish agencies; patients participated in the development process at various points.

What is the date on it, and how recent are the cited research sources?
Issued in January 2010; 90 references with dates through 2008.

What are the main recommendations?
Structured exercise may be considered a treatment.

Credibility

Was the panel that developed the guideline made up of people with the necessary expertise?   Yes __X__ No _____
Could have benefited from a home care nurse.

Was a systematic and comprehensive search for research evidence conducted?
    Yes __X__ No _____
After checking out the online document, we can definitely say yes.

Are the criteria for selecting research evidence clearly described?
    Yes __X__ No _____
Mainly systematic reviews and RCTs, but they were open to considering observational studies. They excluded studies not using the International Classification of Diseases (ICD) definitions of depression and those not using a reliable and validated measure of depressive symptoms. They also excluded studies of persons with severe depression and comorbid psychiatric illnesses.

Is the evidence supporting each recommendation indicated and/or discussed?
    Yes __X__ No _____
Yes, it is clearly set forth for each recommendation.

Is it clear when research evidence was lacking and expert opinion became the basis of the recommendation?
    Yes __X__ No _____
Yes, the differentiation between recommendation and Good Practice Point is explicit.

Was the process for formulating the recommendations systematic and free of bias?

Yes __X__ No _____ Can't tell _____

The process is spelled out in considerable detail. Each person on the panel completed a form indicating their considered judgment of the body of evidence in terms of volume of evidence, directness of applicability, generalizability, consistency, potential clinical impact, and their view of what the synthesis should be (per SIGN Guideline Developer Handbook).

Are the guidelines current?   Yes __X__ No _____

Was the guideline peer reviewed or tested?   Yes __X__ No _____
A draft of the guidelines was reviewed by independent experts and patients (per Section 11.3.2).

ARE THE RECOMMENDATIONS CREDIBLE? YES __X__ NO _____

Clinical Significance

Were all important decisions the nurse would have to make addressed by this guideline?

Yes __X__ No _____

All possible non-pharmaceutical modalities we might use were considered, particularly in the exercise and life style domains.

Were patient concerns and risks associated with the recommendations addressed?

Yes __X__ No _____ Not clear _____

Risk was explicitly taken into consideration. This is seen in the discussion of the evidence regarding exercise.

Is there reasonable certainty (based on the research evidence) that the recommendations, if implemented, are likely to produce good patient outcomes?

Yes __X__ No _____ Not clear _____

Are the projected benefits of the guideline valued by patients?

Yes __X__ No _____ Uncertain _____ Not applicable _____

There is a sizeable portion of our patients who are averse to pharmacological treatments; these folks would value a trial of structured exercise.

Is the intervention or action required by patients acceptable to them?
    Yes __X__ No _____ Uncertain _____ Not applicable _____
55% to 100% of patients in the studies completed the exercise intervention to which they were assigned.* Careful screening to include only those truly interested in an exercise treatment, could presumably push this completion rate to the upper end.

*An issue that was not as clear to us as we would like is whether the studies enrolled only persons who had declined pharmaceutical treatment. Section 1.2 informs us that the intent of the guideline was to evaluate non-pharmaceutical treatments as an "alternative to" (not as adjunctive to) prescribed medication. This suggests that the research studies reviewed had to exclude persons who were taking medication for their depression; however, this is not explicitly stated in Section 1.4. Assuming that the non-pharmaceutical treatments in the SR were studied as primary treatments, the question of whether these non-pharmaceutical management modalities are effective adjuncts to pharmaceutical treatment and how they work in combination with one another remains open-these are different questions from whether they are effective primary treatments.

ARE THE RECOMMENDATIONS CLINICALLY SIGNIFICANT?
    YES __X__ NO _____
For some of the recommendations, the answer is yes, as indicated by the strong (A-level) recommendation. However, other, such as lifestyle modification, the answer is that they probably do no harm, but whether they actually help substantially has not been scientifically demonstrated. The exercise recommendation is in the middle ground-it "may help."

Applicability

[Note: Assume that a community health center is considering what non-pharmaceutical treatments to offer as alternatives to treatment with medication. Effectiveness in reducing depressive symptoms will be a main consideration, but community preference will also be considered.]

Does the guideline address the problem, situation, or decision we are redesigning in our setting?

Yes __X__ No _____

Yes, 18 % of our patients express a wish to avoid prescription medication if at all possible.

To implement the recommendations, what will we have to do differently?

Some of these treatments would be very costly to implement, and others would be rather easy to implement. We will look at each recommendation and rate it in terms of feasibility. We will also consider the Good Practice Points.

Do we have the resources and capability to implement the recommendations safely and accurately?

Yes __X__ No _____

This will be a one-by-one decision-making process.

Which departments or other providers would be affected by this change, and how can we bring them into the change process?

Many of these treatments would require referral to outside providers who have the expertise to deliver them. We would have to identify and vet them. Others could be incorporated into information given to patients when setting up their initial plan of care and conducted within our activities program. Some would require talking with community agencies about the logistics of making them available to our patients (e.g., the community center for exercise and swimming).

How will we know if our patients are benefiting from our new protocol?

We could set up a system for following patients who decline medication treatment, and at 6-month intervals evaluate if they are still participating in their chosen treatment and whether it is effective.

ARE THE RECOMMENDATIONS (ALL OR IN PART) APPLICABLE TO OUR SETTING?   YES __X__ NO _____

Selective ones

SHOULD WE ADOPT ALL OR SOME OF THE RECOMMENDATIONS?
    YES __X__ NO _____

Some recommendations will be feasible; others will not. [Note: In a real situation, these would be spelled out one by one.] We can't offer everything, but the guideline provides valuable information regarding which treatment approaches have established effectiveness and will help us make decisions about what treatment to add to our current offerings. The exercise recommendation is feasible in light of our ability to use the Do Good Works church's hall for exercise classes.

Comments

Completed Appraisal of Conclusions of an Integrative Research Review

Citation: Khraim, F. M., & Carey, M. G. (2008). Predictors of pre-hospital delay among patients with acute myocardial infarction. *Patient Education and Counseling, 75*(2), 155–161.

Synopsis

What topic or question did the integrative research review address?
Predictors of prehospital delay among patients with acute myocardial infarction (AMI).

How were potential individual research reports identified?
Healthcare databases were searched for the years 1995 to 2008. A variety of search terms were used in combination with acute myocardial infarction or heart attack.

What determined if a study was included in the analysis?
Only research articles about prehospital delay were included. Studies about hospital delay were excluded.

How many studies were included in the review?
26

What research designs were used in the studies?
Correlational cross-sectional studies were most common with a few qualitative or mixed designs.

What were the consistent and important across-studies conclusions?

1. The diverse cultural and ethnic populations studied produced varied results regarding several topical areas.
2. Many studies had methodological shortcomings, the most common being low statistical power due to small sample sizes.
3. The nature of and reasons for delay among people who died is not represented.
4. Decision delay was examined exclusively in only one study.
5. Having correct expectations regarding symptoms leads to a shorter delay.
6. Psychological factors, such as denial, fear, and concern about troubling others, lead to a longer delay.
7. Low-level, intermittent symptoms predicted longer delays.

Credibility

Was the topic clearly defined?
Yes __X__ No _____
Yes, the period of decision delay was well defined as a distinct part of pre-hospital delay, and it was differentiated from hospital delay.

Is there a description of the methods used to conduct the review?
Yes __X__ No _____
It could be more detailed in the published report, but adequate when the lead author's addendum is considered.

1. Was the search for study reports comprehensive and unbiased?
   Yes __X__ No _____
   Multiple search terms were used, but the searched databases were not stated. Bias is difficult to evaluate from the information available.
2. Were the included studies assessed for quality?
   Yes _____ No __X__
   At least this is not indicated in the article.

Were the design characteristics and the findings of the studies displayed or discussed in sufficient detail?
Yes __X__ No _____
The design features of the included studies were stated in general, but they were not expanded upon or linked to findings. It would have been inform-ative to know which ones were cohort, correlational, and descriptive

studies, and how big the sample sizes were. It would also have been good to know which findings came from strong studies and which ones were from studies of low quality. The authors note that quite a few studies were underpowered, but they do not say how this was taken into consideration in the synthesis. This casts a shadow on the "no-difference" findings. Evidence tables would have added value to this review.

Was there truly an integration (i.e., synthesis) of findings-not merely reporting of findings from each study?
  Yes __X__ No _____
This is the real strength of this review. The information was organized into useful factor-topics, and the patterns in the findings were described.

Did the reviewers explore why differences in findings might have occurred?
  Yes __X__ No _____
Definitely. Many differences were undoubtedly due to the studied populations, but others were due to differences in the methodologies of the studies. The reviewers did a good job of exploring why differences might have been found.

Did the reviewers distinguish between conclusions based on consistent findings from a sufficient number of studies and those based on inferior evidence?
  Yes __X__ No _____ Varies _____
A few predictor factors had consistent findings (e.g., the influence of denial, fear, and perception of embarrassment; skewness of delay times toward long delays; and the importance of patients having correct cognitive pictures of symptoms). Also, there were some topics with mixed or varied findings (e.g., delay times, differences in delay time in blacks and whites, and influence of age and marital status). The variety of cultures represented in the studies undoubtedly accounts for the lack of consistency of findings. The reviewers explicitly recognized the consistency or inconsistency of findings for each factor in the Results and Discussion sections.

Which conclusions were supported by consistent findings from two or more studies?
We find all the conclusions set forth in the discussion section to be thoughtfully reasoned and well supported. For instance, the findings relative to sociodemographic factors, such as age, gender, and ethnicity, especially lack consistency; the authors recognized this and did not make generalizations regarding these predictors.

ARE THE CONCLUSIONS CREDIBLE?
    YES __X__ NO _____ VARIES _____
Although we would have liked a bit more information about the databases that were searched, evidence tables to better compare the studies, and appraisal of study quality, we find the conclusions of this IRR to be credible. They are credible because of the specific descriptions and strong synthesis of findings and because the conclusions reflect the consistency of findings and number of studies that address each issue.

Clinical Significance

Which conclusions are likely to make a difference in patient safety, comfort, or outcomes?
First, because the time from onset of symptoms to reperfusion of the coronary arteries has important ramifications for patients' survival and future health, this is a very important issue.

Second, some factors are givens (i.e., cultural background, age, and marital status) and thus are not amenable to interventions. However, the role of family members, having correct expectations regarding symptoms of AMI, and how psychological factors affect delay have credible research support- and they are amenable to nursing interventions. Helping patients pre-think or rehearse what could occur in the future has the potential to reduce future delay times and be very reassuring to patients and their families-although this is speculation, not based on the evidence presented.

Are the conclusions relevant to the care nurses give?
    Yes __X__ No _____ Varies _____
The findings relative to prehospital delay, and more specifically to decision delay, have implications for community and patient education. In particular, the following could (and should) be included in primary care, community education, and post-AMI patient teaching: (1) importance of knowing typical and less common presentations of AMI; (2) seek care early rather than waiting to see if symptoms abate; and (3) role of family members in deciding when and how to seek care for symptoms.

ARE THE CONCLUSIONS CLINICALLY SIGNIFICANT?
    YES __X__ NO _____ VARIES _____ NOT SURE _____
Knowing what factors influence delay in seeking help when symptoms of potential AMI occur will help us design our teaching materials. Ultimately,

patients having this awareness of the importance of what they should do could save lives or at least reduce the extent of myocardial damage.

Applicability

[Note: For the purposes of illustrating applicability, suppose that "we" are a small group of RNs and MDs who are on the staff of a 200-bed regional hospital located in a small city in the middle of an agricultural area. We have decided to initiate a community education program regarding the warning signs of a heart attack and the importance of seeking advice or care. We have identified this IRR as speaking to the issue of what information patients need if they experience symptoms indicative of another coronary artery event.]

Does the integrative review address the problem, situation, or decision we are addressing in our setting?

Yes __X__ No _____

Yes, we have had several cases of patients delaying coming to the ED because they thought their symptoms were indigestion or due to dehydration. Others have delayed their decision to contact their primary care provider or come to the ED after quite a long time. We therefore need to get information out to the community about the symptoms of AMI and the importance of seeking care quickly.

Are the patients in the studies similar to those we see, either overall or in a subgroup of studies?

Yes _____ No _____ To a limited extent __X__

Some are; some are not. The fact that this IRR includes quite a few international studies limits the applicability of many of the conclusions to our situation. Clearly, this is an issue that is heavily influenced by national, ethnic, and cultural factors. The conclusions related to the importance of having accurate expectations of AMI pain and psychological factors are relevant to our population.

Are there any reasons why the conclusions might not apply to our setting and patients?

Yes __X__ No _____

Again, most studies in this IRR are done on foreign and urban populations. Our population has many people with a "tough it out" character and are reluctant to seek help and/or miss a day of work, so we will have to keep that in mind. One study (#35) is specific to a rural population. Also, the long transportation times to the hospital for many of our patients will have to be factored into our teaching material.

Are there any organizational, logistical, cost, or time barriers to incorporating into practice a protocol based on these conclusions? Could they be overcome?
Barriers: Yes __X__ No _____
Could be overcome: Yes __X__ No _____
The literacy level of our farm worker group is low, so we will have to consider how to deliver this information. Possibilities include classes or a video at the two community centers in the area and the senior center; articles in the newspaper; and a handout with pictures (Spanish and English versions). If we go with a handout, we should make it available to the primary care providers, the internists, and the cardiologist who serves our potential patients. It should also be given to patients who have been admitted to our cardiac care unit for an AMI or had an AMI ruled out.

What changes, additions, training, or purchases would we need to implement and sustain a clinical protocol based on these conclusions?
There will be some cost associated with producing a locally relevant information handout or video. We will contact the Lions Club, the Elks Lodge, and the Rotary Club regarding donations to the production of these educational materials.

We need to consistently emphasize the various ways compromised coronary artery blood flow can present and the importance of acting quickly. We need to get this information to families as well as persons at risk for AMI. We could also consider giving patients at risk for AMI a heart-shaped refrigerator magnet with a few key points on it. Should it also be given to middle-aged and older diabetics?

How will we know if our patients are benefiting from our new protocol (e.g., target population outcomes)?
We already keep data about onset of symptoms prior to arrival in the ED and then to reperfusion, so we could ask one more question about the decision to seek help. We would expect to see a 5% reduction in pre-hospital delay time after the community education campaign is initiated. To the extent possible, we will keep a list of patients' decision delay times and factors that lengthened them.

SHOULD WE PROCEED TO DESIGN A PROTOCOL INCORPO-
RATING SOME OR ALL OF THESE CONCLUSIONS?
    YES __X__ NO _____

This IRR has several conclusions that we will incorporate into our community campaign and our post-AMI teaching protocol.

APPENDIX E

Completed Appraisal of the Findings of a Quantitative Study

Citation: Evangelista, L. S., Moser, D. K., Westlake, C., Pike, N., Ter-Galstanyan, A., & Dracup, K. (2008). Correlates of fatigue in patients with heart failure. *Progress in Cardiovascular Nursing, 23*(1), 12–17.

Synopsis

What was the purpose of the study (research questions, purposes, and hypotheses)?
"To examine the prevalence of fatigue and identify its demographic, clinical, and psychological correlates in patients with systolic heart failure (HF)." They were also interested in predictors of fatigue.

Who participated or contributed data (e.g., target population, how sample was obtained, inclusion criteria, demographic or clinical profile, and dropout rate)?
150 patients with HF awaiting transplant and being seen at the outpatient clinic of a tertiary referral center. Average age = 55; 73% men; average ejection fraction = 26.7%; 66% had some college or completed college.

What methods were used to collect data (e.g., sequence, timing, types of data, and measures)?
Questionnaires that took 10 to 15 minutes to complete measured fatigue (POM-F); quality of life (Minnesota Heart Failure subscales: total, physical health, and emotional health); and depression (Beck Depression Inventory). The participants were recruited during routine clinic visits.

Was an intervention tested?
Yes _____ No __X__

If yes, answer the following two questions.
    1. How was the sample size determined?
    2. Were patients randomly assigned to treatment groups?
        Yes _____ No _____ Not sure _____

What are the main findings?
    a. *51% of the sample reported a high level of fatigue, and 28% scored in the depression range.*
    b. *Ejection fraction had a low level of correlation with fatigue.*
    c. *Maximal workload, quality of life total, physical health, emotional health, and depression had high correlations.*
    d. *51% of the variance in fatigue was predicted by a model consisting of maximal workload, physical health, emotional health, and depression.*

Credibility

Is the study published in a source that required peer review?
Yes __X__ No _____ Not sure _____

Was the design used appropriate to the research questions?
Yes __X__ No _____ Not sure _____
They were interested in exploring the relationship between clinical and psychological states and fatigue, so correlational design was appropriate.

Did the data obtained and the analysis conducted answer the research questions?
Yes __X__ No _____ Some but not others _____
They obtained data on physiological and psychological variables that could be related to and predict fatigue. Pearson rs and multiple regression are the appropriate statistics for this data and their question.

Was there anything about the way the participants were chosen or their characteristics that could have influenced the findings?
Yes _____ No __X__
Other than to note that they are a sample from a unique subpopulation of HF patients.

Were the measuring instruments valid and reliable?
    Yes __X__ No _____
The instruments are widely used and have reliability and validity histories. The fatigue and depression instruments have normative cut points, however no validity information provided about their validity with HF patients.

Were important extraneous variables and bias controlled?
    Yes __X__ No _____
Controls were not highly important in this observational study, other than defining inclusions: age, diagnosis, and capability to complete written questionnaires.

Was there anything about the way the study was done that could have influenced the finding(s)?
    Yes _____ No __X__
It is possible that asking the patients to complete the questionnaires would make them think about their psychological state more than patients who were not asked extensively about these issues. This could lead to scores that reflect more problems than patients who are not asked extensively about their quality of life, fatigue, depression, emotional health, and physical health. There is no way to get around this, but it could represent a Hawthorne effect.

Also, the lack of control for Type 1 conclusion error, which was a possibility because of the high number of tests of significance that were run, is of some concern. However, when Bonferroni correction was applied to these results, the conclusions of the study did not change in important ways.

If an intervention was tested, answer the following five questions:
1. Were participants randomly assigned to groups and were the two groups similar at the start (before an intervention)?
        Yes _____ No _____ Can't be sure _____
2. Were the interventions well defined and consistently delivered?
        Yes _____ No _____
3. Were the groups treated equally other than the difference in the intervention?
        Yes _____ No _____ Can't be sure _____
4. If no difference was found, was the sample size large enough to find a difference, if one existed?
        Yes _____ No _____ Not sure _____

5. If a difference was found, are you confident that it was due to differences in the intervention?

   Yes _____ No _____

Is each finding consistent with or different from previous findings in this area of study?

Yes __X__ No _____ Can't be sure _____

Yes, as indicated in the Discussion section, the findings are generally consistent with what studies of other HF populations have found.

FOR EACH MAIN FINDING, IS IT CREDIBLE?

   YES __X__ NO _____

We judge all the main findings to be credible.

Clinical Significance

Note any difference in means, r^2s, or measures of clinical effect (ABI, NNT, RR, OR).

The R^2 for the multivariate predictive model is 51%, which is quite substantial.

Is the frequency, association, or treatment effect impressive enough to be confident that the finding would make a clinical difference if used as the basis for a care protocol?

   Yes __X__ No _____

As the authors point out, three of the four independent predictors of fatigue (i.e., emotional health, physical health, and depression) are potential targets for intervention to combat fatigue. This finding could lead to future studies that try to alter the levels of these variables to reduce fatigue. Interventions directed at them could be studied one at a time or as a group of interventions.

   We think these findings establish that fatigue is related to overall physical health and emotional health as well as to heart function. Fatigue is undoubtedly a physical experience, but there is also a response to the experience that affects mental outlook and functional level; this response may be a target for intervention.

IS THE FINDING CLINICALLY SIGNIFICANT?

   YES __X__ NO _____

Yes, we find all the main findings clinically significant, but are surprised at the low correlation between ejection fraction and fatigue.

APPENDIX F
Completed Findings Table

TOPIC: FATIGUE IN PATIENTS WITH CONGESTIVE HEART FAILURE

Author(s) and Date	Questions, variables, objectives, hypotheses	Design, sample, setting	Findings	Notes
Evangelista et al., 2008	*Fatigue-inertia, psychosocial and cardiac variables, QOL, depression, emotional health, physical health*	*Correlational* *150 persons with HF awaiting transplant at tertiary center; mean age = 55; men = 73%; mean ef = 27%* *USA*	*1. 51% had high level of F* *2. Maximal workload, physical health, emotional health, and depression explain 51% of F* *3. Depression in > 28%*	*POMS-F;* *Minnesota Living with HF QOL overall;* *MN QOL physical;* *MN QOL emotional;* *Beck*
Hägglund et al., 2008	*Living with HF* *Experience of F*	*Qualitative* *Interviews and content analysis* *10 women from outpatient clinic; mean age = 83* *Sweden*	*1. Loss of physical energy* *2. Experience of feebleness and unfamiliar body sensations* *3. Experience unpredictable variations in physical ability* *4. Need help from others* *5. Strive for independence* *6. Acknowledge remaining abilities* *7. Being forced to adjust*	

TOPIC: FATIGUE IN PATIENTS WITH CONGESTIVE HEART FAILURE

DATE: JULY 2010

Author(s) and Date	Questions, variables, objectives, hypotheses	Design, sample, setting	Findings	Notes
Stephen, 2008	*F intensity, global fatigue, symptom severity, trait-negativity, functional status, exercise routine, QOL, satisfaction with life*	*Correlational* *53 elders with stable HF; average age = 77; mean = 68%; average ef = 31%* *USA*	*1. F prevalence = 96%* *2. F associated with ↓QOL, ↓perceived health, ↓ satisfaction with life* *3. No relationship between F intensity and functional status* *4. Being married predicted ↓F* *5. Regular exercisers reported less F*	*POMS-F;* *Visual analogue F; HF Functional Status Inventory; MN overall; MN Satisfaction with Life Scale*
Falk et al., 2009	*General F, physical F, mental F, activity, motivation, anxiety, depression, symptom distress*	*Correlational* *112 community-dwelling persons with worsening HF who sought care; average age = 77; men = 60%* *Sweden*	*1. F associated with emotional distress* *2. Most intense symptoms: F; difficulty breathing, insomnia* *3. Depression associated with ↓activity*	*Multidimensional Fatigue Inventory;* *Symptom Distress Scale; Hospital Anxiety and Distress Scale*

Note: F = fatigue; HF = heart failure; ef = ejection fraction; QOL = quality of life; POMS-F = Profile of Mood States-Fatigue; MN = Minnesota Living With Heart Failure Questionnaire; Beck = Beck Depression Inventory.

References

Evangelista, L. S., Moser, D. K., Westlake, C., Pike, N., Ter-Galstanyan, A., & Dracup, K. (2008). Correlates of fatigue in patients with heart failure. *Progress in Cardiovascular Nursing, 23*(1), 12–17.

Falk, K., Patel, H., Swedberg, K., & Ekman, I. (2009). Fatigue in patients with chronic heart failure—A burden associated with emotional and symptom distress. *European Journal of Cardiovascular Nursing, 8,* 91–96.

Hägglund, L., Boman, K., & Lundman, B. (2008). The experience of fatigue among elderly women with chronic heart failure. *European Journal of Cardiovasular Nursing, 7,* 290–295.

Stephen, S. A. (2008). Fatigue in older adults with stable heart failure. *Heart & Lung, 37,* 122–131.

Glossary

Absolute benefit increase (ABI)   The difference between the proportion of persons in one treatment group who attained a clinical milestone and the proportion of persons in another treatment group who attained it.

Across-studies analysis   Comparison, contrast, and pattern searching in findings from two or more studies; the analysis examines the studies as a body of evidence.

Algorithm   A step-by-step instruction for solving a clinical problem; often consists of a series of yes/no questions leading to one of several possible decisions or actions.

Applicability   The relevance of research evidence to a particular setting considering the similarity of the setting's patients to those in the studies, the safety, feasibility, and expected benefit of implementing the findings.

Appraisal   Making objective, systematic judgments regarding the credibility, clinical significance, and applicability of research evidence to determine if changes in practice should be made based on the evidence.

Bias   A study action resulting from preconceptions or false assumptions that produces distorted results, which are results that deviate from the truth.

Blinding   Steps taken in experimental studies to keep study staff and participants from knowing which treatment group a person is in; the function of blinding is to prevent personal predilections from influencing responses to the treatment or rating of responses.

Bonferroni correction   A change in the level at which a *p*-value is considered significant; it is used to prevent a Type I conclusion error resulting from multiple tests on the same data.

Care bundle   A group of evidence-based (e-b) interventions related to a health condition that, when executed together, result in better outcomes than when implemented individually.

Care design   The process of using knowledge, information, and data to develop a plan of care for a patient population or for an individual patient.

Case-control study   A study in which patients who have an outcome of interest and patients who do not have the outcome are identified; then, the researcher looks back to determine exposures and experiences that could have contributed to the outcome occurring or not occurring.

Chance variation   The variability in sample averages that is expected whenever one measures a trait, behavior, physiological state, or outcome in two or more samples from the same population.

Clinical decision support   The function of a computerized clinical information system that uses inputted patient data to retrieve agency protocols, information, and more general knowledge relevant to the care of the patient.

Clinical practice guideline   A generic set of recommendations regarding the management of a clinical condition, problem, or situation. Ideally, the guideline is produced by a panel of experts based on available research evidence.

Clinical protocol   An agency standard of care that sets forth care that should be given to patients   with a specified health condition, treatment, or circumstances. Protocols take a variety of forms including care maps, decision algorithms, standard order sets, clinical procedures, care bundles, and standardized plans of care; they guide care in combination with clinical judgment and patient preference.

Clinical significance   In quantitative studies, an appraiser's judgment that a research finding indicates a large enough intervention effect or association between variables to have clinical meaning in terms of patients' health or well-being. In qualitative studies, an appraiser's judgment that the findings are informative and useful. The term can be applied in a more general sense to recommendations of clinical practice guidelines and conclusions of systematic reviews.

Coefficient of determination (r^2)   The proportion (or percentage) of a variable that is associated with, or explained by, another variable.

Cohen's Kappa   In a test of an observational instrument, a statistic used to establish the degree of interrater reliability (agreement among raters) when classifying observations into categories is required. If all raters assign the same category to all observations, the kappa is +1.00. Generally, kappa values should be above 0.70.

Cohort study   A study in which two groups of people are identified, one with an exposure of interest and another without the exposure. The two groups are followed forward to determine if the outcome of interest occurs.

Comparison group   In an experimental study, the group that was not given the experimental treatment.

Conclusion error   Reaching a wrong statistical conclusion because of: a chance statistical result, a sample size that is too small, large variations in scores, or extraneous variables.

Confidence interval (CI)   An interval that estimates the result that would be found if the whole target population were included in the study; it is an interval around the sample result.

Confounding variable   An influence on the outcome that is present at different levels in the groups being compared. The influence either was not recognized before the study or could not be controlled by study design. Its effect can be statistically controlled or analyzed.

Consecutive sampling   A method of obtaining a sample in which starting at a certain point every person who meets the inclusion criteria is asked to participate in the study and enrollment continues until the predetermined sample size is reached. It is essentially a convenience sample, although less prone to bias than the researcher inviting persons to participate based on his own schedule and inclinations.

Control   Study methods that (1) decrease, isolate, or eliminate the influence of extraneous variables; (2) prevent bias from influencing the results; and (3) limit the role of chance variation.

Control group   See *Comparison group*

Correlation   A relationship between two interval or rank-order variables in which their values move in accordance with one another to a lesser, moderate, or greater degree.

Correlational study   A study in which the relationship between two or more variables is studied without active intervention by the researcher.

Credibility   A characteristic conferred on a finding. The judgment that the finding is trustworthy and not determined by bias, error, extraneous variables, or inaccurate interpretation of the data.

Database   A structured, updated collection of informational records about articles, books, and other resources; access to the records is managed with computer software. Some examples are CINAHL, MEDLINE, and PsycINFO.

Data saturation   In qualitative research, the point in enrollment of study participants at which the researcher is obtaining only redundant information and not learning anything new from the most recently recruited study participants.

Dependent variable   (Also called the outcome variable) In experimental research, the response or outcome that is expected to depend on or be caused by the independent variable. It occurs later in time than the independent variable. (I = Intervention/Independent variable; D = Downstream/Dependent variable)

Descriptive study   A quantitative study that aims to portray a naturally occurring situation, event, or response to illness; data consists of counts of how often something occurs and breakdowns of various aspects of the situation into categories or levels.

Dichotomous variable   A variable that has only two possible values, for example, was readmitted/was not readmitted.

Effect size   A statistical representation of the strength of a relationship between two variables; commonly, the size of an intervention's impact on an outcome variable relative to the impact of the comparison intervention.

Error   Distortion of data or results caused by mistakes in sampling or measuring or failure to follow study procedures.

Ethnographic research   A qualitative research tradition that examines cultures and subcultures to understand how they work and the meaning of members' behaviors.

Evidence   Objective knowledge or information used as the basis for a clinical protocol, clinical decision, or clinical action. Evidence sources include research, agency data regarding system performance and patient outcomes, large health care databases, and expert opinion.

Evidence-based care design   Clinical protocol development that uses all available and credible evidence as the basis for the actions and decisions set forth in the protocol.

Evidence-based practice   The use of care methods that have been endorsed by an agency because available evidence indicates they are effective.

Evidence-based quality management   A comprehensive agency program aimed at improving quality of care and patient outcomes within the agency, institution, or health care system.

Experimental group   In an experimental study, the group that was given the new or previously untested treatment or intervention.

Experimental study   A study aimed at comparing the effects of two interventions or treatments on outcomes. Most experimental studies use random assignment of participants to treatment groups, careful measurement of outcomes, and control of as many extraneous variables as is feasible to achieve maximum confidence in causal conclusions.

Extraneous variable   A variable that is outside the interests of the study but that may influence the data being collected and lead to wrong conclusions. Researchers try to identify them in advance so as to eliminate or control their influence by study design or data analysis.

Findings   The interpretation of study results into statements that are slightly more general than the statistical results.

Generalizability   A judgment about the degree to which the findings of a study will hold up with the larger population

Grounded theory method   A qualitative tradition of inquiry that is conducted to capture social processes that play out in situations of interest; the goal is to incrementally generate a theory that accounts for behavior or decisions.

Guideline   See *Clinical practice guideline*

Hawthorne effect　A change in participants' responses or behaviors because they are aware they are in a study.

Hypothesis　A formal statement of the expected results of a study. Hypotheses are tested by data collection and analysis.

Hypothetical population　Based on the profile of a sample, the population to which the results of a study are believed to apply.

Impact　As used with the Evidence-Based Practice Impact model, it is the effect evidence-based practice has on patients' outcomes and experiences of health, illness, and health care.

Independent variable　(Also called the intervention/treatment variable) In an experimental study, the variable that is manipulated or varied by the researcher to create an effect on the dependent variable. It occurs first in time relative to the dependent variable.

Institutional review board (IRB)　An agency or university committee that reviews the design and procedures of studies prior to their being conducted in the care setting. The purpose of the review is to ensure that the research is ethical and that the rights of study participants will not be violated. IRBs are federally regulated.

Instrument　(Also referred to as a measurement tool) A way of measuring something. The instrument can be a laboratory test, a questionnaire, a rating guide for observations, or a scored assessment form, to name a few.

Instrument validity　The degree to which a measuring instrument captures the concept it is intended to measure instead of another similar concept.

Integrative research review (IRR)　A type of systematic review in which the findings from various studies are integrated using logical reasoning augmented by findings tables and lists. The goal of an IRR is to summarize the research knowledge regarding a topic.

Interrater reliability　The degree to which two or more raters who independently assign a code or score to something assign the same or very similar codes/scores.

Intervention (in the research context)　See *Treatment (in the research context)*

Meta-analysis　A systematic research review involving a statistical pooling of the results from several (or many) quantitative studies examining an issue to produce a statistical result with the larger sample size.

Metasynthesis   A systematic research review in which findings from several (or many) qualitative studies examining an issue are merged to produce generalizations and theories.

number needed to treat (NNT)   A representation of treatment effect indicating the number of persons who would need to be treated with the more effective treatment to achieve one additional good outcome (over what would be achieved by using the less effective treatment).

Outcome measure   The dependent variable in quantitative studies, particularly the condition or state that is affected by the independent variable.

Outlier   Data contributed by a single study participant that is extreme and considerably outside the range of the other scores in the data set.

Phenomenological research   A qualitative research tradition used to examine human experiences. The methods seek to understand how the context of the persons' lives affect the meaning they assign to their experiences; the methods rely on inductively building understanding of the experience across several, a few, or a small number of persons.

Point-of-care design   Care planning for a particular patient that takes place at the bedside or on the clinical unit and includes either modification of a protocol or new courses of action not specified by an existing protocol.

Population   See *Target population*

Power analysis   A way of determining sample size that factors in: effect size, the p-value cut-point, and the risk of reaching a wrong conclusion the researcher is willing to accept.

Prespecification design   Care design for a population of patients that incorporates the best evidence available into a care protocol; it is done away from the demands of moment-to-moment care responsibilities.

Protocol   See *Clinical protocol*

***p*-level**   The prespecified decision point for the level of significance; data-based *p*-values above this level are considered statistically not significant.

***p*-value**   The data-based probability that the obtained result is just the result of chance variation. It is compared to the level of significance decision point   to reach a conclusion about whether the relationship or difference found is statistically significant, i.e., likely to exist in the target population.

Qualitative content analysis   A group of data analysis techniques used by qualitative researchers to derive meaning from the content of textual data. It typically involves developing codes from the data.

Qualitative description   A qualitative research method that produces straightforward descriptions of participants' experiences in language as similar to the participants' original language as possible.

Qualitative research   Inquiry regarding human phenomena that refrains from imposing assumptions on study participants and situations. Its purposes include exploration, description, and theory generation.

Quantitative research   Inquiry that (1) examines pre-identified issues; (2) uses designs that control extraneous variables; (3) uses numeric measures to determine levels of various variables; and (4) analyzes data using statistical or graphing methods.

Quasi-experimental research   A type of intervention research in which either random assignment to control groups or control over the intervention and setting is not possible.

Random assignment   A chance-based procedure used to assign study participants to a treatment or comparison group. Each participant has an equal chance of being assigned to either treatment group. It serves to distribute participant characteristics evenly in both groups.

Random sample   A sample created by one of several methods by which every person in the population has a greater than zero chance of being included in the sample.

Randomized controlled trial (RCT)   An experimental study that involves advanced testing of an intervention using defined study protocols with a large, diverse sample.

Relationship   In research, a connection between two variables in which one influences the other, both influence each other, or both are influenced by a third variable.

Reliability   The degree to which a measuring instrument consistently obtains the same or similar measurement values.

Research evidence   Findings of individual studies, conclusions of systematic reviews of research, and research-based recommendations of soundly produced clinical practice guidelines.

Research-informed practice (RIP)   The use of research evidence by an individual nurse in the care of an individual patient or in her/his practice.

Results   The outcomes of the numerical and statistical analysis of raw data.

Rigor   A quality of a research study that reflects its fulfillment of the recognized standards for its type of study.

Sample   Persons chosen from a population to participate in a study. The ideal sample is representative of the target population.

Scientific knowledge production   The series of inquiry activities that start with a knowledge question and end with clinical recommendations based on conclusions reached by thorough review of all studies about the question. Scientific knowledge production typically plays out over many years and is always considered open to revision.

Scope   The range or breadth of a question, project, review, or guideline including a description of what is included.

Search (in the context of EBP)   A pursuit to identify all research conducted relevant to a topic. More particularly, the use of a computer search engine to comb through bibliographic databases to identify relevant research articles.

Statistical significance   A statistical result in which the probability is small that the result is due to chance variation. Therefore, the result is large enough that a difference or relationship would be highly likely to be found in the population.

Study plan   A term used in quantitative research to describe how the study will be conducted, including how the sample will be obtained; how the data will be measured, collected, and analyzed; and any control that will be used. There are prototypic designs that researchers use or adapt.

Systematic review (SR)   A comprehensive and systematic identification, analysis, and summary of research evidence related to a specified issue. An SR can use statistics, tabulation, compare and contrast methods, or pattern identification to reach conclusions based on the body of studies in the review.

Target population   The entire group of individuals or objects to which the researcher would like to generalize the results. The sample may be randomly drawn from the target population, or the sample characteristics may project a hypothetical target population.

Theory Assumptions, concepts, definitions, and/or propositions that provide a cohesive (although tentative) explanation of how a phenomenon works.

Treatment (in the research context) Clinical interventions, therapies, action, or courses of action that are evaluated in the study. The treatment is the independent variable and its effect on the dependent variables (outcomes) is what is being tested by the study.

Treatment effect measures Various numerical representations of the clinical effectiveness of treatments, therapies, and interventions, including absolute benefit increase (ABI), number needed to treat (NNT), relative risk (RR), and odds ratio (OR).

Type 1 conclusion error The conclusion that there is a significant relationship between variables or a significant difference in groups' outcomes when in fact there is not a significant relationship or difference.

Type 2 conclusion error The conclusion that there is not a significant relationship between variable or a significant difference in groups' outcomes when in fact there is a significant relationship or difference.

Validity See *Instrument validity*

Valid finding A finding of a study or conclusion of an SR that is credible, that is trustworthy, because it was produced by sound methods that controlled possible influences from extraneous variables and bias.

Variable An attribute of a person, social group, thing, or situation that has two or more categories or possible values when measured.

Index